The Skilful Physician

Philadelphia College of Textiles and Science
Paul J. Gutman Library
School House Lane & Henry Ave
Philadelphia, PA 19144-5497

The Skilful Physician

Edited by

Carey Balaban, PhD

and

Jonathon Erlen, PhD

University of Pittsburgh
Pennsylvania

and

Richard Siderits, MD

harwood academic publishers
Australia • Canada • China • France • Germany • India •
Japan • Luxembourg • Malaysia • The Netherlands • Russia •
Singapore • Switzerland • Thailand • United Kingdom

Copyright © 1997 OPA (Overseas Publishers Association) Amsterdam B. V.
Published in The Netherlands by Harwood Academic Publishers.

All rights reserved.

No part of this book may be reproduced or utilized in any form or by any
means, electronic or mechanical, including photocopying and recording, or
by any information storage or retrieval system, without permission in
writing from the publisher. Printed in Venezuela.

Amsteldijk 166
1st Floor
1079 LH Amsterdam
The Netherlands

The original text of THE SKILFUL PHYSICIAN was first published in
1656 by Tho. Maxey, London, England.

British Library Cataloguing in Publication Data

The skilful physician. - 2nd ed.
  1. Herbals 2. Naturopathy 3. Medicine - History - 17th century
  I. Balaban, Carey, 1954- II. Erlen, Jonathon III. Siderits,
  Richard
  615.3'21'09032

ISBN 90-5702-532-9

CONTENTS

PREFACE

The importance of natural foods, minerals and herbs in preventive medicine and healing is a venerable theme in the history of medicine. Since the fifteenth century, natural healing has been featured in a genre of printed self-help medical texts combining principles for preventive medicine and recipes for natural remedies. *The Skilful Physician*, originally published in 1656, is a collection of guidelines for maintaining one's health plus recipes for disease remedies, perfumes and treated wines. Similar to the contents of the seminal 1618 *Pharmacopœia Londinensis*, these recipes use only natural ingredients: herbs, minerals and parts of animals. However, unlike the *Pharmacopœia Londinensis*, which was published by the College of Physicians for a professional audience, *The Skilful Physician* was targeted at the general public.

The book begins with the premise that preservation of good health requires attention to proper diet and life-style. However, recognizing that preventive measures are not perfect, the compiler included recipes for 705 compound medicines to treat a wide variety of illnesses. Instructions for choosing wines, as well as 58 recipes to preserve, "recover and restore" wines are included. Finally, 15 formulas for perfumes are presented. This volume is representative of popular medical texts from the mid-seventeenth century, a genre that includes the well-known *Culpeper's Complete Herbal*, written by Nicholas Culpeper and published initially in 1652. Unlike Culpeper's compendium, which has been reprinted extensively, *The Skilful Physician* has never been reprinted. This new edition makes a fascinating work available to modern scholars and the public.

In addition to the original text, we have prepared an introduction discussing *The Skilful Physician* within the context of seventeenth-century English medical theories and practices by both professional and lay healers, a table of natural ingredients and an index. Since many medical terms are unfamiliar to the modern reader, we have also compiled a glossary of key medical terminology found in the text, with definitions derived from contemporaneous sources. It is hoped that this book will serve as a resource for understanding the preparation of seventeenth-century natural remedies and encourage further scholarship in this important period in the history of medicine and pharmacy.

   The editors wish to thank Idelia Wolfe and Margaret Moran for their
clerical assistance with this project. The illustrations were reproduced
from a copy of the 1633 edition of John Gerard's *The Herbal or General
History of Plants* in the collection of The Hunt Institute for Botanical
Documentation. The editors thank Charlotte Tancin, librarian and senior
research scholar, Hunt Institute, for making this material available for our
use. We appreciate the helpful comments of Norman Gevitz, John
Scarborough and Charlotte Tancin on an earlier version of the manuscript.
We are also grateful to Ruth Kuenzig for providing the original text. This
work is dedicated to the memory of her father Dr. David Eckstein—
physician and humanitarian.

INTRODUCTION

Medicine and health care in seventeenth-century England did not conform
to a simple, strict hierarchical model. Just as English society was
undergoing a series of significant religious, political and economic
changes, organized medicine during this century also was facing severe
challenges to its continuing adherence to Galenic medical dogma.[1] Besides
the emerging threats to traditional medical authority posed by the growth
of Paracelsian chemical beliefs[2] and a new philosophy encouraging
medical experimentation supported by the Royal Society of London,[3]
outside the urban bastion of London a wide variety of healers usurped part
or all of the university-trained physicians' prestige and economic rewards.
The Skilful Physician, published at the midpoint of the century, illustrates
many of the major threads running through the complex pattern of
seventeenth-century English medicine.

Within seventeenth-century London organized medicine was divided
among three groups holding royal charters: physicians (College of
Physicians of London created in 1518), barber–surgeons (Barber–Surgeon's
Company created in 1540) and apothecaries (Society of Apothecaries
created in 1617).[4] The university-trained physicians sought unsuccessfully
to monopolize the practice of physic. Attacks from within their own ranks
by supporters of Paracelsian and Baconian philosophies severely limited
their status in the public mind.[5] A large group of alternative healers, ranging
from non-licensed physicians to quacks, siphoned off many of the traditional
doctors' potential paying patients. Most medical care in London was
provided by domestic healers within a household setting.

The picture of medical delivery outside of metropolitan London is much
more confusing. Ronald Sawyer, in his noteworthy dissertation, discusses
eight groups of popular healers practicing in rural England during this
century: clergyman–doctors, magical healers, medical assistants and
itinerants, bone-setters, itinerants roaming between villages, midwives,
gentlewomen and domestic healers.[6] This varied assortment of popular
healers competed against and, at times, worked with the very few
university-trained physicians who ventured forth from urban centers such
as London, Bath and Norwich.[7] Selection of an appropriate healer was

usually based on one or more of the following criteria: proximity, price, personal ties to the healer, the healer's perceived expertise in handling the patient's particular health problem and the patient's expectations relative to the healer's medical approach.[8]

Throughout the seventeenth century these varied forms of popular medicine provided most of the health care available in rural England. Doreen Nagy, in her insightful examination of this subject, presents compelling evidence about the actual nature of day-to-day medical care during this period. She successfully challenges the earlier Whiggish interpretation of English medical history that focused on London and the power of the university-trained physicians. Nagy convincingly demonstrates that these medical men could not meet the health needs of England's rural populace for several reasons: scarcity of university-trained physicians; their inability to physically reach the far-flung rural citizenry, given the poor road system throughout England; and the lack of financial motivation, as about 85% of the rural population could not afford to pay for a doctor's services. Also, the close tie between healing and religion in the belief system of many of the rural poor provided little motivation to spend any of their meager funds on a doctor's supposed healing powers, when God ultimately decided medical matters. It was well recognized that the basic cures of university-trained physicians were very similar to those used by popular healers, including home cures passed down orally or readily available in the new genre of self-help medical recipe books widely published during the middle of the seventeenth century.[9]

Compilations of medical recipes intended to assist the educated public date back to fifteenth-century manuscripts that provide simple remedies for common ailments. These cures, while couched in Galenic medical theory, employ readily available plants and herbs. The *Short-Title Catalogue* lists 153 medical titles published in English from 1486–1604. More than one-fourth of these English-language publications were collections of remedies. Perhaps the best example from the sixteenth century is Thomas Moulton's *Mirror or Glass of Health*, which went through seventeen editions between 1530 and 1580. Many of these remedy collections were compiled by unknown authors who often cited major figures from medicine's past to lend credibility to the cures found in their pages.[10]

While this type of self-help medical work continued to appear sporadically in the first half of the seventeenth century, the 1650 to 1659 decade saw a sudden outpouring of these publications in England. During these ten years 182 medical books were published, all but 19 in English. Among these titles were a number of medical recipe collections and herbals intended to reach educated lay readers in both urban and rural England.[11] The most famous of these was Nicholas Culpeper's frequently republished *English Physician*, often referred to as *Culpeper's Herbal*.[12] These works, according to Charles Webster, were supposed to foster self-help in medical matters, thus freeing the public from their reliance on Galenically trained physicians and the apothecaries' expensive drug preparations.[13] To illustrate the popularity of this type of text, Nagy cites a 1655 medical recipe book, published under the pseudonym "Philiatros," that contains more than 1,700 remedies. These cures, attributed to well-recognized former medical greats, make use of herbs, plants, common sense, magic, the occult and astrology.[14] *The Skilful Physician*, published one year after this work, represents many basic features of both this style of self-help medical book *and* common English medical and health practices. As Nagy states: "Seventeenth-century medical practice in general was an untidy mixture of folklore, superstition, Galenic theory, herbal tradition, astrology and, eventually, chemical medicine."[15]

    The Skilful Physician follows the general pattern of works in its genre, combining a mixture of symptomatic descriptions of diseases with a list of remedies that may include recipes for medications, directions on diet and discussions of procedures such as setting broken bones and phlebotomy (blood-letting). It may seem peculiar to the modern reader that recipes for perfumes and for preserving and improving wines would be included in a compendium of medicines. It is of interest that Conrad Gesner's classic 1559 text, *The Treasure of Evonymus*,[16] also describes methods for chemical preparations of medicines, spiced wines and perfumes. From the latter text, the contextual link between these products is their common role in the preservation and recovery of health. The preface of *The Skilful Physician* refers to the beneficial aspects of wine for "concoction" (digestion), while Gesner attributes medicinal properties to both perfumes[17] and wines.[18] The medicinal importance of wine is further underscored by the inclusion of seven *Physical Wines* in the compound medicines listed in the 1653 edition of the *Pharmacopœia Londinensis*.[19]

    The compiler of *The Skilful Physician* is anonymous; however, a "Dr. Deodate" is recognized as the author of the preface and a compiler of the text. Dr. Deodate appears to be a pseudonym, probably derived from a seventeenth-century contraction of the Latin phrase *DEO DATUM*, meaning either a Divine gift or a gift to G-d.[20] However, an alternative reading of *DEO* in classical Latin is *Ceres*,[21] a possible allusion to the fundamental role that natural products of the Earth play in the Doctrine of Signatures. Twelve other individuals are credited with contributing to this compendium. This list reflects the influence of three distinct medical traditions. First, the Galenic tradition is represented by Abucasis [written

Albucenses], died c. 1083, the great Islamic physician/pharmacist whose medical encyclopedia contained thirty treatises on a wide range of medical topics, and by the citation of Hippocrates in the Preface.[22] The Paracelsian tradition is represented by Paracelsus, the sixteenth-century medical reformer who openly challenged Galenic dogma. Finally, the tradition of popular healing is represented by the citation of Drs. Powel, Cadaman, Hill, Cranmer, Burroughs, Butler, Stevens and Whead and two wise-women, Mrs. Bill and Mrs. Wing, as sources consulted in the preparation of the book. The latter citations further support Nagy's contention that women played a significant and, at times, well-recognized role as popular healers.[23]

The text of *The Skilful Physician* shows many characteristics suggestive of a compendium from a variety of sources. For instance, there are numerous examples of an interchangeable use of colloquial English, pharmaceutical and Latin synonyms for ingredients, without attempts at constructing cross-references. Thus, the synonyms *Bursa pastoris* and Shepherd's purse, Aron root and Wakerobbin root, Petty moral and Nightshade, Ewfrace and Eye-bright, Alehoofe and Ground Ivy, Herb Bennet and Hemlock or Avens, Borus and Cerus or white lead, and Vermillion and Red Lead are used in different recipes, even on the same page (see p. 64 for Ewfrace and Eye-bright). Although this creates difficulties for the modern reader, the lack of editorial consistency does not necessarily imply a lack of thoroughness on the part of the compiler or printer: the intended audience likely was familiar with these standard terms. The same argument applies to the disease terms in the text. As illustrated by the glossary, *The Skilful Physician* heavily emphasizes the English equivalents of classical Latin and Greek disease terms; this reflects diagnostic criteria from earlier, classic works in the genre such as Sir Thomas Elyot's 1541 *The Castel of Helth Corrected and in Some Places Augmented*[24] and Andrew Borde's 1547 *The Breviary of Healthe*.[25] The disease categories appear to be a simplification of the nosology typified in the latter work, distinguishing between remedies for ring-worm versus tetter and shingles versus St. Anthony's fire, but not providing distinct remedies for different types of leprosies (see Glossary). The entries for different types of fevers provide an example of this simplification: remedies are listed in *The Skilful Physician* for quotidien and continual fevers, but not for the large number of fever categories presented by other works such as those of Borde or Blancard (see Glossary). Given the usage of common colloquial terms for diseases in the text, it seems unlikely that the intended audience would be confused by the relatively infrequent use of synonymous terms such as *lask* and *white flux*, *matrix* and *mother*, *spots* and *pushes* in an eye, *carbuncles* and *botches*, *kidneys* and *rains*, and *red menstues* and *termes in a woman* in this compendium.

Another interesting characteristic of the compiled text is the co-existence of passages describing standard Galenic medicine and passages alluding to superstition and magic, in the same volume. However, despite references to the latter two typical components of popular healing, and to their accompanying exotic ingredients, surprisingly few references are made to these traditional alternative tools of healing. One cure for rabies calls for unicorn horn.[26] Another recipe suggests using the brains of a camel when trying to cure falling sickness, while an alternative remedy for this disease involves ashes of a dead man's skull.[27] Wood betony is strongly recommended to ward off health problems caused by evil spirits.[28] A remedy to "stay the Rhume" calls for three-quarters of an ounce of the skull of a man "that dyed through violence."[29] It is worthy of note, though, that seemingly odd ingredients are not an exclusive feature of popular healing: the College of Physicians included such exotic items as unicorn horn, rhinoceros horn, the skull of a man killed through a violent death, the hoof of a lion, and moss from a dead man's skull in the list of Simples in the 1653 *Pharmacopœia Londinensis*.[30]

Despite the explicit citation of sources consulted for the compilation and the direct attributions of some formulations to specific sources, the compiler of *The Skilful Physician* was apparently not reticent to copy some remedies and related text without attribution. Examples of this practice are especially prominent in the section that describes eye remedies, where other remedies were intercalated between transparently edited text from a mid-sixteenth-century self-help book, Jean Goeurot's *The Regiment of Life*:[31]

For Blood-shotten Eyes.

Take the blood of a stock Dove, or for the want of it, a Pigeon, and drop a little into your eyes, and wet a cloth therein, and lay it on the Eye, helpeth the blood shotten eye, whether by stroak or otherwise. Sometimes the paine cometh of Choler, and then the patient feeleth great heat, sharp prickings, much paine, and commonly there appeareth no gumme in the Eye; if there do, it is yellow: therefore the Patient ought to be purged, as hath been said in the Remedies of the

For bloodeshoten eyes.

The bloode of a stockedoue or in lacke of it an other doue or pigeõ dropped a lytle in the eye and a wete cloute therof layde upon the same, healethe the bloodeshoten eyes whether it be of stroke or any other cause.

Sometyme the sayd peyne cõmeth of cholere, & then the patient feleth greate heate sharpe prycking, & much peyne, & commonly there appeareth no gumme in the eyes, and yf it do, it is head proceeding of the cause of Choler: And in the beginning of the redness, lay Tow or Flax dipped in the white of an egg well beaten with Rose-water and Plantane water.

[*Another remedy*]

yelowe. Therfore ye ought to gyue hym a purgatiõ purgynge cholere, as hath bene sayde in the remedye of the head procedyng of the cause of cholere.

For swelling of the Eyes.

Take a Quince and seeth it in water till it be soft, then pare it, bruise it, and mingle it with the yolk of an egg and the crumbs of white bread dipped in the same Water, and put thereto a little womans milk, and two penny worth of Saffron, bray them together, and lay it over your fore-head and the eyes. Sometime such pain chanceth because of phlegme, and then the Patient feeleth great pain and heavinesse in the eyes, and in this case you must purge the phlegme, as hath been said in the Remedies of the head grieved with excess of phlegme. *The Skilful Physician*, pp. 66, 67.

For swellynge of the eyes.

Take a quynce and seeth it in water tyl it be softe, then pare it & bruse it & mixe it wt the yolke of an egge & the cromes of wheaten or white bread steped in ye said water & put therto a litle womans milke and two peny weyght of safron, braye them al togyther and laye it ouer the forehead and the eyes.

Sometymes suche paynes chaunce bycause of fleume, and then the paciẽt feleth greate heuyness in his eyes, with abun-daunce of gummy matter, or water descendynge into the eyes. And in thys case, ye muste purge the fleume, as it hathe bene sayde in the remedye of the heade greued by the excesse of fleume. Goeurot, fol. xv (b) to xvi (a).

For a great pain in the Eye.

Take half an ounce of Oyl of Roses, the yolk of an egge, and a quarter of an ounce of Barley flower, and a little Saffron mixt together, and put it between two linnen cloths, and lay it to the pain; or else take the crumb of white bread one ounce, and seeth

For very great payne of the eyes.

Take an ounce and a half of oyle of roses, the yolke of an egge, & a quarter of an ounce of barly floure, and a lytle saffron, myxe all togyther & put it betwene .ii. lynnen clothes, and laye it to the peyne.

it with Nightshade, and Morral
water, then mix with the same
bread yolks of eggs, Oyl of Roses
and Camomile of each an ounce
and a half, of Linseed one ounce,
and use it as aforesaid. *The Skilful
Physician*, p. 68.

And other.

Take of crõms of wheaten
breade whyte, an ounce, and seeth
it in nyght shade or morell water,
then myxe with the said bread .ii.
yolkes of egges, oyle of roses, and
comomil, of cene an oũce and a
halfe mseilage of lineseeds and
ounce and use it as is aforesayde.
Goeurot, fol. xvii (a).

For hardnesse that hath been long
in the Eye.

Of hardenesse that hath ben
longe in the eye.

Take a Scruple of Alloes, and
melt it in Water of Cellendine at
the fire, then put of it in the eye.

Or take powder of Cummin
mixt with Wax like a Plaister, and
lay it upon the eye: Or take Roses,
Sage, Rew and Cellendine, of
each alike, mixt with a little salt,
and distil it, and thereof put a
drop or two evening and morning
in your eye. In stead of that water,
it is good to take the juice of
Vervain, Rue, and a little Rose
water. *The Skilful Physician*,
p. 74.

Take a scruple of alloes suc-
cotrine & melte it in water of
celydony at ye fyre then receyue
the fume of it, and afterwarde
wash the eye with fenel water.

An other.

Take poudre of cumyne myxt
wyth waxe lyke a playster, and
laye it uppon the eye.

An other.

Take red roses, sage, rue, cele-
donie of eche a lyke moche, wyth
a lytle salte and distil in water,
and putte thereof a drop or two in
your eye, euenynge and
mornynge. In steade of that water,
it is good to take iuyce of
verueine, rue and a lytle rosewater. Goeurot, fol. xviii (a).

A likely explanation for this example of what is currently termed
plagiarism is that the compiler and/or the intended readership of *The
Skilful Physician* did not recognize Jean Goeurot as a medical authority of

the same stature as the cited sources. Although at least seven distinct English editions of *The Regiment of Life* were published between 1546 and 1596, the most recent edition was published sixty years prior to the appearance of *The Skilful Physician*. We suggest that the publication record of the original text and the unattributed inclusion of these passages are evidence of the perceived efficacy of these (time-honored?) cures. However, the citation of a variety of sources for other remedies and the publication record of *The Regiment of Life* suggest that the invocation of Goeurot's authority was unnecessary in the mind of the compiler to lend credibility to the remedies.

Despite the lack of explicit citations, a Galenic influence is readily apparent throughout the text. Contemporary published sources, such as Blancard's *The Physical Dictionary*, define Galenic medicine as ". . . that Physick which is built upon the Principles of *Galen*, and therefore they are *Galenists*, who embrace the Foundation of the Art which is fetch'd from *Galen*, and the Philosophers (prov'd by Reason, and confirm'd by Experience), found their Principles chiefly upon the four Elements of the Peripateticks; and hence their notions of *Temperaments, Humours, &c.*"[32] This is contrasted with hermetic (or Paracelsian) medicine which, according to Blancard, ". . . refers the Cause of Diseases to *Salt, Sulphur*, and *Mercury*, and prepares most Noble *Medicines*, not only of *Vegetables* and *Animals*, but of *Minerals* too."[33]

The classification of Galenic and Paracelsian components of medicines also extends to their method of preparation. During a discussion of distilled waters, Culpeper writes: "We speak not of strong waters, but of cold, as being to act on Galen's part, and not Paracelsus's."[34] This schema classifies simple distilled waters (and medicines containing them) as Galenic, while hot or sharp distilled waters (e.g., Aqua Vitae and Dr. Stephen's Water) as Paracelsian.

From the perspective of contemporaneous definitions, *The Skilful Physician*—and the 1618 and 1653 editions of the *Pharmacopœia Londinensis*—contain both Galenic and Paracelsian components. *The Skilful Physician* adopts a Galenic humoral framework for the cause of disease. The title page mentions the "several humours,"[35] while Deodate in his preface refers to "discordant humours"[36] and "obstructive humours."[37] References in specific cures also mention "phlegmatick humours,"[38] "superfluity of humors"[39] and "flux of certain humours,"[40] and one recipe for treating head pain blames this condition on the four humours.[41] Further, the vast majority of ingredients (see Table of Ingredients) and preparations are Galenic by either definition listed above. However, the text does include a hermetic component in a small number of recipes. For example, quicksilver is a component of both salves for skin disorders[42] and an orally administered remedy for "leprosy",[43] and vitriol is incorporated in both internal[44] and external medicines,[45] including a preparation to whiten teeth.[46] Further, Galenic and hermetic alternatives appear to coexist without difficulty or contradiction. A case in point is the list of remedies that "stanch" bleeding, which includes (1) a dressing of hysop and cobwebs; (2) a plaister of mastick, hare hair and the white of a newly laid egg; (3) a dressing of a live spider wrapped in linen; (4) a drink of red nettle juice, red wine and vitriol; (5) a powder made of an equal mixture of copperas and bole armoniack; (6) a plaister of roasted salt beef, and (7) a drink of centory, green rue and red fennel.[47] Thus, the selection of remedies in *The Skilful Physician* reflects the Elizabethan compromise between Galenic and Paracelsian medical doctrines.[48]

One remarkable aspect of *The Skilful Physician* is its emphasis on compound medicines. During the seventeenth century, medications were classified dichotomously as simple medicines (commonly termed "Simples") or compound medicines (commonly "compounds").[49] Blancard defines simple medicines as "*Simplicia*, Simples, Medicines unmix'd and uncompounded," while compound medicines are termed "*Composita*, Compound Medicines which are made up of many simple ones, as the Compositions of certain Waters, Syrups, Electuaries, Opiates, Trochies, Ointments, Plaisters, &c. such as we meet with in all the Apothecaries Shops. There are also certain Chymical Compositions, as divers Spirits mix'd, the volatile oleous Salts, Tinctures, Balsams, Essences, Powders, &c. which are all comprehended under the name of Compound Medicines."[50] Simple medicines included fresh and dried plants (roots, bark, wood, herbs, flowers, fruits, buds, seeds, gums/rosins and products from living creatures), juices pressed from plant material, minerals and simple distilled waters.[51] These simple distilled waters were typically prepared by placing a single simple ingredient with water in a vessel termed a 'limbeck' or 'alimbeck,' using methods similar to those described by Gesner in *The Treasure of Evonymus*.[52] *The Skilful Physician*, though, is a compendium of mainly compound medicines, containing multiple simples and/or compounds.

The extensive list of compound medicines in *The Skilful Physician* appears to be an expansion of the standard medicines listed in the 1653 *Pharmacopœia Londinensis*, which presents a variety of treatment alternatives for specific diseases. The Preface of *The Skilful Physician* lists three criteria that were used to select formulations for the compendium: "[in selecting and publishing the remedies] I have taken care 1. of interfering with any others, and 2. lest I might delude and deceive thee with impertinencies, or anything picked out of others of the same nature; and 3. that I might avoid that general defect of all hath hitherto come forth of this useful Subject, especially in the Cure Of Internal Distempers, by varying the Administrations according to the Complexion, Strength, and Constitution of the Patient."[53] In

modern terms, the initial two criteria are an assertion of the relative
uniqueness of the listed remedies compared to standard texts. One obvious
feature that emerges from a comparison with the *English Physician*[54] and the
1653 *Pharmacopœia Londinensis* is that *The Skilful Physician* utilizes a
greater variety of herbal ingredients, most of which are listed in the 1633
edition of Gerard's *History of Plants*.[55] *The Skilful Physician* even includes a
description of White Dothet because ". . . no Herbal maketh mention of this
Dothet."[56] Secondly, there are many more specific compound medicines
listed in *The Skilful Physician* than in either the *English Physician*[57] or the
Pharmacopœia Londinensis. These additional medications include both
compound medicines for specific diseases and formulations for oils and
syrups that are not found in the 1653 list from the College of Physicians.
Finally, variant recipes for named formulations in the 1653 *Pharmacopœia
Londinensis*, such as Aqua Vitae, Aqua Mirabilis, Dr. Stephens Water, Lac
Virginis and Cordial Water, are presented in *The Skilful Physician*. The
recipe for Doctor Stephens Water from *The Skilful Physician* is one example
of an augmented formulation of a recipe from the 1653 *Pharmacopœia
Londinensis*. The *Pharmacopœia Londinensis*[58] states:

Take of Cinnamon, Ginger, Galanga, Cloves, Nutmegs, Grains of Paradice, Seeds of
Annis, Fennel, Caraway, of each one drachm; Herbs of Time, Mother of Time, Mints,
Sage, Penyroyal, Pellitory of the Wall, Rosemary, flowers of red Roses, Chamomel,
Origanum, Lavender, of each one handful; infuse them twelve hours in twelve pints of
Gascoign Wine, then with an Alembeck, draw three pints of strong Water from it.

The formula from the *The Skilful Physician*,[59] though, contains additional
ingredients:

Take a gallon of good Gascoigne Wine, then take Ginger, Gallingal, Cinnamon,
Nutmegs, Graines, Cloves, Mace, Anniseeds, Fennel seeds, Carraway seeds, of
each a dram, then take red Mints, red Rose leaves, Garden Time, Pellitory of the
wall, Smal Marjerom, Rosemary, Peniroyal, Sage, Wild Time, Camomile,
Lavender, Avens, of each one handful, then bruise them all in a Mortar, and beat
your Spices small, then put your Spices and Herbs into your Wine, and let it stand
twelve hours, stirring it oftentimes, and then still it in a Limbeck. The first pint is
the best, the second is good.

Other formulations, such as Aqua Mirabilis, differ in the substitution of
the ingredients Galingale (the English herbs *Cyperus longus* and *Cyperus
rotundus vulgaris*[60]) for Galanga (true Galingale [*Galanga major*, a root
from the East Indies, and *Galanga minor*, a root from China][61] or
Galangal[62]) and squills (sea onions) for cubebs (a type of peppercorn) in
The Skilful Physician:

Pharmacopœia Londinensis, p. 67: Take of Cloves, Galanga, Cubebs, Mace, Cardamons, Nutmegs, Ginger, of each one drachm; Juyce of Sullendine half a pound; Spirit of wine one pound; white wine three pound; infuse them twenty-four hours and draw off two pound with an Alembick.

The Skilful Physician, p. 25: Take Gallingale, Cloves, Squills, Ginger, Melilot, Cardomons, Mace, and Nutmegs, of each one dram; of the juice of Cellendine half a pint; mingle all these made into powder with the said juice and a pint of Aqua-vitae, and three pints of good White-wine, and put all these into a Stillatory of glasse, and let it stand all night, and on the morrow still it with an easie fire.

Finally, a major augmentation is shown in Dr. Walmseley's formulation of the decoction Lac Virginis [or Lac Virgineum] from *The Skilful Physician*:

Pharmacopœia Londinensis, Lac Virgineum, p. 74: Take of Allum four ounces, boyl it in a quart of spring Water, to the third part: Afterwards, Take of Litharge [marginal footnote: 'Beaten into very fine pouder'] half a pound, white Wine Vineger a pint and a half; boyl it to a pint, strain both the waters, then mix them together, and stir them about till they are white.

The Skilful Physician, p. 82: Take of Alumen Plumosi half an ounce, of Camphire one ounce, of Roach Allome one ounce and dram, Sal gemmi half an ounce; white Frankinsence two ounces, Oyle of Tarter one ounce and a half; make all these into most fine powder and mix it with one quart of Rosewater, then set it in the Sun and let it stand there nine dayes, often stirring it, then take Littarge of Silver half a pound beat it fine, and searse it, then boil it in one pint of White Wine Vinegar, until one third part be consumed, ever stirring it with a stick while it boileth, then distil it by a Filter, or let it run through a thick Jelly bag, then keep it by itself in a glass Vial, and when you will use these Waters, take a drop of the one, and a drop of the other in your hand, and it will be like milk which is called Lac Virginis, wash your face or any part of your body therewith. It is most precious for the same. Probatum Dr. Walmesley.

Thus, the presentation of modified formulations for 'standard' medicines, the use of an expanded list of ingredients and the extensive instructions for making specific compound medicines are all consistent with the author's prefatory remarks in *The Skilful Physician*.

The relationship between the compiler's third criterion for selection of recipes (". . . that I might avoid that general defect of all hath hitherto come forth of this useful Subject, especially in the Cure Of Internal Distempers, by varying the Administrations according to the Complexion, Strength, and Constitution of the Patient"[63]) and the emphasis on compound medicines is less clear. The author of *The Skilful Physician* clearly follows the Galenic doctrine that heating, cooling, drying and moistening of the body (and specific organ systems) can transform the constitution of individuals; for example, he writes that ". . . immoderate Watching [wakefulness] dryeth the body too much, it turneth a sanguine constitution to be cholerick, and it turneth a phlegmatick constitution to be melancholick, it overdryeth the braine; it wasteth the spirits, it weakneth the digestive faculty, enclineth the body to consumptions, &c."[64] Since individual simple medicines were characterized by both organ-specific effects and heating, cooling, drying or moistening properties,[65] they could both cure patients and produce such side effects as alterations of complexion or temperament. Is the author asserting that the doses of the compound medications in this volume avoid these potential problems?

Most of the text and recipes in *The Skilful Physician* combine herbalism with folklore and common sense. Thus, these medical recommendations would have been easily acceptable to both the educated public who could read this volume and to the remainder of the populace with access to these remedies by word of mouth. Many recipes call for combining various ingredients with wine or ale, the common beverages of the public. Though a few exotic plants and herbs are prescribed, most remedies call for easily obtainable items, such as onions,[66] parsley,[67] wormwood,[68] wheat,[69] sage,[70] garlic,[71] and honey.[72] Several of the recipes simply say to add herbs to the drug mixtures.

Dr. Deodate's preface makes it clear that this volume was published primarily for lay readers rather than for professional healers. Strong emphasis is placed on activities to preserve one's health. The author details what he believes to be appropriate actions concerning diet, sleeping, exercise and other daily functions. He states that if an individual were to follow these suggestions, he would not have to consult a physician or refer to the medical cures in this volume. *The Skilful Physician*'s compiler summarizes this approach to health care when he says: "So doubtless, if men in the government of their Health would use Reason more, they would need the Physician lesse: For Intemperance, which is the great enemy of Reason, is the chief Cause of the Maladies."[73]

NOTES

1. Lester S. King. "The Transformation of Galenism," in A. G. Debus (ed.) *Medicine in Seventeenth Century England: A Symposium Held at UCLA in Honor of C. D. O'Malley* (Berkeley: University of California Press, 1974), pp. 7–31.

2. Allen G. Debus. *The English Paracelsians* (London: Oldbourne Book Co., 1965).

3. Harold J. Cook, "Physicians and the New Philosophy: Henry Stubbe and the Virtuosi-Physicians," in R. French and A. Wear (eds.) *The Medical Revolution of the Seventeenth Century* (Cambridge: Cambridge University Press, 1989), pp. 246–271.

4. Charles Webster. *The Great Instauration: Science, Medicine and Reform 1626–1660* (London: Duckworth, 1975), pp. 250–256.

5. "Introduction," in R. French and A. Wear (eds.). *The Medical Revolution of the Seventeenth Century* (Cambridge: Cambridge University Press, 1989), pp. 1–9.

6. Ronald C. Sawyer. "Patients, Healers and Disease in the Southeast Midlands, 1597–1634." PhD Dissertation, University of Wisconsin–Madison, 1986, pp. 126–192.

7. Doreen E. Nagy. *Popular Medicine in Seventeenth-Century England* (Bowling Green, Ohio: Bowling Green State University Popular Press, 1988), pp. 4–19.

8. Sawyer, pp. 196–204.

9. Nagy, ch. 4.

10. Paul Slack. "Mirrors of Health and Treasures of Poor Men: The Use of the Vernacular Medical Literature of Tudor England," in C. Webster (ed.) *Health, Medicine and Mortality in the Sixteenth Century* (Cambridge: Cambridge University Press, 1979), pp. 237–274.

11. Webster, pp. 270–273.

12. F. N. L. Poynter. "Nicholas Culpeper and His Books," *Journal of the History of Medicine and Allied Sciences* 17(1962):152–167.

13. Webster, pp. 270–273.

14. Nagy, pp. 47, 48.

15. *Ibid.*, p. 2.

16. Conrad Gesner. *The Treasure of Evonymus, contyninge the vvonderfull hid secretes of nature, tochinge the most apte formes to prepare*

and destyl Medicines, for the conseruation of helth: as Quintessĕce, Aurum Potabile, Hippocras, Aromatical wynes, Balmes, Oyles, Perfumes, garnishyng waters, and other manifold excellent confections. Wherunto are ioyned the formes of sondry apt Fornaces, and vessels, required in this art. Translated (with great diligence, & laboure) out of Latin, by Peter Morvving felow of Magdaline Coleadge in Oxford. (Iohn Daie, London, 1559) Fascimile edition of copy from Beinecke Rare Book and Manuscript Library, Yale University. Da Capo Press/Theatrum Orbis Terrarum Ltd., Number 97, The English Experience, New York, 1969.

17. *Ibid.*, p. 367.

18. *Ibid.*, pp. 383–401.

19. Nicholas Culpeper. *Pharmacopœia Londinensis: or the London Dispensatory: further adorned by the studies and collections of the Fellows, now living of the said Colledg.* Printed for Peter Cole, London, 1653, pp. 71, 72.

20. Oxford English Dictionary (OED2).

21. Oxford Dictionary of Classical Latin.

22. *The Skilful Physician*, pp. 2, 14.

23. Nagy, ch. 5.

24. Sir Thomas Elyot. *The Castel of Helth Corrected and in some places augmented* (London, 1641) Facsimile edition, New York: Scholars' Facsimiles & Reprints, 1937.

25. Andrew Borde. *The Breviary of Helthe* (London, 1547) Facsimile edition of British Museum Shelfmark: C.122.d.1., Da Capo Press, Amsterdam, 1971.

26. *The Skilful Physician*, p. 30.

27. *Ibid.*, pp. 156–157.

28. *Ibid.*, p. 176.

29. *Ibid.*, p. 56.

30. *Pharmacopœia Londinensis*, p. 53.

31. John [Jean] Goeurot. *The Regiment of Life, wherunto is added a treatyse of the Pestilence, with the booke of children newly corrected and enlarged by T. Phayer.* Facsimile edition of London 1546 imprint, Bodleian Library (Oxford) Shelfmark 8°.P.24 Med. Walter Johnson, Inc./Theatrum Orbis Terrarum, Ltd., Number 802, The English Experience, Amsterdam, 1976.

32. Stephen Blancard [Blankaart]. *The Physical Dictionary. Wherein the Terms of Anatomy, the Names and Causes of Diseases, Chirurgical Instruments, and their Use are accurately described. As also the Names and Virtues of Medicinal Plants, Minerals, Stones, Gums, Salts, Earths, &c. The Method of Chusing the best Drugs: The Terms of Chymistry, and of the Apothecary's Art: The various Forms of Medicines, and the ways of com-*

pounding them. London, John and Benj. Sprint and Edw. Simon, Seventh Edition, 1726, pp. 167, 168.

33. *Ibid.*, p. 182.

34. Nicholas Culpeper. *Complete Herbal* (London: W. Foulsham & Co. Ltd., 1923), p. 405.

35. *The Skilful Physician*, p. 1.

36. *Ibid.*, p. 5.

37. *Ibid.*

38. *Ibid.*, p. 13.

39. *Ibid.*, p. 33.

40. *Ibid.*, p. 78.

41. *Ibid.*, p. 79.

42. *Ibid.*, pp. 46, 93, 96, 104.

43. *Ibid.*, p. 99.

44. *Ibid.*, p. 95.

45. *Ibid.*, p. 78.

46. *Ibid.*, p. 161.

47. *Ibid.*, pp. 30–32.

48. Debus.

49. Culpeper.

50. Blancard, pp. 99, 313.

51. *Pharmacopœia Londinensis*, pp. 3–66, 187–[189, misnumbered 185].

52. Gesner.

53. *The Skilful Physician*, p. 13.

54. Culpeper.

55. John Gerard. *The Herbal or General History of Plants. The Complete 1633 Edition as Revised and Enlarged by Thomas Johnson.* (Facsimile of Edition published by Adam Aslip, Joice Norton and Richard Whitakers, London, 1633) Dover Publications, New York, 1975.

56. *The Skilful Physician*, p. 111.

57. Culpeper.

58. *Pharmacopœia Londinensis*, p. 69.

59. *The Skilful Physician,* p. 164.

60. Gerard, pp. 30–31.

61. *Ibid.*, p. 33.

62. Blancard, pp. 166–167.

63. *The Skilful Physician*, p. 13.

64. *Ibid.*, p. 8.

65. *Pharmacopœia Londinensis*, pp. 36, 38, 40, 43, 45, 47–48.

66. *The Skilful Physician*, p. 16.

67. *Ibid.*, p. 17.

68. *Ibid.*
69. *Ibid.*, p. 18.
70. *Ibid.*, p. 19.
71. *Ibid.*, p. 20.
72. *Ibid.*, p. 39.
73. *Ibid.*, p. 2.

SKILFUL PHYSICIAN:

Containing

DIRECTIONS for the Preservation of a Healthful *Condition*,

AND

Approved Remedies for all Diseases and Infirmities (outward or inward) incident to the Body of Man.

With

A right manner of applying them to the several Humours, Constitutions, **and** Strength of every Patient, for their better **and more** successful Operation.

Whereunto is added,

Experimented Instructions for the compounding of PERFUMES.

ALSO

For the Chusing and Ordering of all kinds of W I N E S , both in preserving the Sound, and rectifying those that are Prick'd.

Never before imparted to Publick View.

London, Printed by *Tho. Maxey*, for *Nath. Ekins*, at the Gun neer the West end of *Pauls*, 1656

1

The PREFACE.

It is the Physicians care to recover Health: but it ought to be every ones care to preserve their Health; and if we were careful to keep out Diseases, we should not be troubled to drive them out. Reason tells us, that it is better to keep out an Enemy, then to let him in, and then to beat him out. So doubtless, if men in the government of their Health would use Reason more, they would need the Physician lesse: For Intemperance, which is the great enemy of Reason, is the chief Cause of those Maladies, wherewith the bodies of men and women are afflicted; and they must needs act contrary to Reason, who do any thing that is contrary to the course of Nature; as to eat, or drink, or sleep, or stir the body more then Nature requireth, or less then Nature requireth. The good old Physician Hypocrates saith, That fulness or emptiness, or any thing else which is otherwise then Nature would have it, should be shunned as hurtful. For this is the thing that maketh work for the Physician; and he is more employed in helping the bad Effects of too much, then of too little; and the Cause of this is the abuse of Reason; when we make it the work of our Reason to find out ways of Intemperancy; and we make Reason a Slave to Appetite: where as if we would live like Rational People, we should rather imploy our Reason in observing our owne Nature, and observing what is agreeable to it, and what is not agreeable to it. And so we might by our own experience find out many things, which would make much both for the preserving of our Health, and prolonging of our Life. Certainly, we might easily keep our selves in Health, if we were as careful to keep when we have it, as we are to regain it, when it is lost: and it is a strange over-sight not to prize our Health until we are tormented with Diseases; to throw away our Health unreasonably or carelesly, and then to lament our loss too late, and to be in long torture, and at great charge before we can regain. Therefore those who rightly prize their Health, which is indeed a great Treasure, let them live temperately, observe diligently their own Natures, and follow exactly these Rules for the preservation of Health, which have been found out by the great industry, judicious enquiry, and long experience of Learned Men: the which Rules you have set down here as followeth, in some few and plain Directions.

The DIRECTIONS for the Preservation of HEALTH.

I. Of DIET.

1. OPpress not your stomack with immoderate or unseasonable eating or drinking. If you be in Health, do not eat or drink unlesse you have an appetite to it, and bee sure that you have an empty stomack before you eat, and to eat to fulness and overcharging of the stomack is not good. It is better to rise from Table with an appetite to eat more, then to sit down to Table without an appetite.

2. Judg those meats most agreeable to your body, which you desire most, and digest best, without any trouble to you; but eschue those meats as hurtful to you, which you have eaten upon an empty stomack being in health, if after the eating of them, they cause soure and ill savoring belchings, with heaviness in your stomack.

3. Observe this order in eating, if you have several dishes before you, first eat that which is of easiest digestion, and then eat that which of harder digestion.

4. If any do change their course of Dyet which they have used for a long time, as they who by high feeding and continual fulness, come to have a very fat and gross body, they resolve to use a more sparing Diet; or they who have been accustomed to a very sparing and low Diet, if on a sudden they come to have fulnesse and variety of Dyet; or they who have much used anything, as Tobacco, &c, which they resolve to forbear, let them observe these following Cautions: 1. Not to do it suddenly, but by little and little; for all sudden changes are hurtful to nature. 2. That they do it not, but in time of perfect health, because they are then best able to undergo such change. 3 That they do it not when they are much disturbed with businesse or otherwise; because when the mind is much disturbed, Nature is easily drawn to irregulate working to cause Diseases, and especially by a sudden change from that to which hath been accustomed. 4. If a man hath accustomed himself to anything the most part of his life time, howbeit this custome is bad, ye[t] he cannot safely begin a change in his old age.

5. Fasting from meat and drink in some cases is good, as in the increasing of acute Diseases, or if there be much crudity in the stomack; but fasting unadvisedly used is hurtful; as to those who have melancholick or cholerick dry bodies, much fasting is very injurious; but to those who are

3

phlegmatick, plethorick, fat, full of moist humours, temperance in their Diet, with often and seasonable fasting is very good. Likewise those who drink so much as to be distempered thereby, if they eat before that drink be well digested, they undoubtedly wrong their bodies: and howbeit they are not then sensible of it, having a strong Constitution; yet certainly this will be a foundation of the decaying of nature. Extraordinary drinking doth very much diminish the strength of Nature; and much more, if you add eating to excessive drinking. Experience maketh it appear to us daily in many, that excessive drinking or eating doth oppresse Nature, and causeth the decay of Nature even in the strongest constitutions. This is certain, that excessive fulnesse, or too great want of what we should have, or anything else which is not according to the course of Nature, is hurtful.

6. Some use only one meal in a day, which is not to be commended, unlesse their digestive faculty be very weak and slow in its operation. Some use two meals in a day, others take three meals in a day, the which custome, as it is most generally received, so indeed it is most to be approved of, if it be done with Discretion; viz. if you take such things as are most agreeable to you, and so much at a meal as may be easily digested before the next meal. It is a good rule of Diet, to eat often and a little at a time, not to let the stomack be long empty, nor to eat again before it be empty; for to eat or drink (when we have meat in our stomack half digested, or almost digested) before the digestion be finished, it doth much to disturb the digestive faculty, pervert its operation, and so is the cause of many Diseases: but to keep the stomack alwayes in working, and to give it that whereupon it can work most easily, and to give it so much work as it can quickly performe: this doth encourage Nature to follow its work, it strengthneth the digestive faculty, and preserveth it in its strength. By this rule, every one may order their own Diet well, if they rightly consider their strength and constitution, and condition of life. As those who stir much may feed oftner then they who use a sitting life; and those who have hot, cholerick, slender bodies, may feed oftener than they who have gross, fat or phlegmatick bodies. For they who have gross and ful bodies ought to use a sparing Diet, & to use such meats and drinks which are of a little nourishment and of a drying faculty. But if you would know what time of the day you may feed most largely. I answer, In the forenoon or in the morning, if you purpose to sup at night, that it may be well digested before supper time; for they who dine largely at noon, it is not probable that their dinner can be wel digested before Supper time, unlesse they be of a cholerick, hot constitution, for such have a quick digestion, and cannot eat much at a time. Now whereas many put the question, whether it be better to sup largely or dine largely[?] or if it be better to

dine largely, and not to sup at all, where as the common custome is to dine largely, and to use a light supper. I answer, If your stomack be not empty, if that which you have eaten before be not well digested, it is better not to sup at all, for the reasons already mentioned: but if your stomack be empty, and you have a good appetite to your supper, you may sup as largely as may you dine, so as you refrain from going to bed three or four hours after.

7. To eat of one sort of meat only at a meal, is best; but if you eat of several dishes, let them be such, as are neer of a Nature: for to eat of several dishes of disagreeing Natures, as to eat fish and flesh at the same meal, &c. it overthroweth the digestive faculty, filleth the body with discordant humours, and produceth strange bad Effects.

8. To drink too sparingly at meals doth very much hinder concoction, to drink great draughts and seldom, doth weaken the stomack, which then is in concoction, and driveth down the meat too hastily, and corrupteth the whole body with over much moisture and crudity; wherefore it is best to drink often at meals and a little at a time, and to swallow it down, not hastily, but leisurely; for the drink being mixt with the meats, by divers little draughts leisurely taken, tempereth them wel both for concoction and distribution. Ordinary Beere is best at meals, and at the ending of your meal take some strong drink, viz. Wine or strong Beere to help concoction. Drink not betwixt meales, if you can possibly forbeare it, unless great thirst and drought of the stomack require it, and then only a little is to be taken.

   As for that custome commonly used, to drink fasting in the morning, it is not good for any but those who have a hot and dry constitution, or subject to obstructions, to allay the drought of the stomack, and to cleanse away slimy or obstructive humours, which are in the Stomack, Liver, Veines or Reines.

9. It is a common custom and commendable, to set first on the Table bread and salt, and to take them last away, thereby shewing the necessary use of them at meals; and indeed they are to be reproved who use not (as some do) bread or salt at their meals. For Salt helpeth concoction much, and preventeth the crudities of the stomack, and therefore it is good to eat much salt with fresh meats, or to have your meats powdered.

   As for Bread, we may very well give it the first place at meales, for it yeildeth a nourishment very familiar to our Natures. Let your bread be of the flower of the best Wheat, let it be fitly leavened: for so it is more easily digested, and yeildeth better nourishment; but if it be too much leavened, it is of heavy digestion, and of no commendable nourishment.

Let it be temperately seasoned with salt, let it be light, well wrought, well baked, and eat it not over new, nor too stale. When you eat flesh, eat twice so much bread as flesh. When you eat fish, eat thrice so much bread as fish, especially if the fish be of the moister sort, that the superfluous moisture of it may be tempered by the driness of the bread; for they who eat little bread with their meats, commonly are troubled with windy crudities, watrish and impure stomacks.

10. That you may know what kind of meats is best for you, take this general rule, use such meats as are most agreeable to the constitution of your body, to your age, and season of the year. Those who are of a hot cholerick constitution, should use meats of a moistning cooling nature. Those who are of a cold, dry, melancholick constitution, should use meats and drinks of a moistning and heating faculty. Those of a phlegmatick constitution, should use meats and drinks of a heating and drying faculty. Those of a sanguine complection, should use a Diet of a temperate nature. And to those who have strong stomacks, meats of strong nourishment, and of slow concoction are most agreeable: but to them who have weak stomacks, as old or sickly people, &c. meats of lighter substance and of easier concoction are best.

In respect of the season also, you must alter your Diet; in the Spring and Summer use a more sparing Diet then in Harvest or Winter. In the Summer use meats and drinks of a cooling and moistning faculty, in the Winter let them be heating and drying; in the Spring let them be of a temperate nature, and not too nourishing; in the Harvest, let them be moistning, and moderately heating.

I cannot here shew you particularly what things are cooling, or moistning, or heating, &c. because I must be short being in a Preface, and I refer you to those who have treated largely of these things; viz. Muffets Improvement of Health.

Of Sleep and Watching.

Life cannot continue without food, and Health cannot be preserved without moderate sleep; for this refresheth the wearied spirits, and repaireth the decayed spirits, it furthereth the concoction, and is a present help for Crudities; but if it be immoderately used, it is hurtful, it causeth defluxions, heaviness of the head, dulness of wit; cold plegmatick Diseases, &c. therefore that you may use sleep comfortably and profitably, have a care, that your sleep be seasonable, for as you should not watch when you should sleep, so you should not sleep when you should be awake; and therefore eschue noonsleeps, and too long morning sleeps, as great enemies to health; for whatsoever is not according to the course of Nature, is contrary to Nature, and so will by little and little weaken Nature, and in the end overthrow it. Now we see it natural to all living and sensitive creatures to observe this rule, To sleep in the night time, and in the day to be provident to supply their wants; and therefore they who do contrary to this rule, are contrary to the course of nature, and wrong themselves, howbeit they are not at present sensible of it. And without doubt these two (which are both contrary to Natures rule) viz. unseasonable sleeping or watching, and unreasonable eating and drinking are the great causes which deprive us of Health, and shorten our lives, as those especially who are rich find it by experience, who stay out of bed very late, and lye long in the morning, a bad custom: but as you tender health, sleep not in the mornings too long, unlesse honest occasions, or an ill disposition of body causeth much watching in the beginning of the night; then it is needful that you make amends by sleeping so much the longer in the morning: neither should you sleep at noone, for sleeping after dinner (if it is constantly used) causeth superfluous moisture of the braine, and causeth cold Diseases of the braine, as Palsies, &c. puffeth up the Spleene with wind, prepareth the body for Agues, Imposthumes, &c.

Yet in some extraordinary cases sleeping after dinner may and ought to be used;

1. If you have not slept well in the night nor in the morning.

2. If you be faint with excessive heat of the Season.

3. Old people, because of their weaknesse, may sleep after dinner, or any other time when they can.

4. Those who have slender and dry bodies, receive great benefit by sleeping after dinner; for it moistneth their bodies, and refresheth their bodies, and refresheth their spirits. But those who have full gross bodies, or who are of a sanguine or phlegmatick complexion, let them beware of sleeping after dinner.

Now those who would sleep at noon must observe these things following.

1. That they sleep not immediately after Dinner, but an hour after, or half an hour at least.

2. That they sleep not lying, but rather sitting with the body upright.

3. That they sleep not over long, not above half an hour, or an hour at most.

4. That they sleep not in a place too hot (especially in the Summer time) but rather enclining to cold: the most convenient place for any to sleep in at any time, is that which is not too hot nor too cold, not too close nor too open; and above all, it must not be dampish, for that is very hurtful

to the body, especially to the head: you must have care a to keep your head and neck wel from the cold when you sleep.

When you sleep, lye upon your right side; and not upon your left side, unless it be to ease your body, when you are wearied with lying on your right side: lye upon your left side as little as you can; for to lye upon the left side, hindreth concoction, encreaseth the Diseases of the Spleene, causeth troublesome Dreames, &c. So likewise to lye upon your back when you sleep, is very unwholesome; it causeth troublesome sleeps, it causeth the Night-mare, it occasioneth the Lethargy, Palsies, Cramp, it heateth the Raines; it is very bad for those who are troubled with the Stone, or are inclined to it.

Now if you would know how long you ought to sleep, observe this rule, That you should sleep, until you find the concoction of the stomack and liver be finished, the spirits well refreshed, and you find a lightsomnesse in the whole body, especially in the stomack and head. But if you find heavinesse in the body, head, and eyes, or stomack, or if you have ill savoured belchings, or &c. they signifie that you have not yet slept enough.

Again, the time of your sleep must be determined according to your strength and constitution; as those who are weak and sickly, or aged and children, must take longer time of rest, then those who are strong, or young, for whom seven or eight hours sleep is enough. And those who have dry, cholerick or melancholick bodies, need longer sleep then the phlegmatick or sanguine, or those who have grosse fat bodies; for it very much refresheth and moistneth dry bodies, to whom there is nothing more hurtful then too much watchfulness. But too long sleep to phlegmatick, grosse bodies is very hurtful.

It is a custome to warme the bed before we go to bed, which should not be used by those who are healthful and strong (unlesse fresh sheets be layed upon the bed) for it weakneth their bodies, and maketh them tender. But it is good for them who are aged, or are weak by Nature, or lead a tender course of life, for such cannot well endure a cold bed, it may wrong them much: weak or tender Natures, are by very small occasions overcome and put out of their right courses.

I conclude concerning sleeping and watching with this, That immoderate and unseasonable Sleeping weakeneth the natural heat, filleth the body with bad humours, and enclineth the body to cold, phlegmatick Diseases, dulleth the spirits and wit.

And immoderate Watching dryeth the body too much, it turneth a sanguine constitution to be cholerick, and it turneth a phlegmatick constitution to be melancholick, it overdryeth the braine; it wasteth the spirits, it weakneth the digestive faculty, enclineth the body to consumptions, &c.

Of Exercise.

The stirring of the body by walking, riding, some pastime, &c. If it be moderate and in fit time; it encreaseth natural heat, refresheth and quickneth the spirits, maketh the body lightsome and nimble, helpeth concoction, furthereth the expulsion of the Excrements and bad humours, &c. In any stirring industrious course of life, for the most part they live longer and healthier then those who use a sitting restful life.

But you must have a care, that you use not too much stirring or motion of the body to weary your selfe too much; for this will consume the natural moisture, and waste the spirits, encline the body to a Consumption,&c.

Those who would use any kind of Exercise only for their Healths sake, let them not do it upon a full stomack, or immediately after eating, for the most part of Physicians do agree in this, that wee should not go about any exercise of the Body until the first and second digestion is compleated, when the stomack is light and almost empty.

It will be good also to disburden your selves of the excrements of the belly, and of the urine, before you begin your Exercise, lest the Excrements by the violence of the heat of the Exercise, be drawn into the veines, or &c whereby the blood may be corrupted, obstructions caused, @c. And if you use any exercise or violent motion of the body immediately after meales, or while there is meat in the stomack not digested, it marreth digestion, and causeth crudities and bad humours; whereupon will follow Scabs, Ulcers, Imposthumes. This is to be understood chiefly of those who use a restful life, and live tenderly. But those who live in continual exercise of their body, as labouring men, they need not be so cautious for the time or manner of their Exercise (for that to which our Natures are constantly accustomed, will not do us harme;) if men keep themselves to one constant course of Exercise, and not at any time to exceed their ordinary custome: but if they do things rashly and immoderately, otherwise then they use to do; as if they fall upon any work upon a full stomack; or if violent hot working they are carelesse of themselves, and keep not themselves warm, &c. Thereupon certainly will follow alterations of the body and Diseases. For that to which we are not accustomed, if it be violent and oppresserh Nature, it must of necessity work dangerous alterations in us. You must be very cautious in doing of any thing to which you are not accustomed, until by tonstant use it becometh familiar to our Nature, and then it may be used safely, howbeit at first perhaps it was dangerous, if not used with great caution.

A constant custome in any thing prevaileth much with Nature, so that a man may safely do that to which he hath been accustomed, which would be very dangerous to another. And therefore violent stirring of the body to

those who have a restful life, or untimely exercise immediately after
meales, is hurtful; but to rise up after meal, to stand or to walk softly is
good: and if it be in cold seasons of the year, let the place be temperate,
not too hot nor too cold; if it be in the hot seasons of the year, walk in the
open fields, nigh to some pleasant rivers after supper; but after dinner in
some shadowed place, or some cool Arbour, &c. Observe this general rule
concerning the place, after meals to stand or walk in, That it incline more
to cold then to heat. For as the heat of Exercise immediately after meals,
so the heat of a hot place by drawing our natural heat from the inward
parts of the body to the outward, it marreth digestion, and filleth the body
with crude humours, therefore after meals let your place be pleasant and
moderately cool, your exercise gentle walking and pleasant discourse with
merry companie; spend an houre so, and thereby you shall find digestion
furthered, your body much refreshed, natural heat and strength cherished
and encreased. But when you use great motion of the body, as in travel,
pastime, &c. do it moderately, so as you do not weary your selves too
much, and oppresse the strength of nature: and in this moderate beneficial
stirring of the body there may be several degrees observed, according to
the constitution of the body, and season of the year.

1. Those who have a gross or phlegmatick body, should use much
exercise, and should exercise themselves so, as thereby to provoke sweat;
but they must have care that they provoke not sweat immoderately, nor
proceed to extreme wearinesse, for thereby the spirits and good humours
of the body will be too much wasted, and the fat of the raines melted.

2. Those who have dry slender bodies, must use easie exercise: They
must stirre their bodies no longer then the colour and the flesh is
somewhat ruddy, and the sweat begins to come out; too much motion of
their bodies will bring them to a Consumption.

Again, your Exercise must bee according to the season of the yeare; for
as the season is colder, so you may use stronger and more laborious
exercises, and oftner: and as the season inclineth more to heat, so the
exercise or motions of your body must become more moderate and calme.

One thing I will add here, viz. Rubbing of the Body, which is much
commended to us by all Physicians, and is found by the experience of all
who have used it, to be a thing very beneficial to the body, and it may well
stand in stead of all other Exercises or motions of the body, to those who
cannot have such Exercises, either because of their weaknesse, or &c. It
stirreth up and encreaseth natural heat, it quickneth the blood, it strengthneth
the parts, it drawes humours from the higher parts of the body to the lower
parts, it concocteth crude humours, it strengthneth digestion, it draweth bad
humours from the principal parts of the body; there is not any one thing

which may be more commended then this, for the preservation of the strength of Nature. But as all other Exercises of the body, so rubbing of the body must be used with caution, viz. That those who have gross or phlegmatick bodies must rub over their bodies until they provoke sweat; but those who have hot bodies, or dry slender bodies, they must rub their bodies until the flesh beginneth to swell, and groweth ruddish, and no longer. So likewise according to the Season, we must use rubbing more or lesse; as the season is colder, so must we use rubbing more, and less in hot seasons.

The manner how it is to be done, is thus. Rub with your hands, or rather with a warme linnen cloth your shoulders, armes, breast, sides, thighes, Legs and feet; but the belly, stomack, and back, especially neer to the reines must not be rubbed. If you can your selves do it, and not to have another to do it, it will be so a great deal better. You must do it when you lye downe at night, but then more gently; but in the morning before you rise do it more strongly; and when you rise, have a care to keep your selves well from the cold. Begin your rubbing easily and softly, afterwards faster and harder; and while you are rubbing, lay a double cloth warmed to your stomack and belly. After you are risen, and have combed your head well backward, then rub your head and your neck with a warm linnen cloth, and (if it be a cold season) before the fire, remembring the Cautions concerning rubbing before mentioned. This rubbing of the Head and Neck, is especially to be commended to those who have moist heads, Students, and such as are troubled with Rhumes, Palsies, &c.

Of Excrements.

1. To go to stool twice or once in the day at least, preventeth those many inconveniences which are caused by the too long stay of the Excrements in the body; but if you cannot do so by reason of costiveness, which is very hurtful, and hath many inconveniences following it, therefore drink much, especially at meals, that thereby the stomack and intestines may be well moistned: this will keep the Excrements soft, and will make passages slippery. But if Nature is dull and slow to evacuation, it will be good to use some gentle loosening thing, at first once in two dayes for some time, then use it once in a day: and when you have accustomed your self to go to stool so once in the day, Nature it selfe will afterwards observe that custome.

2. Sweating is very good for gross phlegmatick Bodies; but those who have dry slender bodies, must use it very moderately; and those whose bodies are too much dryed by a Disease, or are enclining to a Consumption must eschew sweating as much as they can.

3. Keep not Urine or Wind in your body, when Nature would void them, for they are very hurtful, if they be kept long in the body; and if you cannot break wind upward when it is in the stomack, or break it downward when it is in the belly, then use something which is good against the wind: let it stay in your body as little time as you can, especially if it be bred (as most commonly it is) of Crudities; but when your body is free from Crudities, do not accustome your selfe to break wind, refraine from it then as much as you can; for if we bring Nature to a custome to break wind much, it is the way to make it breed wind.

4. To use any thing to provoke the evacuation of phlegme at the mouth or nose, is not to be approved of; it is best to let Nature follow its own course, unlesse those Excrements of the mouth or nose be obstructed: or abound exceedingly by reason of a cold, or some other Cause.

Of Passions of the Mind.

Eschew all excessive Passions, as excessive joy, excessive anger, excessive fear, &c. for they oftentimes cause weaknesse of the body, and Swounings, and oft times sicknesse, and sometimes sudden death. Likewise envy, extreme cares, continual fear and continual sadnesse, are great enemies to health and shorten life: but a quiet contented, cheerful mind, free from all these Passions, is a great supporter of Health and prolonger of Life.

Of the Choice of Aire.

The best Aire is that which is pure, clean, and temperate, not too hot nor too cold, nor too moist, nor mixed with grosse moisture, or corrupt noisome vapours. Therefore shun that Aire which
1. Evaporateth from corrupt Ponds, standing Pools, impure places, as nasty Ditches which are full of impurities, &c.
2. Which is in Valleys or low places, which are shut up about with Hills, so as no wind can come to it to purifie it.
3. Shun the Aire of Marish and moorish grounds.
4. Shun foggy mists.
5. Stay not in the night Aire; nor in any moist or dampish Air, as a moist Easterly Air, or a moist Westerly Aire
An impure Aire which ariseth from corrupt impure places, infecteth the body, and causeth dangerous Diseases.
An Aire which is too moist, or a Night aire encreaseth phlegm, and causeth Rheumes.

The Aire of low and marish places, fill the body with gross phlegmatick humours, causeth paine in the joints, Cramp, Palsie, and other cold Diseases of the braine, &c.

An Aire extreme cold (if we continue long in it) it weakeneth the brain and sinews, causeth Rheumes and Coughs, weakneth natural heat, &c.

An Aire too hot spends our spirits, weakneth concoction, dissolveth and draweth out natural heat, it burneth the blood, &c.

That Aire then is most wholsome which is temperate and clear; and therefore those dwellings are commended as the best, which are seated on high dry grounds in open Aire, far from low, marish or filthy places, for there the aire is most pure, subtile and temperate.

REader, I have here given thee some plain useful Directions for the preservation of thy Health, as fully to this businesse as the bounds of a Preface permitteth. I now proceed to give thee Remedies for the regaining of thy Health if lost; and I assure thee they are such as are not taken upon trust, but often tryed and approved. In the publishing of them, I have taken care 1. of interfering with any others, and 2. lest I might delude and deceive thee with impertinencies, or anything picked out of others of the same nature; and 3. that I might avoid that general defect of all hath hitherto come forth of this useful Subject, especially in the Cure Of Internal Distempers, by varying the Administrations according to the Complexion, Strength, and Constitution of the Patient. And that thou maist not be much troubled in finding out what thou desirest for thy present condition, I have put them in such an order, that thou maist easily find every thing under its proper Letter, the several Letters of the Alphabet referring either to the Diseases, the Remedies, or the parts of the Body Affected. If these shall be successful and acceptable to thee, I trust ere long, to gratifie thee with more complete Directions for the Preservation of Health, and to impart such Secrets, as few in the world have been acquainted with to this day.

In the mean time, I have here presented to thee (toward the latter end of this Treatise) a few Instructions for the Choice of all sorts of Wines, and how to Order them, both for the preserving of those that are Sound, and to chuse such as will last; as also how to recover and restore those that through defect of Substance, or by long keeping are decayed and prick'd. I think I may truly affirm, they are the first of that kind that have come to publick view.

A Hearty Well-wisher
of thy Health,
D. D.

The Names of the most Eminent Persons
whose Skil hath contributed any thing to this Book.

Dr. Powel.
Dr. Deodate.
Dr. Cadaman.
Dr. Hill.
Paracelsus.
Dr. Cranmer
Dr. Burroughs.
Dr. Butler.
Albucenses.
Dr. Stevens.
Dr. Whead.
Mrs. Bill.
Mrs. Wing:

THE
SKILFUL
PHYSICIAN.

ACHES.

A Soveraign Medicine for any Ache.

TAke Barrowes grease, a lapful of Archangel leaves, flowers, stalks and all, and put it into an earthen pot, and stop it close, and paste it; then bury it in a horse dunghil nine dayes in the latter end of May, and nine dayes in the beginning of June, then take it forth and strain it, and so use it.

A Receipt for all cold and raw Humors;
and Aches in mens bones.
Proved by Doctor Powel.

Take two ounces of Mastick, two ounces of Vermillion, half a pound of Frankinsence, one penny worth of Rosen, beat every one of these into fine powder by it self, then mingle them altogether; and if they look not red enough, put in more Vermillion; and when you will use this Medicine, take a spoonful of this Powder, and put it into a chafing dish of quick coals, and let the Patient sit on a stool close covered, and the chafingdish put under the stool, which must be shifted three times before the Patient rise from the stool; and the Patient must sit Evening and Morning upon the stool (as aforesaid) all naked, saving a sheet about his neck to cover him before, even to the feet, and another behind him of like length, and upon the sheets two blankets; and by that time two spoonfuls of the Powder be spent, the Patient will sweat and be faint, and when the Patient hath sate

15

out the third chafingdish, he must go to bed, and lye in the same cloathes, and never change them in three dayes. He may eat and drink what he list, so his Drink be warm.

For all manner of Aches, and the Sciatica.

Take a handful of Herb-grace, and bray it smal in a Mortar, then take one ounce of Frankinsence, and one ounce of Commin, and beat them to Powder severally; then take one pound of black soap, and seeth it on the fire till it be melted, then put in the aforesaid things, and let them boile together, till it be thick; then take and spread it like a Plaister upon a cloath, and lay it to the Grief as hot as may be suffered, and so let it continue twelve houres, then take it away, and if the place be blistered, lay that to it no more, but prick the blisters with a needle; and if it be not blistered, then lay on a fresh plaister, and let it ly twelve hours more, and keep the place grieved and the Patient very warm. Probatum est.

For any Ache whatsoever,

Take two great Onions, and make holes in the tops, and put into each one dram of Camphire, so much of Frankinsense as a Walnut, one pennyworth of English Saffron; roast the Onion in the fire; then pill it, and strain it to an Oyle, and put thereto so much of the marrow of a dead horses haunch bone, and mingle it well together, and annoint the place pained therewith.

A precious Remedy for any extreme Ache.

Take a Whelp that sucketh (the fatter the better) and drowne him in water, then take out his guts clean, and fill his belly with black Soap, and put him on a spit and roast him well, and take the dropping thereof, and put it in a Vessel, and then lay the Patient in a sweat, and annoint him therewith, and cover him warm with clothes, that he may sweat well, then make a fire of Charkcoals in a pan, and lay thereon a good handful of Sage, and let him take the aire thereof in a close room; and do this five times.

For all manners of Aches in Bones, Joints, or Sciatica.

Take Balme and Cinqfoil; but most of all Betony, Nep and Fetherfew, stamp them, and drink the juice with Ale or Wine. Probatum.

A very good Plaister for any Ache or Swelling in the Joints.

Take of Stipticum Paracelsi, and Calcithers, of each alike, spread it upon Leather and make a Plaister thereof, then annoint the place grieved with Oyl of Roses, and after lay on the Plaister.
Mr. Smart.

For an old Ache or Sciatica.

Take Harts-horn, and chop it in reasonable smal pieces, then put it in a Pipkin, cover it with water, and stop it close, and set it in an Oven with Bread, and when it is baked, take out the Pipkin, and when it is cold, it will be a Jelly; then warm some it, and annoint the grieved place with a warm hand, and chase it in often.

For an Ache.

Take Aqua composita and Neatsfoot Oyle, warm them, and annoint the place therewith, and lay warm cloaths thereon.

Another.

Take Parsly and Wormwood, of each a handful, and seethe them in a quart of Ale, with a quantity of sweet Butter, and wash the place therewith, and bind the Herbs to the place, as hot as may be suffered.

Another.

Take Smallage stampt, and put it in to Aqua vita, and strain it, and put thereto Boars grease, and straine them together, and annoint the place there with morning and evening.

For an Ache or the Sciatica.

Take Neats foot Oyle and Aqua composita, and annoint the place therewith, then take wool newly taken from the Sheep and put thereon with warme cloathes.

Another.

Take the juice of Smallage, Sorrel, and of Woodbind leaves, of each alike, then take Honey and the white of an egg, of each alike, and mingle it together till it be thick, and lay it on cold without any boiling at all.

Another.

Take as fat a Goose as you can get, and when she is ready drest, then take a couple of the fattest young sucking Cats you can get, and slay them, and cut them into gobbets, and put them into the belly of the Goose, and so roast it as long as it will drop, then take the liquor and annoint the place pained therewith, and bathe it wel before the fire, as hot as you can suffer it, and dip a brown paper therein, and lay it hot thereunto with warm cloaths bound fast to it all night. Do this for the space of three or four nights together.

AGUES.

For a Quartain Ague.

Take a quart of Ale, one ounce Cene, half an ounce of Licoras, half an ounce of Anniseeds, a few Raisons of the Sun, boil these together till your Ale be more then halfe consumed, then give it to the Patient to drink, as warme as he may, when his Fit is upon him, and go to bed, and keep him warm. This is to be used three several times, if his Fit go not away at the first. Probatum.

For an Ague.

Take the Root of a blew Lilly and scrape it clean, and slice it, lay it in soak all night in Ale, and in the morning stamp it and strain it, and give it the Patient to drink, an hour before the Fit cometh.

For the Feaver Cake.

Take Barley meal, or else the flower of wheat, and make a cake and bake it, and then take the juice of Hemlocks, and annoint the belly with it: Also you may take Oyle of Exceter, or Sallet Oil, and fry a few Oats therein, and lay it to the Patients stomack as hot as he can suffer it. Probatum.

For a hot Burning Ague.

Take Succory roots and leaves, Parsley roots, Endive leaves, Borrage leaves and Sorrel leaves, seethe all these together in a pottle of running water, and when it is sodden, strain the water from the Herbs, then put to it a good piece of Sugar to make it pleasant, and two spoonful of Vineger, that it may be somewhat sharp: you may also put in Buglos.

An excellent Medicine for an Ague.

Take a handful of good Bay Salt, and put it into a Mortar and bray it very small, then put thereto as many of the biggest Cobwebs that you can get, as the quantity of four fingers, and beat them a good while, then put into them a good handful of Smallage clean picked, and so beat them all together very well into one substance; then take it out the Mortar, and put thereunto two ounces of the best Venice Turpentine unwashed, and temper them well together, and two hours before the Ague fit cometh, divide it into two parts, and bind it equally to both wrists on the place where the Pulse beateth, and roll it up well with a linnen cloth, that it stir not from the place, and tack it fast with a needle and thred, and so let it lye four and twenty hours, and it will alter the Fit of the Ague and drive it away; but if not, try the second time, and no doubt but it will help. A little fresh butter will get off the Medicine from the wrists.

A good Medicine to remove or avoid a Burning Fever.

Take of Dragon Water, of Angelica Water, of Red rose Water, of each three spoonfuls, three grains of Bezar Stone, the quantity of a Nutmeg of Mithridatum, or else a spoonful of Jean Treakle, half a penny worth of English Saffron; Mingle all these together, and take it fasting, and sweat after it, and use this two or three mornings together.

For the Ague.

Take one penny worth of Gore Turpentine, of Rye Leaven the quantity of a Hasel Nut, being somewhat stale, a little course Mastick, and a little bay salt, both beaten small, one handful of Smallage, and a few Cobwebs shred smal; mingle all these with the Turpentine, and spread the same upon a piece of white Sheeps leather on the rough side, being pricked full of holes, and three hours before you think your fit will come, bind it to your wrists, and let it continue nine dayes or more.

Another.

Take a pottle of Ale, seethe it, and skum it, then put to it the tops of Centory, Mints, Sage, Wormewood and Hysop of each a handful; boil all in the Ale, till half be consumed, then take the Herbs out with a spoon, then put a quantity of Sugar in the Ale, to allay the bitternesse of it, and so let it boil a little while again, then strain it through a faircloath; that done, put thereto as much Treakle as the biggnesse of a bean and then keep it in a fair glasse, and let the Patient drink thereof first and last, and drink not after for the space of an hour.

For all Feavers and Agues of sucking Children.

Take powder of Christal, and steep it in wine and give it the Nurse to drink: also take the root of Morsus Diabili with the Herb, and hang it about the Childs neck.

For an Ague.

Take Bur-roots and red Nettle crops, and seethe them in Stale Ale, and clarifie it, let the Patient drink it a little before the cold fit cometh, and when he beginneth to sweat, give him a posset of Ale made with Marigolds, and Fennel being clarified, and it helpeth in four or five Fits.

Another.

Take of Smallage and Fetherfew, of each a handful stamp them, and straine them, and take half so much (as the juice thereof) of small Ale, being mixt together, drink it in bed before the Fit cometh, cover your self warm.

Another.

Take Endive, Sowthistle, Dandillion, Lettice, Sorrel, of each alike, stil them altogether, and the water thereof is very good for an Ague.

Another.

Take Soot and yolks of Eggs, and bay Salt, and pepper, being mingled wel together, lay it to both the wrists, and drink warm Ale.

Another.

Take three cloves of Garlick, and bruise them, a penny worth of Aqua vitae, and half a pint of Ale, seethe them together; and drink it before the Fit cometh, as hot as you may.

Another.

Box leaves dryed and made into powder, and Sheeps trecklings put in soak in strong Ale, and drunk, is very good.

An approved Medicine for an Ague.

Take a red Fennel root, and cut it very smal, and take six and fifty cornes of Pepper beaten very small, and mingle them together, and bind them to your wrists half an hour before your Fit cometh.

AQUA COMPOSITA.

How to make a Special Aqua Composita to take for a Surfet or cold stomack.

Take a handful of Rosemary, a good root of Enula campane, a handful of Hysop, half a handful of Thime, six good crops of Sage, as much Mint,and as much Penniroyal, half a handful of Horehound, two ounces of Liquorice well bruised, and as much Anniseeds; Then take two gallons of the best strong Ale, and take all the Herbs aforesaid, and wring them asunder, and put them into an Earthen pot wel covered, and let them stand a day and a night; from thence put all into a brasse pot, and set it on the fire, and let it stand till it boil, then take it from the fire, and set your Limbeck on the pot, and stop it close with paste that there come no air out of it, and still it out with a soft fire. There is to be added to it by a new counsel, one handful of red Fennel.

A Receipt of G.K. to make Aqua composita.

Take of the best strong stale Ale, three gallons, of Licoras clean scraped and bruised half a pound, of Aniseeds clean dressed and bruised one pound.
Of each smal cut one ounce.
    Fennel seed
    Carraway seed
    Sassafras seed
    Piony seed
    Winter savory seed
    Seed of Anodinum
    Seed of Ameos

Of each One ounce.
  Ginger
  Nutmegs
  Gallingal
  Great Gallingal

Bruised, of each half an ounce.
  Cloves
  Long Pepper
  Cubebes
  Callamint aromaticus
Of each two ounces.
  Cinnamon bruised
  Ivy roots sliced
  Enula campana roots dried and thin sliced
  Roots of Tussilage.
Of Bay berries bruised, first blanched, one ounce.

Of each a quarter of an ounce.
  Setwal
  Spiknard
  Mace
  Lignum Aloes
Of each a handful.
  Roots of Angelica sliced, and of the seeds bruised
  Ligna Cassia sliced
Of each a handful
  Juniper berries bruised, or the Wood thin sliced
  Red Rose flowers
  Flowers of Sticardue
  Saint Johns wort
  The Herb Canapitis
  Diptamnus Cretius.
  Pimpernel
  Phillipendola
  Scabious
  Betony
  Egrimony
  Planteane
  Camomile flowers

of each an ounce
  The Wood or Tree called Tamariscus

The roots of Sassaparilla bruised
The roots of Orpine

The Roots of Gentian sliced two drams.

one ounce.
    Of the Gum of Mirrh
    Of Olibanum
    Of Mastick

Of Alkanite one ounce.
Of Sugar four ounces.

The order of drawing this Aqua Composita.

Half your Cinnamon, your Lignum Alloes, the roots and the seeds of Angelica must be reserved out of the Brasse pot, and knit in a linnen bag, and laid in the Receiver, whereinto your Liquor must run; and by and by the Alkanite must be put into the Receiver. Also receive out of your brasse pot all your Herbs and Flowers until the last draught come; your other Spices, Seeds, Roots and Gums must be put with your Ale into your brass pot, then set on your Limbeck, and close it fast with a paste, and keep the head therof always cool with cold water, and draw it so long as it wil run good, which is tried by casting a little of it into the fire, if it burn, it is good; if not, take off your Limbeck charily, and powre out all your stuff that is in your linnen bags in the receiver, and all the rest of your flowers and herbs, and put to them a gallon and a half of fresh Ale, and set on your Limbeck again, and draw it as before; and the Cinnamon and the Sugar that is left, must be put into the Receiver again: and when all is drawn out, put your first draught and your last together, and keep it for your use.

The best way to make Mrs. Bells Aqua composita.

Take six gallons of the best strong Ale, the Ale wort must be so strong, that it will bear an Egge, and the Ale must be at least a week old, then take two pound of Anniseeds, two pound of Licoras scraped and bruised, Fennelseeds, Coriander seeds, Carraway seeds, Parsley seeds and Gromel seeds, of each a good handful, and (for any other Seeds or Spices use your discretion) then take of Lavender, Rosemary, Sage, Hisop, Savory, Sweet Marjerom, Standing Time, Mother-Time, Running Time, Burrage, Buglos, Succory, Endive, Lettice, Violet leaves, Strawberry leaves, Mugwort, Red Fennel, Peniroyal, Red

Mints, Herb-grace, Germander, Avens, Wormwood, Bay-leaves, Nep, Clary, Horehound, Comfrey, Marigold leaves, Mercury, Sowthistle, Sorrel, Plantane, Ribwort, Angelica, Carduus Benedictus, Wood-Betany, Scabious, Balme, Liver-wort, Long wort, Saint Johns-wort, Saint Peters-worts, Parsley, Dandillion, Basil, Lavender Spike, Blood-wort, Egrimony, Burnet, Garden Gallingale roots, Setwal-roots, Polipodium of the Oak, Pimpernel, Clivers, Shepherds-flowers, Knot grasse, Cinqfoil, Long-debeeff, Sparragus, Water-cresses, Spinage, of each of these two handfuls, two or three heads of House-leek. Put all the seeds, Herbs, and Roots to the Ale, and let them lye a steeping, all night, then still them in a Limbeck and draw of it so long as it runneth good; which is tried by casting a little of it into the fire; if it burn, it is good, or else not.

To make another Aqua composita.

Take a brass pot of four gallons, and rub it very clean within side, then take three Gallons of a good strong Ale, and a gallon of Wine lees, so that your pot be not full by three fingers with your Herbs and Spices, as followeth. Take a pound of Anniseeds well bruised, and half a pound of Licoras scraped and bruised, and put it into the pot, then take a handful of Rosemary, and a handful of Hisop, a good root of Enulacampana and scrape it well and slice it; half a handful of Unset Time, half a handful of Mints, a handful of red Fennel, a handful of red Sage, six good crops of Marjerom, and as much Peniroyal, a quater handful of Hartstongue, half a handful of Horehound; gather not the Herbs till the dew be off them, then wring all your Herbs asunder, and put your Spices and all in your pot, and let them stand all night, then set your pot upon a fire of Charcoals, and set on your Limbeck upon the pot; and stop your pot round about with paste, so that no air come forth; then make a little fire under the pot, and put cold water in the top of the Limbeck, and be sure you keep it alwayes full with cold water; and as soon as it begins to drop into the Receiver, abate the fire a little, and keep it so that it drop not too fast nor too soft; for if it drop too fast, it will be too hot of the fire; and if too soft, it will be too weak: you can draw but a quart of the best, and a quart of the second.

Another way.

Take three gallons of Claret-wine with some Lees amongst it; for want of Wine, take very strong Ale, then take two pound of Anniseeds bruised, and four pounds of Licoras clean scraped and bruised, one pound of great Raisons stoned; Parsley and Fennel roots, of each a good handful, scraped and the pith taken out, with a root of Angelica, then stop it very close, and let it stand three dayes and three nights, then still it in a Limbeck, and keep the best by it self, and you must put as much Sugar candied into the glasse as is worth a shilling, and hang two grains of Musk in a cloth in it.

AQUA VITAE.

To make Aqua Vitae for a cold stomack.

Take Rosemary and Hisop, of each a handful, Sage and Horehound, of each half a handful, one root of Enula campane, Marjerom and red Mints, of each six crops, Licoras and Anniseeds well bruised, of each two ounces; then take three gallons of strong Ale grounds, and set all these on a fire in a pan til it begin to seethe, then take it from the fire, and put it in a brasse pot, and set on your Limbeck, stopping it close with paste, and keeping a soft fire under it.

To make Aqua-vitae to avoid Flegme.

Take of Peniroyal a handful, of Strawberry leaves two handfuls, and Pimpernels three handfuls, and add these to the former Receipt.

AQUA MIRABILIS.

How to make a precious Water, called, Aqua Mirabilis.

Take Gallingale, Cloves, Squills, Ginger, Melilot, Cardomons, Mace, and Nutmegs, of each one dram; of the juice of Cellendine half a pint; mingle all these made into powder with the said juice and a pint of Aqua-vitae, and three pints of good White-wine, and put all these into a Stillatory of glasse, and let it stand all night, and on the morrow still it with an easie fire.

This Water is good, for by a secret nature it dissolveth the grief of the Lungs without any pain, it purgeth Melancholy, it expelleth the stopping of the Urine, and it marvellously profiteth the stomack, conserveth Youth in his own state long, and preserveth memory, destroyeth the Palsie: it being given a man or woman labouring for life, one spoonful relieveth him: Of all Artificial Waters I think none better: In Summer use one spoonful thereof, in Winter two.

BACK.

A good Medicine to strengthen the Back.

Take Oaken leaves and buds, Knot-grass, Comfrey, and Clary, of each alike, and still them: this must be taken every morning two spoonfuls, but let it be a fortnight old, or else the fire will not be out of it.

Another.

Take Comfrey, Knot-grass, and the flowers of Archangel; boile them in a little milk of a browne Cow, and drink of it every morning; it is very good.

For the Rains of the Back and Stomack.

Take of the Fern that groweth on a house, and Camomile of each a handful, two or three slips of Unset Hysop, bruise all these together, and seeth them in a quart of Rhenish or White-wine, with a handful of Currants, till it come to a pint; and after it is sodden, put into it an ounce and a half of white Sugar candied, and let it melt of it self, then strain it through a fair cloath, and give it the Patient to drink warm morning and evening.

To strengthen the Back.

Take a handful of Knot-grasse, a handful of Archangel flowers, nine branches of Gromel, and stamp it a pint of Ewe milk, and warm it bloud warm, and let the Patient drink it an hour before he riseth for nine dayes together.

For the Raines of the Back.

Take your own water, and boil it well and scum it well, then take a quarter of an ounce of Oile of Bayes, and an ounce of Oyle of Roses, and boil it from a pottle to a pint or a quart, and annoint therewith the rains of the back, and also the Spleen vain in the foot.

For the pain of the Back, and heat of the Back.

Take Rose-water, and put thereunto Sanders and Rose-leaves, and lay them in steep in your Rose-water one whole night, and it (being drunk) will take away the heat, and greatly comfort the Reins: or wash the back therewith.

To cleanse the Back, and purge the Raines.

Take one Fennel root, and two Parsley roots, and pick out the piths of them, and put thereto one handful of Pellitory of the wal; and all these things being washed clean, seeth them in possen Ale, and drink thereof when you go to bed, and if you awake at midnight, drink of it also.

A good Medicine to strengthen a weak Back.

Take a good handful of the pith of the back of a young Ox or Heifer, slice it, and take out the stuff in it, and put it in a fair dish, put thereunto one, two or three of pure Dates, the skin within side taken off, and minced as fine as may be; then boile them in two or three spoonfuls of Rose-water, then look what quantity of Dates, so the like of Raisons of the Sun, and red Currants, your Raisons must be minced smal, and the stones taken out, then boil your Raisons and Currants and Rose-water together till they be tender, and put in some crumbs of Bread, Cinnamon, and Sugar, and Saffron small beaten to powder, then temper all these together in a fair dish, and have ready Pastionel, which is made of Sugar and yolks of Eggs, fine flower and butter, these work together into paste, and roll it as thin as you can, and make it into pieces, the fashion of a Pease cod, and bake them slenderly, and reserve them to your use, and when you list to eat of them, take one and heat it by the fire side in the morning, and eat it, and another at noon.

For the Back.

Take some Comfrey roots, Knot-grasse, Clary and Shepherds purse, stamp them and strain them, with a little Muskadine, and put thereto the rest of a pint of Muskadine, one Nutmeg grated, and two yolks of Eggs, and so drink of it cold.

To cleanse and comfort the Back and Reins.

Take a pottle of fair Spring-water, and put thereinto halfe a pound of Eringo roots, as new as you can get them, and meerly of themselves as they grow, without any candying or confectioning, only bruise them very well before you put them into the pipkin of water, then take three good sticks of Licoras, and bruise them, and put them into the same water: let all these boil together over a temperate fire until half be consumed, then it take off, and every morning drink a pretty draught thereof for seventeen or eighteen dayes together.

A Conserve to strengthen the Back.

Take Eringo roots, and conserve them, as you do Damask white and red
Roses, in every respect, the pith being taken out, one pound and half of sugar
is enough for every pound of Roots, and three pints of water, and stew them
closely at the first, as you do your Roses; if you will add to them five or six
graines of Ambergreece beaten to a fine powder, it will be more cordial.

A good Drink against the heat of the Back.

Take Fennel, Comfrey and Plantane, of each a handful, Anniseeds,
Fennel seeds and Licoras, of each an ounce, Mastick two drams, Lapis
dactilus two drams, boile these in two quarts of new milk till half be
consumed, then strain it and drink of it morning and evening. After this
drink, the space of an hour,take on the top of a knife this Electuary:
Diatragacanth, frigid. one ounce, of Sirrup of Violets one dram, mix
them together, and take it as aforesaid.

For paine and heat in the Back.

Take Sage, Rosemary, Camomile and Maudlin, of each one handful,
stamp them together, and frye them in May butter, and annoint the back
with it warm.

Of the pain in the Back.

This pain proceedeth of Rheumes that fall into the sinews of the
Muscles, or of great labour, and such like occasions.
Seeth Nep in your broth, which draweth the noisome and grieved matter
out of the neck, and driveth away all pain in the shoulders and back bones.
Also silver Mountain seeds sod in water and drink thereof twice a week
every time three or four ounces. It is very good against all weakness of the
back and raines.

BALM.

To make an excellent Balm.

Take a pottle of the best White wine, three pints of Oyle of Saint Johns-
wort, of the blossomes of Saint Johns-wort, Carduus Benedictus, Sage,
Valerian, of each two pound, of Marjerom and Comfrey one pound, chop
them, and stamp them small, and put them into the Wine and Oyle; then take
new Wheat four ounces, dry it well and bruise it, and put it into the Wine

and Oyle, stir it well and seeth it four and twenty hours upon the embers close covered, sometimes stirring it, then boile it and stir it well, and when you perceive the wine is almost consumed, take it off and strain it, then set it on a soft fire, and take Venice Turpentine, Mirrhe, Incense, and Mastick, of each four ounces, Olibanum five ounces, Sanguis Draconis one ounce, beat all these to fine powder, and searse them through Lawn, put in the Turpentine a little before the rest, stirring it exceedingly well, then set it a little on the fire, and off and on, keeping it stirring till it be almost cold, then put it in a glasse bottle for your use. It is good for all manner of wounds.

BELLY.

For a swelling in the Belly.

Take Sassafras, Hartstongue, Betony, Centory, of each two handfuls, Pelitory of Spain, Cinnamon, Ginger, Cloves, of each one ounce, Licoras two ounces, Spinark one ounce, put all these in a gallon of White wine; and let it stand three dayes, and then drink of it the space of eight dayes.

Another.

Take a quart of Spring-water, and about some twenty leaves of a weed called Dithander, and put thereinto some ten or twelve Cloves, and boyl all these together till it come to a pint, and drink thereof.

An Oyntment for a great belly, whether it be by reason of an Ague, or Wormes, or the Spleen.

Take Romane Wormwood, common Wormwood, Garden Tansie, Fetherfew, Sowthernwood, Unset Leeks, Peach leaves, Herb-grace, of each one handful, wash them, and wring them, then take a pound of Barrowes grease or May butter, stamp all the Herbs in a Mortar very small, then mingle them with the grease, and make it up into balls as big as Tennis Balls, then put them in the Cellar seven or eight daies till they be all hoary, then break them into an Earthen pot, and boil them on a soft fire till the juice be consumed, then take it up and strain it, and keep it for your use: And when you use it, warm some it, and annoint the belly before the fire morning and evening.

For a pain in the Bowels through hot Choler.

The party must be purged with Sirrups which do cool, and Glisters. For a Purge, take eight and twenty damask Pruins, and five or six

Figs, Seeth them in water, and take of this Decoction three or four
ounces, temper Cassia therein, and Oyl of Sweet Almonds five or six
ounces tempered with sugar, and drink the same at once. It looseneth
the body very gently, and may be given to children newly born.
Likewise Manna decocted with sowre Dates, Pruins and Sugar, is good
to give a stool.

BITING.

For the Biting of a Mad Dog.

Take Garlick, Salt and Rew, stamp them altogether, and in the manner
of a Plaister lay it to the sore, and give the Patient Treakle to drink three
times in a week till the danger be past. Probatum.

Another.

Take a handful of Box, and stamp it, and strain it with a draught of
milk, put into it a pretty quantity of Lobsters shell beaten to powder, and
some Unicorns horn, if you can get it, and drink thereof and wash the
wound therewith.

Another.

Take Betony, Wild Sage, and Night Shade, of each a good handful, and
a pint of running water, stamp the Herbs, and strain them therewith, and
put thereto a penny worth of Treakle, and give the Patient to drink two or
three mornings fasting.

BLEEDING.

To stanch the bleeding of a Cut.

Take Hysop, and cut it as small as you can, and put it into the wound,
and put Cobwebs thereupon, or a linnen cloth clean washed and dryed
and burnt to tinder, and laid to the cut, doth stanch it without a doubt.

To stanch the Bleeding, and to heal.

Take Mastick and the hair of a Hare mixt with the white of a new laid
Egg, and make a Plaister thereof, and lay it to the wound.

Another for the same.

There is not a better thing then the powder of Bole Armoniack for to stanch the bleeding of a wound, the powder to be laid upon it; or for the Nose, to be put in with the blast of a quil.

Another for the same.

Take the shavings of Parchment, and lay it to the wound, it stancheth and healeth.

Another.

Take dried Vervain and make it into powder, and so lay it in the wound.

To stanch bleeding at the Nose, Vein, or Wound.

Take a piece of linnen cloth, and a Spider, kill it not, but wrap it in the piece of linnen cloth, and put it up the Patients Nostrils.

Another.

Take Orpine, which is chiefe of all Herbs to stanch blood, beat the Herb in your hand, chafing it till it be warm, it will stop all manner of bleeding.

Another to stop bleeding at the Nose, mouth, Wound or bloudy flux.

Take the juice of red Nettles, with a little red Wine, and a little Vitriol, burnt or unburnt, and drink it.

Another for the same.

Take a little lint, and make it round like a pease, and dip it into ink, and put it into the Nose, and it will stanch bleeding straightwayes.

Another.

Take the Mosse of a Crab tree, and let the Patient smell it as it cometh from the tree.

Another.

Take a quantity of green Coperas, as much Bole Armoniack beaten to fine powder and cast it into the wound.

Another.

Take Wine Vineger and the white of an Egg, and beat them together, and spread them on a linnen cloth, and for a man lay it on his privy members, and for a woman on her brest.

Another for a Wound.

Take wild Tansie and bruise it small, and lay it on the wound, or make powder of it, and fill the wound full of it.

For bleeding at the Nose.

Take Betony and stamp it with as much salt as you can hold between your two fingers, and put it in your Nose.

To stanch Blood.

Take the lean of salt Bief, so much as you think will goe into the wound, and lay it in the Embers of the fire, and let it roast till be red hot, and thrust it into the wound hot, and bind it up fast, and if the wound be in the foot, bind him about the Anckle; if in the legg, about the knee, if in the knee, bind the thigh; if in the hand, about the wrists; if in the arme, about the bought of the arme with a good list or Garter two or three times about, and it will stanch bleeding.

To stop Bleeding.

Take Centory, green Rew, and red Fennel and stamp and strain them and drink it warmed.

Another.

Take an old clean linnen cloth, and wet it well in Vineger, then burn it, and take the powder thereof, and if it be a wound, cast it therein, and it will stop the bleeding immediately; but if the Nose bleed, then snuff up the powder into the Nose, and it helpeth.

Another.

Take the crops of Southernwood, and crush them in your fingers and put it into the nose.

Another.

If your Nose do bleed unmeasurably, then tye your little finger very hard about the lower joint, and for the most part, it faileth not, but stayeth the same.

For spitting of Blood.

Take the juice of Betony, and temper it with Goats milk, and give it the Patient to drink three dayes together.

Another.

Take Smallage, Rew, Mints and Betony, and seeth them well in good milk, and sup it warm.

To stanch blood.

Take an Herb called Periwinkle, and hold it between thy teeth, and it helpeth.

For pissing of Blood.

Take Ambrosia and Bursa pastoris of each a handful, Parsley seeds the like, stamp them together, and drink the juice thereof with Goats milk.

The cause of pissing of blood may be superfluity of Humors, Sharpness of Urine, Winds, Tumors, Impostumations, debility of the Kidneyes and Bladder, then is there a pain about the Privities, and the blood is congealed and separated from the Urine: In case the blood be much and runneth out swiftly, then it signifies a broken Vein, otherwise an Ulcer; but if the Urine be like water that flesh is washed in, then it is of a weak liver; but if from superfluity of blood, then it is to be seen by the fulnesse of the body; if through sharpnesse of Humours the Patient is ever burning, therefore he must avoid all sharp, tart and salt things.

Of letting Bloud.

Phlebottomie is needlesse to those that be of so strong a nature, that (being overladen) are able to expel all superfluity through natural passages, as by bleeding at the Nose, & c.

Quest. But why is Phlebottomie used?

Ans. When blood aboundeth, it is commonly in those that have a hot liver, full veines, a high colour and brownish, and not fat and corpulent: Also in those that eat and drink abundantly, live at ease, and use meats that ingender much blood, which when Nature cannot digest, it corrupteth the braines, from which issueth dangerous Diseases; and in these cases, this is a more sure remedy, then to admit of inward Physick.

Also letting of blood doth strengthen the brain, comfort the sight, warmeth the marrow in the bones, freeth the inward parts of many infirmities, stayeth vomiting, oftentimes helpeth the flux or lask, cleereth the senses, restoreth sleep, reneweth the spirits, because melancholy blood is thereby diminished, cureth deafness, reduceth lost voices, augmenteth the powers and vertues of all the body, being thereby rid of superfluities; the abundance of blood is known, no less by the thicknesse and troubled matter consisting of the Urine, then by the signes before mentioned. And though the blood be not inflamed, but superabundant, it causeth many dangerous diseases; and if any in the mornings about the dawning of the day do commonly sweat, it is a sign of Superfluity in the Veines.

Thirdly, Where cold and bad blood is, there must be a Purgation precede Phlebottomie, or else the cold blood will remain.

Lastly, Its good sometimes to be let blood that the blood may be led or drawn from one place to another.

BONES.

How to use Fractured Bones: four kind of Factures.

First, when it is broken in length: Next, when it is broken overthwart. Thirdly, when it is oblick and crooked. Fourthly, when it girded and broken, and shivered in divers pieces, either legs or armes.

Albusences, and others later Writers, make the difference of Fractures; not according to the bone fractured, but after the place affected; as if the Nose be broken, brain-pan, jawes, ribs, backbone, armes, legs, or other parts, which be not differences of Fractures, but of the place affected, according to nature.

Four Directions in the Cure of Fractures, according to the place fractured.

First, to respect, that the bones be put again in their former place. Secondly, to be reduced to their natural, and so conserved and kept without motion or hurt.

Thirdly, That the bone broken may be ingendred and conglutinated together by ingendring of Callus.

Fourthly, To correct the Accidents that do come after the Fracture of the bones.

How the Bones out of joint ought to be put together.

Be sure of help to hold the party at need; for the Legg or Arm let him sit in a Chair, and with the annointing draw it out till the place be met, as tenderly as you may, having respect to the party grieved his complexion and nature.

How Bones may be conserved after they be set in their natural place.

Look well to your rolling. First, it is very good to take the white of an egge and Oyle of Roses mixt together, and wet therein the linnen Cloathes which may cover the place broken, and somewhat more of the other, and roll it not too hard, for it may cause dolour and flux of humours.

How the Rollers must be used.

The first Roller upon the Fracture three or four times, and so to the second part upwards; the third Roller leek downward, and it must be half as low as the first; these Rollers should be wet in water and wine before you use them. If the pain be vehement, then the member would be wrapped about with fine wooll well carded, or else with stuff wet in Oxicrotium.

A defensive Medicine.

Take Unguentum Populeum two ounces, Bole Armoniack one ounce, mix these together with Oyle of Roses, and a little Vineger.

If the place appear blistered.

Take half a pint of running water, and set it on the fire, and put in fine Wax, a little Oyl of Roses and fine Barly meal, seethe them altogether, but not very thick, then make thereof a Plaister or Cere-cloth; strike it upon the cloth, upon the bottom of a Pewter dish, over a Chafingdish and coals, and lay it lukewarm to the arm or leg, a night and a day and it will asswage the humour of boyning.

For the Wound of Broken Bones.

Take luke-warm Mell Rosarum, and Oyle of Roses, and stamp of flax dipped in the Whites of Eggs, and so bind it upon the sore; Also apply about the place Bole Armoniack, Sanguis Draconis, and Olibanum, beaten with a little Oyl of Roses, Barley meal and Vineger round about the sore, and so comfort the Patient.

A Defensive against Boyning of a broken Bone in the Leg.

Make your Plaister of Oyle of Roses and Oyle of Mirtle melted together with a little wax, and when it is cold, put to it Bole Armoniack and Pompuleon, of each one ounce, of Wine two ounces, and lay it a handful broad upon the hurt and let it lye.

A Poultice for any Boyning inward.

Take a pint of new Cowes milk, a pint of Rye-bread crumbs, a handful of French Poppy leaves shred small, two ounces of Oyle of Roses, three yolks of new laid eggs, and as much Saffron as the weight of a Groat, First boil the milk, the crumbs and the Poppy together a good while, and then put in the rest, and spread it upon a faire linnen cloth.

To asswage the swelling upon any broken Bone or out of joint.

Take Unguentum Pompuleum one ounce, Bole Armoniack one ounce, mix them together with a little Oyle of Roses, and a little Vineger.

For the Bone ache.

Take the leaves and flowers of Henbane, and put them in an earthen pot and with May butter, and close the pot, and set it in a dunghil three months, then annoint the grieved place therewith.

BODY.

To distil a Cock, good for any weak Person.

Take a red or black Cock, and pluck him quick, and whip him alive with small twigs a pretty while, then cut off his head and gut him, and cut him in quarters, and wipe him very dry with a fair cloth; then take an earthen pot and lay four or five splints to keep it from the bottom of the pot; then lay in the four quarters upon the splints, and lay between every quarter some of these Roots and Fruit following, Fennel roots, Parsley roots, Succory roots of each two or three, two or three slips of Rosemary, two or three Dates quartered, half a handful of Raisons of the Sun the stones taken out, six spoonfuls of Rhenish Wine, Malmesey or Muskadine, three or four whole Mace, cover the pot, and stop it close with paste, and set it in a pot or kittle of hot water, and let it boil softly with a temperate fire four hours, then take it up and let it run through a fair cloth without any forcing, then put it in a fair glasse or pot, and keep it close covered, and give to the Patient two or three spoonfuls at once, or in quantity as the stomack is able to take it, in some broth made of Mutton or Veal, first in the morning, and as often in the day besides as he hath a stomack to take it.

To preserve the Body.

Take a pottle of fair water and six Calves feet, and put therein Betony, Long-wort, Liver-wort, Knot-grasse, Clary, Balm, with a quantity of Mace, Cinnamon and Ginger, and six Dates; let all these be sodden together till it come to a Jelly; and then take a quart of White-wine, or very pure Claret, and put therein, and eat it at your pleasure.

Another.

Take the marrow of Venison, a pint of running water, three leaves of Clary, three leaves of Comfrey, one handful of Archangel, a handful of Charnel, threee Dates, a handful of small Raisons, seeth altogether till it come to half a pint, then strain it, and put thereto a pint of white Bastard, and a quantity of Manus Christi.

Another.

Take a pint of Muskadine, and put thereto Hemp-seed and blanched Almonds, and Cap Dates, two or three whole Mace, and a Nutmeg, and three crops of Rosemary, and a little Saffron and red Rose-water, and boil them all together till half be boiled away, and after they be boiled, put thereto Mithridatum about the quantity of a hasel Nut, but let it not seethe after, and let the party drink thereof at his going to bed at night.

Another.

Take a pottle of water, and a Chicken, and two Fennel roots, two Parsley roots, three Dates, a handful of Currants, and boile them altogether, from a pottle to a pint, then take two spoonfuls of Hasel Nut kernels, and eight blanched Almonds, stamped together with the Nuts, and strain them into the broth, and so drink it morning and evening.

For avoiding gravel in the Body.

Take a couple of eggs, and boil them hard, then take the shells only, and stamp them very small, then take six Dates stones, and one Nutmeg, and stamp them likewise, then take of Cene as much as the two former things do weigh, then searse it through a very fine Searse, then take the weight of four pence or six pence and drink it in a quantity of White Wine, Ale or Beere, in the morning as long as the things do last, and it will break it away, with hot broth within one hour after.

A Medicine for a weak Body.

Take a Legg of Veal, and wash it very clean, and put it into a gallon of fair spring water, set it over the fire, and skumme it very cleane, and then put in a quarter of a pound of the best red Currants you can get, and half a handful of the Roots of Orpine, the skin being clean pick'd off, and some grated bread to thicken; let it boil softly over the fire till it cometh to a pottle, and then put in half an ounce of Coral very finely beaten, and half an ounce or Cinnamon finely beaten, and let it be stirred when the Spices be put in; and this you must drink three times a day, being boiled three or four walmes after the Spices be put in. You must drink this in the morning fasting, and an hour before Dinner, and an hour before Supper. It must be very warm when you drink it, and in the morning fast two hours after you have taken it. This is good for a weak back, for the Mother, and for the Whites, and for the running of the Rains.

To comfort the Spirits of one that is weak.

Every two or three hours give the Patient a spoonful of Syrrup De Corticibus Citri, and therein three of four drops of Aqua Coelestis.

A very good Glister for a weak body that is troubled with the Cholick.

Take a piece of a knuckle of Veal, set it on the fire in a convenient quantity of water, one Fennel root scraped, and the pith taken out, one Parsley root scraped, the pith taken out, Camomile, Penniroyal, Burrage and Bugloss, of each a handful, Raisons of the Sun stoned, three pieces of large Mace, and a piece of Cinnamon bruised a little, one Nutmeg quartered: Let these boil till it hath a good taste of the meat, then strain out a pint of this Broth in a Bason, and put to it four spoonfuls of Oyle of Rew, the yolk of one new laid egge, three penny worth of Sugar candied; stir all these well, and give it with a Glister-pipe bloodwarm, about eight of the clock in the morning and four in the afternoon.

BRAINES.

A Gargarism to purge the Braines.
By Dr. Deodate.

Take six spoonfuls of Wine Vineger, and twelve spoonfuls of water, and two spoonfuls of Honey, clarifie them together, and add thereto one spoonful of Mustard.

BREST.

To heal a sore Brest when it is broken.

Boil Lillies in new milk, and lay it on to break it, and when it is broken, tent it with a Mallow stalk, and lay on it a Plaister of Mallowes boiled in Sheeps tallow. These are to be used if you cannot keep it from breaking.

For a womans Brest not broken.

Take Oyle of Roses, Bean flower, the yolk of an Egg, a little Vineger, temper all these together, then set it afore the fire that it may be a little warm, and then with a feather strike it upon the Brest morning and evening or any time of the day when she feels the pricking.

A Drink for a sore Brest or Wound.

Take of Avens, Plantane, Ribwort, Bugloss, Primrose leaves, Cuckoe Sorrel, Bramble leaves, and a yellow flower like to Dandillion, but somewhat less, Daisies, roots and all, Sanacle, Worm-wood, Strawberry leaves, Herb Robert, Egrimony, Cinqfoil, of each a good handful, not too much wormwood, for making it bitter; boil all these in a pottle of White-wine, and make it somewhat sweet with Honey, then strain it and wring out all the juice as neer as you can, then drink a good draught thereof in the morning and at night, till it is done, and lay to the sore a Primrose leaf, or a

Plantane: And when the brest is sore or hard, take Polipodium, Plantane and great Raisons, beat them smal, and lay it all about the Brest upon a cloth.

For an Ague in the Brest.

Take Groundsel, Daisie leaves and roots, course Wheat chessel, make a Poultice thereof with the parties owne water, and lay it warm to the Brest.

A Drink to purifie the Brests from Rheume

Take Hysop, Figs and Honey boile them in Wine, from a pottle to a quart, drink it in the Evening hot and in the morning cold.

For a sore Brest, or to dry up a womans milk, or to asswage the hard swelling, if it lye not too long.

Take stale strong Ale or Beer grounds, a small peece of Allome, and a little Honey, and boil them together, then take a piece of woollen cloth, and cut two holes in it for the two nipples, and dip it in the liquor, and lay it to the brests very hot, lay a piece of black wool upon the nipples.

For stopping in the Brest.

Take Rew and seethe it in Verjuice, and so to drink it.

For a heat and swelling in a Womans Brest.

Take the white of two new laid eggs and beat them very well; also take a handful of Violet leaves, and pound them very fine, and put them to the whites of the Eggs, and take as much wheat- flower as will make it as thick as a Plaister, and temper it well altogether and spread it upon a cloth, and lay it upon the brest, and it will ease the pain, and take away the swelling. Also Snow-water and Sallet Oyle, &c. Probatum.

If a woman want milk in her Brests.

The cause may be of heat or drowth, or of some cold quality of the brest, that the blood which should alter into milk be dried out.

Again, the want of milk, may be for want of meat, or use of such meats as may dry out the blood; or by bad digestion of the stomack, &c. use a good Diet, and eat green Marjerom in the morning fasting.

BRUISE.

For a Bruise.

Take running water a gallon, Ferne roots scraped clean, and sod in the water till it be halfe consumed, and then stamp them and strain them, and then put it between a linnen cloth, and lay it to the bruise or squat as hot as may be suffered, and it will help: you may wash the place pained with the liquor so that the skin be not broken.

A soveraign Medicine for bruised blood congealed in the body.

Take Lyons Claw, that is Predalian, or our Ladies Mantle, and Sage, and Parsley, of each one handful, of Anniseeds, Fennel seeds, Hysop seeds, and the root of Elicampane about two ounces, seethe them in two pound of water until the third part be consumed; drink this, and it loseth all congealed blood in the body, and expelleth it in the Urine.

An excellent Balme to cure any bruise, though Bones be broken therein, and it is very good to cure wounds.

Take of Scala Coeli one pound, Rosemary flowers four ounces, Pomgranat rinds two ounces, Sallet Oyle two pound, White Wine halfe a pint, bruise the Scala Coeli and the Pomegranate rinds, and in the Oyle and the Wine with the Rosemary flowers, infuse them ten dayes in the Sun; after that, boil them till the Wine be consumed, then strain it, and unto the Oyl being strained, put these things following, Mastick, Olibanum, of each four ounces, Aloes one ounce, Cassia four ounces, Venice Turpentine twelve ounces, Verdigrease one ounce; boil these in the Oyle until the Gummes be dissolved, then strain it, and keep it to use, and remember that in the end of the boiling the Verdigrease be put in, and let the Turpentine be put in last, not letting it boil after, but only with the heat dissolve it self.

For any Bruises, Aches, or any such like pain.

Take Rosemary tops, Toutswaine leaves, Plantane leaves, of each two handfuls, Stone pitch and Turpentine, of each one pound, a pint of Sallet Oyl, a quarter of a pound of Wax, two ounces of Olibanum; the Herbs must be beaten very small in a Mortar, and then boile them together in a Pipkin six or seven hours till it come to be as stiff as Soap, and when it is so boiled, it must be strained through a linnen cloth, and so put up into Gally pots, the Olibanum must not be put in till the other be boiled sufficiently.

For a Bruise, or Strain, or Green Wound.

Take half a pint of Sallet Oyle, a quarter of a pound of White-lead, two ounces of Cerus. First, set the Oyl on the fire in an earthen pan, and when it is ready to boil, put in the White-lead, being in fine powder, so let it boil a quarter of an hour, then put in your Cerus being beaten small, and stir it while it seethes, then drop a drop in cold water, and if it will roll, it is boiled enough; then powre it all into a Bason of cold water, and when it is cold enough to touch, annoint your hands, and roll it up in little rolls.

An excellent Remedy for Bruises and Aches which come of cold.

Take young Bay-leaves and Wormewood, of each a quarter of a pound, a pound and a half of Suet of a Loyne of Mutton, a quart of Oyle Olive, of Oyle of Spike two ounces, shred your Herbs small and your Suet, the put them in a stone pot, and powre the Oyles upon them, and cover it very close, and so let it stand close covered two dayes; then boil it till the Liquor be very green, that the goodnesse is out of the Herbs, then strain it, and reserve it for your use.

Another.

Take a pound of Butter out of the Charn-milk, and set it on the fire, and clarifie it, then take a handful and a half of red Sage, as much Camomile, as much Herb-grace, and half as much Smallage, some young Bay-leaves, chop all the Herbs small, and put them into the clarified butter, and boile them on a soft fire, stirring it until it be green, then strain it, and keep the Liquor for your use.

For a Bruise or Strain.

Take the grounds of Ale or Beere, Wheat Bran and Chickweed, and lay it to the grief three of four times a day upon a red cloth.

For a Bruise or Sore unripened.

Take Oatmeal and seethe it in sweet Cowes milk, until it be as thick as pap, and put it into a pan with a quantity of Sheeps suet, and boile them well, and then make a Plaister thereof, and lay it to the grief as hot as you can suffer it.

BREATH.

A good Medicine for a stinking Breath.

Take two handfuls of Cumin seeds, and seeth them in good Wine from a pottle to a pint, and then drink of it fifteen days together morning and evening.

Of a stinking Breath, how it cometh.

This Infirmity proceedeth, First, when the Gums are putrified: Secondly, from hallow teeth: Thirdly, Stinking humors that fall downe from the head to the Pannicles of the mouth, and make the spettle to stink. Fourthly, Stinking slime of the stomack. Fifthly, the corruption of the Lights. Sixthly, Stinking matter and purulency. Seventhly, stopping in the Nose, or some exulceration of the same.
If it be from any of these causes proceeding from the Head, then it is of heat; then purge the head, and wash the mouth often with Plantane water.
Also take green Oaken leaves, and dry them, and beat them to powder, and take one dram sod in Wine.

BURNING.

An excellent Medicine for Burning or Scalding.

Take Sage and seeth it in running water, and wash the wound with the water as hot as you can suffer it, and it will take away the heat immediately, then take Sage, and Harstongue leaves, and Sheeps dung, and fry it with Sheeps suet, and annoint the place therewith with a feather, and let it lye still; then take Sheeps dung and dry it to powder, and strew it twice a day, and annoint it twice a day; but take heed of picking any of it away, lest there be holes in the skin ever after: And to asswage the stiffness, when you can abide it no longer, then bathe it a little in Sage water; but the less bathing, the sooner it will be whole.

For a scalding or burning with fire.

Take black Soap, about the bignesse of the sore, and spread it upon a linnen cloth like a Plaister, and so lay it upon the sore, and within half a day it will draw out the fire, and then lay healing Salve to it.
The Oyle of Cream and Snow water, is good to wash the place so hurt.

For Burning or Scalding.

Take the whites of two Eggs, and one yolk, and beat them well together and scum off the froth, then melt three spoonfuls of Barrowes grease, and take three spoonfuls of the juice of Sage, and put thereto, and stir it well together till it be cold, then make thereof a Salve.

To heal a Burning or Scalding.

Take the fat of dryed Bacon, and hold it between a pair of Tongs red hot, and let it drop into a pot of faire water, and of the dropping make your Plaister.

For Burning in the fire.

Take the second pill of a young Elme tree, and lay it in fair water the space of twelve hours or more, then fill out the water and warm it on the fire, and annoint the Patient therewith, and let it drink in the water, and when it is dry, then take new with the juice of Plantane as much of the one as of the other, and then annoint it therewith after the first water.

To make Oyle of Cream for Burning or Scalding.

Take a quart or a pint of new Cream, and boil it in a cleane Vessel, and ever stir it till it become curdy, and that it turne into an Oyle, then straine it through a cloth, and the Oyle will come from the curd.

For Burning with Fire, Gun-
powder, Scalding or the like.

Take Snow water, or running water, and put thereinto fine Sallet Oyle, and beat them well together, so done, bathe the place grieved twice or thrice, and so rest that the fire may be taken out: Then make this Oyntment following: Take of Daisies, roots and leaves, of Balme, and of Alehoofe, of each two handfuls, of Valerian and Orpine leaves, of each one handful, beat all these together very fine in a stone Mortar after they have been well washed and dryed, then take of fresh Butter unsalted two pound, of Barrowes grease one pound, and a pint of Neats foot-Oyle; boil all these together, till the water of the Herbs be consumed, by which time it will be a perfect Oyntment, then take it from the fire, straine it, and presse it well out, and keep it well in an earthen pot, it will last seven years, and when you use it, take Primrose leaves and pare away the ribs, and after the sore place is well annointed, lay the smooth side upon the place grieved all over, and so lay on fine linnen, and change it often.

For a Burning.

Take half a pint of Cream, two handfuls of Wild Daisies, with their roots, a few Rosemary tops, and a little Sugar, boil them together till they become an Oyl, then strain it, and annoint the place therewith; but first wash it with Whey.

For a Burning or Scalding.

Take Maiden wort and stamp it, seeth it in fresh butter, and strain it, and annoint the place.

Another.

Take one handful of Barrowes grease, and two handfuls of Groundsel, and two or three handfuls of Houseleek, stamp the Herbs together, the put to them new sheeps dung two handfuls, of Goose dung two handfuls, and stamp them altogether, and being hot, strain them through a cloth into an Earthen pot, and with the liquor annoint the burned place.

Another.

Take Plantane, Waybred, Daisies, and the green bark of Elder, and green Goose dung, and Oyl Olive, stamp them together, and wring them through a cloth, and bath the hurt with a feather.

CANKER.

To kill the Canker.

Take Herb-grace, Ribwort, Fetherfew, Groundsel, Parsley, Sorrel, leaven, Boares grease, of each a handful, and a little bay salt; shred all these together, and seeth them in the dregs of Ale with some Verjuice.

For a Canker in a Womans brest.

Take the dung of a white Goose, and the juice of Cellendine, and bray them well in a Mortar together, and lay thereof to the sore, and this will stay the Canker, and heal it.

For a black Canker in a womans brest.

Take pild Garlick and Rye meal, beat them together, and boile them in Wine Vineger till it be thick as pap, then lay it on the sore, and change it three times a day till it be white, then take Pimpernel and stamp it with a little Honey, and lay it to the brest, and it will heal it.

For a Canker in the Nose, Mouth, or Throat.

Take of Rosemary stripped from the stalks, and of red Sage leaves, of each a like; dry them, and burn them in a clean chafingdish, then take a pretty piece of Allome, and burn it very fine, and make your Herbs very small, and then with some Honey temper it altogether; and make it pretty soft, and annoint the place with it three times a day, in the morning fasting, after dinner, and after Supper; let the water out of your mouth if you can, but if it go downe it will not hurt you; and before you annoint it, wash it with Orange pils cut in pieces, and laid in water; if you make it bleed it is the better. This Medicine will look very black, but it is very good.

For a Canker in the mouth.

Take six spoonfuls of honey clarified, with as much water, boil it over the fire till the water be consumed, still stirring it; and when it is clarified, put to it a pint of the best and strongest White Wine, and a piece of Roch Allome of the bigness of a Hasel Nut, and a spoonful of Bay salt, let all these seeth together the space of a quarter of an hour, then take dry Rose leaves, Woodbind leaves, and Sage, of each a handful, and let them seeth a quarter of an hour more together upon a Chafingdish and coals, and let the Patient wash the sore with the liquor, and lay the leaves upon it, and if the Liquor be too thick to wash your mouth, take fair running water, and White Wine Vinegar, and a spoonful of Honey to be sodden together with the Herbs aforesaid.

For a Canker or Itch over the Body.

First take of Quicksilver, of Sallet Oyle, of Oyl de Baies, of each two pennyworth, a quantity of Quicksilver; to kil the Quicksilver, add a little bay salt, or Salt peter, mingle all these together and so use it.

CAUDLE.

To make a Caudle of great virtue.

Take a pint and a half of the strongest Ale may be gotten, twenty Jordan Almonds clean wiped, but neither washed nor blanched, two Dates minced very small, and stamped, then take the pith of a young Bief, the length of twelve inches, lay it in the water till the bloud be out of it, then strip the skin off it, and stamp it with the Almonds and Dates, then strain them all together into the Ale, them boil it until it be a little thick; give the party in the morning fasting six spoonfuls, and as much when he goeth to bed.

CHILDREN.

For a child that is Jaw fallen, or Roof fallen.

Take a handful of Chickweed, and lap it in a red Cole leaf, or else in a linnen cloth, and roast it in hot embers, and it will be a green Salve, then lay thereof to the bone in the neck, as hot as may be suffered. Also take sowr leaven of white bread, and crum it on the mould of the Childs head as a Plaister, and by Gods grace it will raise up the bone or mold within nine hours.

For scowring of a Child that will take nothing inwardly.

Take a handful of Pimpernel, and dry it between two tiles, and lay it to the soles of the feet.

An approved Medicine to cure Children that are weak limbed, and cannot go. By Dr. Deodate.

Take Sage, Sweet Marjerom and Dane wort of equal quantity, beat them a long time together, and strain the juice out of them, which juice put into a double Vial glass, so that the glasse be full of it; then stop it with paste very close and cover it with thick paste all over, then set it in an Oven, and there let it stand so long as a great loaf requires time to be throughly baked, then take it out and let it be cooled, then break the paste round about it, and if the juice be grown thick, break the glass and take it out in another dish, and keep it in a gally pot, and when you will use it, take of it the quantity of two spoonfuls at a time and as much marrow of an Ox leg, melt it together and mingle it well, and morning and evening annoint, (as warm as can be suffered) the hinder parts of the Childs thighes and legges, and also his knees, chafing it well with your warme hands; and in a short time his limbs shall be exceedingly strengthned, and be enabled (by Gods blessing) to go and walk.

To loosen the Belly of young Children.

Tye a Nutshel full of the Salve of Mallowes on the Navel, and let it lye thereupon til it be soaked in. Do this once, twice thrice, till it be amended.

The Salve of Mallowes is thus made: Take Mallow leaves and pound them, then melt fresh Butter, and boil the Mallow leaves therein till it be green, then strain and use it.

Or give the child Sirrup of Violets, being heat, or Sirrup of Damask Roses, a quarter of an ounce at a time.

For the Lask of young Children.

Give to the child both morning and evening a spoonful of Plantane water to drink; if the Child be old, give it the more, and give it no drink but such wherein Gold hath been three times quenched, Also annoint the stomack with the Oyle of Mastick and Oyl of Mints, towards his navel downewards.

Also take the juice of broad Plantane, and Wine Vineger, of each a like quantity, and mix therewith Barley meal till it be somewhat thick, then cool it a little, and spread it upon a woollen cloath, and apply it upon the belly warm and when it is cold, heat it again.

Also take a new laid egg, and take a way the threeds (as some call it) the two white spots that are joyning to the yolk, and beat it a good while, then with meal make a Cake and bake it in a pan, then beat it in a Mortar, and put powder of Cinnamon unto it, and bake it again, and let the child eat thereof now and then.

COLICK.

For the Collick and Stone.

Take a handful of Stone crop, Wild Time, Garden Time, Parsley, Saxifrage, Pellitory of the wall, of each a handful, four or five Rhadish roots, a little Philip Pimperlow, scrape the roots, and slice them, and put all these into a gallon of new milk of a red Cow, and let it stand twelve hours, and then distil it with a soft fire, and take five spoonfuls of this Water, and put it into a good draught of Rhenish or White Wine, then warm it milk warm, and with the juice of a Lemmon and some Nutmeg and Sugar, drink this fasting in the morning, and fast four or five hours after, and walk up and down; take this every third day. Probatum.

A good Medicine for the Wind Collick.

Take a flint stone, and cast it into the fire until it be red hot, then put it into a pot of drink, and there will arise a great foame, let the Pateint drink thereof.

Another.

Take the Herb Eve, and Holly without prickles, dry them by the fire upon a paper, and being well dryed, make them into a powder, and drink so much thereof at a time as will ly upon a Groat in White Wine or Ale, it is exceeding good.

For the Collick in the stomack.

Take a quantity of Conserves of Red Roses, three Pepper cornes, and beat them small; also take the seeds of Unset Time, with Anniseeds, beat them small, and put them into the Conserve of Roses, and mingle them well together, then put into a Gally pot, and when your pain first cometh upon you, take the quantity of a small Walnut, and presently after as much Green Ginger as a Hasel Nut.

For the Collick and Stone.

Take Parsley, Pellitory of the wall, Saxifrage, Wild Time, Eyebright, of each two handfuls, twenty Rhadish roots scraped and sliced; steep all in a pottle of Red Cowes milk all night, then distil them in the hottest of May, and use it as followeth, Take nine spoonfuls of the water, and nine of Rhenish Wine, the juice of Lemmon, half a Race of Ginger finely minced, and sugar it as you please for a draught: drink this thrice a week fasting and use presently moderate excercise.

A Preservative against the Collick and Stone.

Take a quantity of Parsley roots about two handfuls, boil them in running water till they be soft, then take out the pith and stamp them well, and put them in a pottle of stale Ale, then strain them from thence, and drink thereof for the space of nine dayes at the least.

Another.

Take a quart of White Wine, and boil it in an earthen pot, and when it begins to boil, put into it a handful of Mother Time, and let it boil half a quarter of an hour, then put unto it a head of Garlick stamped in a Mortar, then boil them together a little space, then strain it, and give the Patient to drink, and let him drink as much as he can when the grief is upon him; but if it cease or break not, then take about a penny worth of Honey unto halfe a pint of the Drink, and by Gods grace it will help.

For the wind Collick.

Take a good quantity of Wormwood and tops of Rosemary as much, and boile them in Sack, and put them in a linnen cloth, and lay it warme to the belly where the griefe is, and (by Gods grace) it will help presently.

Another for the same.

Take a spoonful of the powder of Holland, which is to be had at the Apothecaries, and put it into a good quantity of stale drink, and make it luke warme, and so drink it. Or else take the weight of a French Crowne thereof in some warm broth after the manner of a Purgation; for it is not only good to break the wind presently, but it will purge also, and cause some stools. Probatum.

To break the Wind Collick.

Take Wormwood and Tansie, of each three branches, seven or eight leaves of brown Sage, stamp all these together and strain them into a quantity of Ale, and then drink it luke warm twice if it be need.

For the Collick and Stone, and burning Fever.

Take some leaves of the Herb called Dandillion, and pound them small and strain them into stale Ale or Beere, and so drink some three or four times: It is not only good against the Collick and Stone, but also against a hot burning Fever.

An approved good Medicine for the Collick and Stone.

Take Coriander, Caraway, Fennel, Spicknard and Anniseeds, of each one ounce and a half, of Grommel seeds and Licoras one ounce; beat all these into fine powder, and let the Patient drink a scruple in White Wine a little warmed, and walk one hour after it fasting, and do this every morning and evening; and put thereto six drops of the juice of Juniper berries, and you shall find it excellent in operation. Probatum.

Another.

Take Parsley roots, Marsh Mallow roots, and red roots, of each alike stamp them, and put them into a pint of White Wine, and strain it, and let the Patient drink a good draught for three mornings together, and it will cause the Stone to break, and provoke Urine abundantly.

For the Stone Collick.

Take half penny worth of Summer Savory seeds, and of Parsley seeds, of Bay berries, of Gromel, of each half penny worth, and boil them in a posset of White Wine, and drink.

For the wind Collick.

Take the water of Heraff and the root of a red Dock, the inner pith taken away, and the neather bark of an Ash of one years growth, and pound them, and strain them with the said water, and so drink it first and last.

Another.

Take Parsley seeds and bruise them, and seeth them in Sack, and drink it warm when you have your pain. Also Carduus Balsam is excellent.

An excellent Medicine for the Collick or Stone.

Take Pellitory, Unset Leeks and Mallowes, of each a like, stamp them, and put thereto a pennyworth of Neats foot Oyl, and fry them well together in manner of a Plaister, put them in a linnen bag, and apply it to the Raines of the back, but for the Collick apply it to the Navel, and it will help within an hour.

CONSUMPTION.

For a Consumption.

Take a couple of Marrow bones and seeth them, and put in a great handful or two of Unset Leeks cut small, with the roots and blades fair washed, and when they be washed and sodden, take them forth and strain them, and take out the Marrow, and put it into the broth, then take a half pennyworth of Ginger, as much Pepper, a penny worth of Cinnamon, a half penny worth of Cloves and Mace, a quarter of a pound of Sugar; let all be very small beaten, and put into the broth, and drink it warme morning and evening as the stomack will bear it.

A Soveraign Medicine for man or woman in a Consumption.

First take a red Cock and kill him, and flea him, and cut him in four quarters, but wash them not, then take six cap Dates, and cut them in four quarters, and take half a score of large Mace, and six whole Cloves, then put in three or four pieces of old Gold, and stamp the bones of the Cock, then take a pewter pottle pot, and lay in one quarter, and lay upon it some of every Spice, and a piece of old Gold, and so upon every quarter until the last be put in, and you may (if you will) put to the said Ingrediants, Amber, Coral and Pearle, but no kind of Licoras neither first nor last, and when it is perfectly boiled, put thereto a dozen or sixteene Raisons of the Sun, the stones taken out; Then take so much Rye dough as will stop the pots mouth close, and thick enough of the paste, so that no water may enter into it; then take a good great brasse pot, and set it on the fire, that the pewter pot and the ingredients that is in it may stand covered with water at least two handfuls, and put some heavy weight upon the pewter pot that it be not thrown over in the boiling, and let it seeth continually from five of the clock in the morning, untill eight of the Clock at night; then take it off and open the Pewter pot, and let the Patient take of that Syrrup a spoonful at a time.

And when you make it for a woman, you must use these Herbs, Hartstongue, Motherwort, Mugwort, Mother Time and Comfrey, but no Herbs must be used for a man. And if the woman be hot in the liver, take Liverwort; and if troubled with the Stone, take a little of Pellitory of the Wall.

A very excellent Water for a Consumption.

Take a red Cock, and pluck him alive, then quarter him and take out his bowels very clean, and wipe him very dry with a linnen cloth; then put the quarters in to a pottle of the best Sack, and put into them Rosemary, Time, Penniroyal and Pimpernel, of each of these one small handful, of Dates, the stones being taken out, half a pound, of Currans one pound, let then lye and steepe in the Sack two houres then still them in a Stillatory, and of the water thereof use two spoonfuls one hour before you go to Dinner, and so likewise before Supper, and it will much restore your body. This was used by the Lord Chief Justice Popham.

For a Consumption.

Take a pound and half of Pork, fat and lean, and boil it in water, and put in some Oatmeal, and boil it till the heart of the meat be out, and then put in two penny worth of milk, and boil it a quater of an hour, and give the Patient a draught in the morning, in the afternoon and at night, and now and then some Barley water, and by Gods grace it will help.

Another.

Take a fair earthen pot, and put therein a gallon of Claret Wine, and then take a Capon well flesh'd, but not fat, and gut him, and put in his belly half a handful of Mace, and as much Raisons and Currans, then cover the pot and set it on the fire, and let it seeth till the half be consumed, then put the Capon into a Mortar, with some of his broth, and bray his bones and all, then let it seethe one walm after, and passe it through a Jelly bag into a close Vessel, then take a Goblet full, and put thereto the yolks of six new laid Eggs, the strainet taken away, and seethe it well, and then give the Patient to drink as hot as he can suffer it, in the morning fasting, likewise before noon, and before he goeth to bed; and ere three Capons be spent, by the grace of God he shall be much amended.

To restore one that is in a Consumption.

Take three pints of new milk, and one pint of very good Red Wine, and four yolks of Eggs, beat them with the milk, and Wine, and put to it as much fine Manchet crumbs as will make it thick like thin batter, and put in one quarter of an ounce of beaten Mace, and distil all these with fire, and draw a pint of water out of it, and take one spoonful of the water in Pottage or drink morning and evening.

To nourish one in a Consumption.

Take a Chicken, and take out his bones, and wash it in White Wine, and put it into a pipkin without liquor, with a few Currans, and then still it five or six hours upon Embers without coals, then take a spoonful thereof and drink with thin broth.

For a Consumption.

Take Coltsfoot, Burnet leaves, Wood-Betony leaves, red Rose leaves, Comfry roots, of each a handful pick'd and sliced, boil them in running water, from three quarts to three pints, then strain them, and put into the liquor two pound of good Sugar, and the whites of two new laid eggs, then boil it a quarter of an hour, and take off the skum, and take of this Sirrup seven spoonfuls in the morning fasting, and at night to bedward. Probatum.

For a Consumption or Cough of the Lungs.

Take three spoonfuls of English Honey, and three of fair water mixed together, set it on the fire till the skum arise, then take off the skum, and take it from the fire, then put thereto the powder of Coltsfoot, and make it as thick as Conserve of Roses, which use at your pleasure.

A precious Water for a Consumption.

Take a quart of Rosewater, as much of womans milk, Goats milk, or Cowes milk, put unto it twenty yolks of Eggs, and mix them well together, and thereof distil a Water, and give the Patient therof to drink first and last, with a Cake to eat made with Gold and Pearle.

A Water good for a Consumption or weaknesse.

Take a gallon of new milk of a red Cow, and the yolks of twenty eggs, beat them very wel together and put thereto a pint of good Red Wine and two Manchets sliced; so mingle all these things together, and put them in a plain Still, and still it with a soft fire, and now and then stir it, or else it will have crust on it; the Water may be taken at any time three or four spoonfuls with some Sugar, the oftner the better.

COUGH.

For the Cough, be it never so extreme.

Take a quart of new milk, and a pint of strong Ale, and make a posset thereof; then take off the curd, then take a quarter of a pound of Raisons of the Sun stoned, and two big sticks of Licoras, and two spoonfuls of Anniseeds, bruise them, and seeth all in the posset Ale, until half be sodden away, then take it from the fire, and put therein so much sweet Butter as the bignesse of a Hasel Nut, but let it not seeth after; and let the party drink thereof evening and morning six or eight spoonfuls at a time as hot as he can. Probatum.

For the Cough.

Take a head of Garlick, and prick it full of Cloves, then take half a handful of three leaved grasse, and as much Goats grease, and put the Garlick head therein, and wrap it in russet paper, and so roast it in the ashes till it be soft, then beat it in a Mortar and straine it, then drink it in some Ale or Beer, it is good for the Cough.

A Tisan for the Cough.

Take a quart of good old Ale, and set it on the fire and skim it clean, then take half a dozen of good Fennel roots, and scrape them, and take out the pithes, and bruise them in a Mortar, and put them in the Ale; then take a quantity of licoras scraped and bruised and put it to the rest, then take a handful of Anniseeds, and sift them cleane, and bruise them in a Mortar, and put it into the Ale, and let it seeth together a pretty while, then take a handful of small Raisons, wash and pick them clean, and bruise them in a Mortar, and put it into the Ale and let it seeth a walme or two after, then take a penny worth of Sugar candied and put into it, when it is almost sodden from a quart to a pint; and when it is full sodden to a pint, take it off and strain it, and drink it at times convenient, and put to this Tisan, Sugar, Honey, and Powder of Elicampane root, of each a little, and some great Raisons, the stones taken out, and Parsley roots, and two or three figs.

For the Cough, if it be of the Lungs.

Take half a pint of Aquavitae, of Anniseeds a half penny worth, and as much English Licoras, scrape it and slice it thin, rub the Anniseeds very well, and fan the dust out of them, and put them in together, and let them boil on a soft fire till half be consumed, then strain it out, and wipe the pot, and put it in again, and put to it three ounces of brown Sugar candied, and set it against the fire till it be melted, then take it off, and use as often as you will drink.

For the Cough or Cold.

Take a quart of Ale, and put thereto a good sprig of Rosemary, and boil it, then put to it a spoonful of Sugar, and as much butter as an egg, and brew them together, and let the Patient drink thereof to bedward, and keep warm.

For the Cough.

Stamp two handfuls of Centory, and seeth it in three quarts of Ale to the half, then stamp it again and seeth it, and put thereto a pint of honey, and so take every morning thereof three spoonsfuls.

Another.

The Cough is a Messenger of all Diseases of the Lights and Brest, through the grosness, drought, moisture, spittle, and other excrements; for the Cough is a motion of the Lights the which by the aire and moving vertue of the Muscels that are within the brest is meet, and made for to cough up all that which hurteth the lights, and the Rhume provoketh the Cough most of all. There are often perillous Coughs through Rhume that falls down out of the head upon the lights, and into the brest, which is very ill to get out. It is good to purge the head with Cochia Pills, and to drink sometimes a draught of Barly Water in the morning, and eat something after it. Then take this Potion, Take Syrrup of Endive, Honey or Roses, and the Sirrup of Steches, of each half an ounce, Water of Succony and Endive or each one ounce and half, tempered together.

This Powder is approved to stay the Rhume; Take Spica of the Indies one quarter of an ounce, Cinnamon one quarter of an ounce, of the Scull of a man that dyed through violence, three quarters of an ounce: take every time it cometh, one dram after meat in Wine or any decoction.

Physicians do commend Barly Water mixt with Julip of Violets.

CORNES.

For to take away Cornes.

First cut away the Corne and root him out, then drop into the hole a drop or two of a black Snail, and put thereto the powder of Sandyfer, and it will wear the Corn away.

Also cut your Cornes away, and lay a little piece of the red Cerecloth upon the hole, and in three months it will wear clean it away.

CRAMP.

For the Cramp.

Take the little bones of the Hares hinder legges which are in the knee joints, if you touch the place grieved therewith it helpeth.

Also take Hollioaks, Oyl of Violets and Swines grease of each a little quantity and make an Ointment of them and annoint the place.

Another.

Take the Flank wool of a sheep carded in flakes, and dipped in Sallet Oyle, and wrap it about your leggs, or where it taketh you, and it will heat the cramp and ease it.

DEAFNESSE.

For Deafnesse an excellent Medicine.

Take the juice of Betony with the most part of Camomile, wet in it a lock of wool, and stop it in the deaf ear: and Water stilled of the same Herbs, to be powred into the ears, is a help for deafness.

For the Hearing.

Take Oyle of Roses and White Wine Vineger, of each alike, and mingle them together, and at night in bed put one drop into the ear, and stop it with black wooll, and lye on the other side.

DROPSIE.

A very good Drink to cure the Dropsie.

Take of Peperitis Roots, otherwise called Horse Rhadish, three ounces, slice them by the length very thin, of Licoras scraped and bruised two ounces, Winter Savory, Time, Penniroyal, the tops of Nettles of each a small handful; of Smallage roots, Fennel roots, of each one ounce, of sweet Fennel seeds bruised three ounces, infuse all these things one night in two quarts of fairwater, and three pints of Canary Wine, then boil all together the next day one quarter of an hour, then take it from the fire and let it run through a clean cloth and so drink a small draught thereof in the morning fasting, and as much in the afternoon at three a clock and fast two hours after it, and so continue taking it until you be wel. Mr. Smart.

An excellent Medicine for the Dropsie.

Take Scruvey grasse otherwise called Sold Mella, and stamp it and straine it with White Wine, drink every morning some four or five spoonfuls blood warm, and fast one hour of two after it, and do the like every evening; this you must do two or three months together, taking now and then a little Mithridatum upon the point of a knife, and keep yourself very warme, and wash those parts of your body that are swelled with this that followeth: Take Watercresses and Brooklime, and boil them, and wash the places therewith that are detected, and let it dry in.

For the Dropsie.

Take a pitcher full of two gallons of new Ale, then take Setwal, Calamus Aronatics and Gallingale, of each two penny worth, of Spikenard four penny worth, stamp all, and put them into a bag, and hang it in the pot, and when it is four dayes old, then drink it morning and evening.

A Dyet Drink for a Dropsie, Timpany, or other Swelling.

Take one ounce of Sassaparilla, cut in small pieces, a quarter of an ounce of Sassafrasse, Hermodactulus half an ounce sliced, Anniseeds and sweet Fennel seeds of each half an ounce beaten, Licoras one quarter of an ounce, Raisons of the Sun two ounces, the stones taken out; boil all these in three quarts and a pint of fair water, Wine measure; then take it of the fire, and put to it one ounce and a quarter of Cene, and let it stand twelve hours, then strain it, and take at your rising in the morning, and a little before Dinner and a little before supper, and at going to bed, a quarter of a pint to a draught, and use it three dayes together, or more if need require.

DRINK.

Dr. Deodates Scurbuttical Drink.

Take Roman Wormwood, Carduus Benedictus, Scurvy-grasse, Brooklime, Water-cresses, Water Trifoil, of each one handful, Dodder, Cetrach, Scolopendria, Burrage, Buglos, Sorrel, Vervain or Speedwell, of each one handful, Elicampane root one ounce, Raisons of the Sun three ounces, slices of Oranges and Lemmons of each fifteen, boil, or rather infuse these in a double glasse, with so much white Wine, as will make a pint and a halfe of the liquor when it is done.

An excellent Drink for the Stomack
and Brest, grief of the heart, the Palsie,
Jaundies, the Rhume, the soreness of the Throat, the Ptisick, all
faintnesse about the Heart and Stomack, and
to make a good digestion, and to be of a
good colour.

Take the Powder of Pellitory of Spain, and of Centory, Anniseeds, Licoras, Graines of Paradise, Callamus, Ginger, Cinnamon, mix all of these, and use them evening and morning the quantity of halfe a spoonful in Wine or Ale.

A Dyet Drink to be taken in the Spring.

Take a quarter pound of a Madder roots, two ounces of red Dock roots, of Scabious, Egrimony, Carduus Benedictus, Liverwort, of each a handful, of Cene two ounces, of Licoras, Anniseeds, Sassaparilla, Sasafrass wood, Lignum vitea and Hermodactilus, of each one ounce, put all these together into a rundlet of two gallons; bruise all the Herbs and Spices, then put to it two gallons of Beer or Ale, and let it lye five or six dayes; then take Rubarb the weight of a Groat, and put it in cloth, and steep it in a draught of Beer all night, and wring it into the Beer before you drink it.

A most excellent Diet Drink for the French Disease.

Take of good White Wine ten quarts, of good strong Beer as much, put thereto of the Bark Guacum, two pound of Cene, one pound of Licoras scraped and beaten to powder, one pound of the root of Sassaparilla scraped and cut in pieces an inch long, and slit in the midst, one pound of Apples of Colliquintida, the kernels taken out; put all these things together into ordinary stone pots such as their mouthes may be so little, as may be stopped close with corks or dough, and being so stopped, boil them in such a Vessel, as they may be hanged in, and not touch the bottome in the boiling, and so let them be kept boiling continually without ceasing for the space of four and twenty hours from the time they begin to boil, which you may do by having seething water ready in another vessel, and being so well bruised, strain the liquor from the dregs, and put therein one ounce of pure Mithridatum, and so let the Patient drink so much as he can possible, and no other drink till he hath made an end of it, and let him not eat any bread but bisket made without salt, and every day a few Raisons of the Sun, and nothing else for the space of ten dayes; then if the Patient hath not drunk all this potion of drink, let him (if he be weak) eat of a Chicken roasted or a rib of a neck of Mutton dry roasted once in four and twenty hours, until he hath made an end of this quantity of drink, the which being drank, the Cure (by Gods help) is perfectly wrought; This quantity of Drink hath been drunk in six dayes, and it hath done the Cure: after the Cure is done, in any case keep a good Dyet for a quarter of a year, and abstain from women, and over much drink.

An Excellent Drink to prevent Physick, being taken
and used in the Spring and Fall, and approved by
many who have found the successe to be accordingly.

Take a gallon of Wort made of Malt, and put into it a good handful of Egrimony, and as much Goose-grasse, let then seeth in the Wort almost an hour, then strain it out, and put into the Wort of good Cene clean picked, and Anniseeds, both bruised, of each one ounce and half, and let them seeth one hour, and remain in the Wort, after take a good pot ful of the Wort, and put into it ten penny worth of the best Rubarb thin sliced, then close up the pot with paste, and let it stand to infuse upon embers twelve hours, then put it again to the rest of the Wort; and tun it up as other Ale, and at the bunghole put in a good hanful of red Dock roots scraped and sliced; Drink of this in the Spring and Fall of the leaf, a draught or two in the morning, and fast after it two hours, and use it for three weeks or a month at both times of the year as you see cause, and take it every day or second day as you finde it work.

A Dyet Drink to heal Wounds.

Take Egrimony two handfuls, of Daisie leaves and roots, Wild Angelica, Ribwort, Mugwort, Wormwood, Comfry, Mints, Canapit, Speedwel, Avens, Bramble leaves, Arcamilla or Sincle, Scabious, Betony and Dandillion of each of these a handful, boil them all together in two gallons of running water some three hours till it be half consumed; then put into it a pint of White Wine, and half a pint of honey, then strain it out, and so keep it, letting the party drink thereof two or three times a day.

EYES.

A good Medicine to preserve the Eyesight.

Take green Barly before it be eared, and distil it, and use daily now and then, to lay a little on your eyes of that Water, and it will continue the sight.

A special good Poultice for sore Eyes, that be much swelled and cometh by the Rheume.

Take a quantity of Bean flower, some of an Apple finely scraped, a little womans milk, of Sorrel Water, red Rose-Water, Plantane Water, of each a little quantity, mix all these together, and make a Poultice thereof, then spread it upon a fine linnen cloth somewhat thick, and put it to the Patients Eyes cold.

A Plaister for sore eyes.

Take the pap of a roasted Apple two spoonfuls, the like quantity of new laid eggs, of Saffron thirteen chives dryed and made into fine powder; work these together to one substance, and put thereto of Womens milk of a maiden child one spoonful, of Rose water the like quantity; of these make your Plaister, and lay it to your eyes morning and evening, and have in a readiness the powders of these stones following, Lapis Calaminaris quenched nine times in White Wine, Aloes Hepatica, white Sugar candied, Tucia prepared, Camphire, of each of these half a dram, made fine to powder, sow these in a fine cloth or fine silk, and put it in a glasse of water, and of this Water drop into your eyes morning and evening and lye upon your back when you drop it into your eyes. Make your Water as followeth, Take Roses, Marigolds, Plantane, brown Fennel, Eyebright, Cellendine, Tormentil, Betony, Scabious Fumetory, Oaken buds, of each of these two ounces, mix all these in a glasse, and put in the powders above said.

A very good Medicine for Eyes that be troubled with Pin or Web, or other dimnesse.

Take the yolk of a new laid egg or two, and beat it well until it cometh unto a great froth, then let it stand so a little while, and let the Oyl run into a sawcer, and put the juice of Daisies, with the blossomes, leaves and roots, being stamped and strained, into the Oyl of Eggs, and put a little clarified honey unto it, and mix these well together, and let the Patient take every morning and evening into the ey that is grieved, a drop put in with a feather, let this be used so long as the pain lasteth.

Another for sore Eyes.

Take a little Rosewater and womans milk, and mix them together, where of the Patient may use a drop at a time as above said. And if the

Patient be a man the womans milk must be of her that hath a daughter; and
if the Patient be a woman she must have the milk of her that hath a son
sucking upon her.

For a Pearle, Pin or Web in the Eyes.

Take a little Hony clarified as it cometh from the Hive, and so drop it
into your eye evening and morning, and it will help. Probatum.

A very good Medicine for sore eyes that
cometh of the Megrim.

Take the white of an egg, and beat it well, then skim it, and put to the
Oyle some case Ginger finely beaten, and some White Wine Vineger, then
take Flax and dip it into the Oyl, and lay it on your Temples, and take heed
that no part thereof come into your eyes. Do this four or five nights or
more, when you go to bed, and everytime wash your eyes with the water
that cometh of cutting of Vines. Probatum.

A Water very comfortable for the Eyesight.

Take of Rose leaves, red Fennel, Vervain, Rew, Cellendine, and
Eyebright, of each a handful, and so still them all together, and you shall a
good Water for the eye sight. Probatum.

To recover the Eye sight.

Take Smallage, Rew, Fennel, Vervain, Egrimony, Betony, Scabious,
Avens, Houndsdtongue, Eyebright, Pimpernel and Sage, of each a like
quantity and distil all these together with a little Urine of a man-child, and
five grains of Frankinsence, and drop of this water every night into the
eyes, and the sight will recover by Gods grace. Probatum by Mr. Whaley.

For sore eyes and blind.

Take the white of a new laid egge, strained from the yolk, beat it
well to an Oyl, and take off the froth, and put to the Oyle a spoonful
of good White Wine Vineger, and a spoonful of Rose water, beat them
all well together,and with a little flax, lay to each temple a Plaister,
but take heed it touch not the eyes; use this three or four times to
bedward, it hath brought them to sight that that were seven weeks
blind. Probatum.

For red Eyes.

Take a new laid egg or two, and roast them very hard, then without taking away the shels cut them in sunder, and take out the yolks, and scrape a little white Copperas, and put it where the yolks were, as much Coppereas as little pease is enough for one egg, then strain the whites with the shels through a cloth into a sawcer, and with this Oyl annoint your eyes when you go to bed.

For Eyes that be Bloodshed, or have Pushes in them.

Make a toast of fine leven bread, and lay it in Wine till it be soft, then put it in a cloth, and to bedward lay it in the cloth to the eyes, and it will heal them.

For an Eye that hath been hurt, so that the Ball was ready to fall out, being swolne as big as an egge.

Take a rotten Apple that is throughly rotten, and take it from the core, then beat the white of an egg well, and drop the juice of the Apple therein, and bind it with a cloth to the eye, and so dress it twice a day till it be whole.
The gall of a Hart and clarified Hony well mingled together is very good for the Web in the eye; it must be laid on with a feather.

For a Pin or Web in the eye.

Take White Wine and put it in a Bason that is bright; and put Bay salt unto it , and let it stand for nine dayes, two of the dayes shake the Bason, and at the ninth dayes end put into a glasse and keep it for your use; it is also good for red eyes.

An excellent Water for sore Eyes, by Pearle, Pin and Web, Lash or Prick.

Take of Cellendine, Herb-grace, Betony, brown Fennel, Eyebright, red Rose flowers, Maidenhair, or as many of those as you can get, distil of each alike much apart by themselves, and not altogether, then take of each water a like a quantity, and put them together in a glasse, and let the party grieved lye upright one half quarter of an hour in the morning at noon and at night, and drop into his eyes at each time one or two drops, and close the eys afterwards.

For sore Eyes.

Take a rotten Apple that is throughly rotten, and cut out the core, and then strain it through a fine cloth into some fair thing, and of the juice of that Apple drop into your eye that is sore morning and evening.

A precious Water to clarifie the Eyes and to take away the Pearle in the Eye.

Take red Roses, Smallage, Rew, Vervain, Maidenhair, Ewfrace, Endive, Seagreen, red Fennel, Hillwort, and Cellendine, of each like quantity, then wash them clean, and lay them in good White Wine the space of a day, and then distil them, the first water will be the like Gold, the second like silver, and the third like Balme for any sore, and it is precious for Ladies in stead of Balm water.

For heat in the Eyes.

Take a new laid egg, open the top, and let out all that is in the shell, and divide the yolk from the white, and then put in the white again into the shell, and put thereto as much of the juice of Houseleek strained, as there is of white of the egge, and so much Roach Allome as a hasel nut; then set the egg shell with the things aforesaid in it, upon some embers, and so let it boil, and when it is boiled, the white will be somewhat hard; then take it off, and let all the water run from it, and that water drop into the eye that be sore morning and evening.

The juice of Slowes, being dropped into the eyes, is as good a Medicine as may be, and so is the juice of Cellendine; but they must be severally used.

A very good Water for a Blast or Rheume in the Eyes.

Take Callaminaris stones, and burne them well in the fire, and when they be very hot, quench them six or seven times in pure White Wine and Rosewater, then leave the stones in the liquor two or three dayes, and after apply it to your eyes. Mrs. Meggs Receipt.

An Oyntment for sore eyes, and such as be blasted.

Take the powder of Callaminaris, and put thereunto the grease of a fat Pullet that never laid egg, and some White Sugar candied finely beaten to a powder, and some Oyl of Almonds, mix all these well together, and use it as occasion is offered. Mrs. Meggs.

For a Pearle in the Eye.

Take a quantity of Pearlwort, as much Heyhowd, and a less quantity of Ground Ivy, and stamp them, thereto put a spoonful of life Honey, and about two or three drops of Rosewater, strain these, and drop the juice often in the eye.

Another for the same.

Take white Hemlock, and Ground Ivy a little quantity, sowre leaven and a little Bay salt, and stamp them, then put thereto a little Vineger, and thereof make a Plaister upon Sheeps leather, and lay it to the wrist of the contrary side.

To stay the hot Rheume in the Eye.

Take Bole Armoniack powdered, the white of an egge well beaten, and thereof make a Plaister, and lay it to the temples.

Another for the same.

Wet a Cloth in the juice of Houseleek, and lay it upon the brow.

For heat in the Eyes.

Take White Wine, wherein Lapis Calliminaris hath been seven times quenched, and drop it into the eyes when you go to bed, with a feather.

For the black or White Pearle in the Eye.

Take a handful of Ground Ivy, and stamp it, and strain it with some fasting spettle, and temper it with a little clarified Honey, and drop it into your eye. Take Sugar candied, and beat it small, and searse it fine, and blow it with a quill into the eye. Take Coperas, and beat it very fine, and blow it in the eye. Take Wormwood and beat it, then take the white of an egg and beat it, and take off the froth, then make a pellet of flower, and wet it, and warm it, and lay it to the eye,

For sore Eyes.

Take the whites of two eggs, and beat them with a spoon till they be as thin as water, then take away the skum with a feather, then take a piece or rough canvass, as broad as ones forehead, and put upon your canvass Tow or Flax, then powre your egge upon it, then take Bole Armoniack with Terra Sigillata, and so bind it fast to your Temples when you go to bed, lye not upon the sore eye side, and in the morning when you rise take it off suddenly, but soak it first with fair water, lest it grieve you when you take it off. Do this three nights together.

Another.

Take the Oyle of a Goose wing, a little English Honey, and beat them well together in a sawcer, then strain it through a clean cloth, and drop it into the eye with a feather. Probatum.

For heat in the Eyes.

Take a piece of new white loaf, and put it into running water, and wrap it in a linnen cloth, and lay it to the Eyes.

For a Pin or Web in the Eyes.

Boil in egg-shell water, the stones of Raisons of the Sun, and Goose dung new taken and strained therein is very good.
Capons grease washed in Plantane water, and Tutia prepared mixt in it is very good for a sore eye.

For Bleare Eyes.

Take the juice of Wormwood and mingle it with the water aforesaid, and put into your eye will take away the blood and aking.

For Blood-shotten Eyes.

Take the blood of a stock Dove, or for the want of it, a Pigeon, and drop a little into your eyes, and wet a cloth therein, and lay it on the Eye, helpeth the blood shotten eye, whether by stroak or otherwise.
Sometimes the paine cometh of Choler, and then the patient feeleth great heat, sharp prickings, much paine, and commonly there appeareth no gumme in the Eye; if there do, it is yellow: therefore the Patient ought to be purged, as hath been said in the Remedies of the head proceeding of the cause of Choler: And in the beginning of the redness, lay Tow or Flax dipped in the white of an egg well beaten with Rose-water and Plantane water.

To recover the sight

Take three drams of Tuttie made into a very fine powder, as much Alge Epatum, or Epaline in powder, two drams of fine Sugar, six ounces of Rose-water, as much pure White Wine mixt all together, and put it into some clean Vessel of Glasse; and being well closed and stopped, let it in the Sun a month together, stirring it once every day; then take four or five drops of the same water, and put it into the Eyes morning and evening; this in short space will cause the sight to come again as faire as ever before.

For swelling of the Eyes.

Take a Quince and seeth it in water till it be soft, then pare it, bruise it, and mingle it with the yolk of an egg and the crumbs of white bread dipped in the same Water, and put thereto a little womans milk, and two penny worth of Saffron, bray them together, and lay it over your forehead and the eyes. Sometime such pain chanceth because of phlegme, and then the Patient feeleth great pain and heavinesse in the eyes, and in this case you must purge the phlegme, as hath been said in the Remedies of the head grieved with excess of phlegme.

To clarifie the sight, or for redness of the eyes

Take Salt and Ginger, and make it in a fine powder, and temper it in White Wine, and let it so stand a day and a night, then take of the thinnest, and wet your eyes with a feather, when you go to bed: to resolve the Gum, you must wash your eyes with houseleek; sometimes the pain cometh because of ventosity or wind, and then the Patient feeleth such pain as it were beating between the ears with a Hammer, for which it is good to make a Decoction of Camomile flowers, Mellilote and Fennel seeds in water and White Wine, and therein wet a fourfold linnen cloth well pressed down and lay it upon the eyes often. Otherwhiles there chanceth pain in the eyes by outward accidents, as wind, dust or heat; milk well beaten with the white of an egge is good: and sometimes the same pain cometh of striking, and then drop in your eye the blood of a Pigeons wing, which blood will take away spotted marks and rednesse of the face.

For a great pain in the Eye.

Take half an ounce of Oyl of Roses, the yolk of an egge, and a quarter of an ounce of Barley flower, and a little Saffron mixt together, and put it between two linnen cloths, and lay it to the pain; or else take the crumb of white bread one ounce, and seeth it with Nightshade, and Morral water, then mix with the same bread yolks of eggs, Oyl of Roses and Camomile of each an ounce and a half, of Linseed one ounce, and use it as aforesaid.

A very good Water to strengthen the sight and to prevent a Catherick.

Take Eyebright, Vervain, Tormentill of each two pound, Cellendine, Egrimony, Wood Betony, Honeysuckle flowers, White or Red Roses, Vine leaves, Pimpernel, Fennel, Rue, Oculus Christie, Chickweed, Smallage and Clover of each a pound, beat them small, and steep them in a gallon of White Wine twelve hours, then fill your Still reasonable full, and put to it three great spoonfuls of Honey, a pint of new milk, and half a pint of Urine of a man child, then still it, and draw about a pint and a half of a Still.

For an Eye that it very full of pain.

Take of Violet leaves a quarter of a handful, and Daisies roots and all, half as many, wash them and dry them very well in a cloth, then stamp them, and put to it a spoonful of red Rose water, and strain it, then take the white of a new laid egg well beaten, and take away the froth, then put that to the things aforesaid with half a quarter of a spoonful of Honey, and drop this in the eye morning and evening, and twice or thrice a day; and at night lay on the eye the pap of a well roasted Apple, or of a rotten Apple, and put a little juice of Houseleek amongst it, and a little fine Sugar candied, lay it upon the Eye two or three nights; if the pain be great, lap upon it a piece of fresh Bief, two or three hours, and so again as you feel cause. Lay to your neck behind, Elder leaves and Wood betony dryed between two tiles sprinkled with a little Vinegar, and strew on good store of beaten Pepper; when it is hot, lay it on a thin cloth, and so lay it to the neck night and morning four or five times. Also make blisters behind the ears if you see cause. If there grow any skin upon the eye, put in Allome Water with the juice of Cellendine in it, or if it be much, the juice of Ground Ivy; drop this in twice a day, and the white powder once a day.

For Blood-shotten Eyes.

If the Violet Water will not help take five or six cornes of Cummin seeds bruised, as many blades of Saffron put in a fine rag, let it soak in a spoonful of red Rose water, strain it, and put to it a spoonful of Womans milk, and drop this often into the eye.

For a very great Pearle in the Eye.

Put in the eye a little clarified Honey, and a little fine Ginger in it, and sometimes the powder of white Sugar candied: half an hour before you put in either, put in a little fresh grease.

For a Rheume in the Eyes.

Make Eggshell Water, with the juice of Houseleek, as much white Copperas as a pease, twice as much Honey; this is good if you perceive the Humor to be very hot; also it is good with Snow water: and if the Humour be cold, make it with half stilled water, and half Eyebright Water; if between both, make it with fair water.

To stay the Rheume in the Eyes.

Take Woodbind bruised, and lay it to your Temples.

For a Pin or Web in the Eyes.

Take Herb Christopher, stamp it, and strain it, and put in a little honey, drop it in twice a day; also; lay on his eye white bread, milk and Violets made in a poultice; also take Cellendine, Daisies, roots and all, brown Fennel, Cliver, Betony, Plantane, Sorrel twice as much as the rest, there must be of each a handful, a pint of new milk and a dram of white Coperas in powder, two great spoonfuls of Honey, do not draw it dry: drop it in the eye three or four times in two hours, and lay a wet cloth upon the eye.

To bring away the Rheume from the Eye.

Set the feet in Camomile sod in water two houres if you can, then lap them in a blanket two hours keeping it warme with warm clothes.

For any spot in the Eye.

Take the scraping of a whetstone and Bay salt very fine, and put thereof twice a day into your Eye.

For a Pin and Web.

Roast an egg, and put in a piece of Copperas as big as Pease, and nine Cummin seeds, strain it, and put in a little Honey; Alloes Sicatrina made in powder, and strained with a little Rose water, is very good for any sore eyes. Capons grease washed with Plantane water, and Tutia prepared and mixt together is very good for sore eyes to annoint them with them.

To stay the Rheume in the Eyes.

Make water seething hot, and wet a good big cloth in it, and lay it all over the forehead, when it beginneth to wax cool, wet another, and lay to it hot, and do so half an hour together against the fire.

For a prick in the Eye, with a thorne, and to drive out the thorne or stubble.

Take the treddle of an egg, and put it in your eye, and bind it in.

For a Bruise in the Eye.

Lay to the Temples a piece of raw fresh Bief, and to the eye put in Violet water, and lay on the Eye the pap of an Apple, with some of that water, a little Sugar, and the yolk of an egg boiled together.

For an Ague in the Eye.

Lay on the eye a piece of fresh Bief two hours, and drop on the Eye Allom water, and lay in the Temples leaven, Rosewater, Vineger and Nutmeg to stay the Rheume.

For a Pin and Web.

Take Ground Ivy, stamp and strain it with red Rosewater, and drop it often in the eye.

A very good Powder for a spot in the Eye.

Take of Alloes Sicatrina, Sugar candied, or very good Sugar, of each a like quantity, and make it into a fine powder, and put it often into your eyes when you go to bed, and Eyebright water in the morning, and once more in a day.

For red or yellow Eyes.

Take the juice of Parsley and the white of an egge mingled together, and a little Rosewater, dip flax therein, and lay it over your eye, and it will help you.

For Eyes that be blasted.

Take Plantane Water and the white of an egg, mix them well together, and wash your eyes therewith, and lay it on your eyes.

To clear the sight.

Take Cellendine, Eyebright, red Fennel, Roses, Seagreene, Maidenhair and Rue, of each two ounces, then put thereto half an ounce of Alloes, stilling all these in a Stillatory, then wash your eyes therewith.

For red Eyes, and for the Pearle.

Take white Ginger, and rub it on a whetstone into a dish; then take as much salt as you have powder, and put them in White Wine, and let them stand a day and a night, then take the juice and liquor thereof with a feather, and annoint your eyes.

To take away the Web in the Eye.

Take the gall of a Hare, and a little quantity of purified honey, temper them well together, then take a feather, and annoint your eyes therewith.

A Water for the Eyes.

Take of Tutty and Alloes Sicatrina, of each six ounces made in fine powder, four drams of fine Sugar in powder, of white Rosewater, and of the best white Wine unchanged, twelve ounces mixt all together in a glasse, stop it close, and let it stand in the Sun a month, let not your glass be ful, shake it once a day, turning the bottoms upwards, then strain it through a fine cloth from the dregs, and when you use it, one drop is sufficient at a time; use it morning and evening, and if one drop be too little, take two.

For sore Eyes.

Take the whites of two eggs, and beat them with a spoon till they be as thin as water, then strike away the froth with a feather, then take a piece of rough canvass tow or flax, then powr your whites on it, then take Bole Armoniack with Terra Sigillatum, and scrape them both upon it and with a knife spread it Plaister wise, as much of the one as of the other, and so fast bind it to your forehead, and in the morning when you rise take it not off suddenly, but take it off with fair water. Do this three nights together.

For Blood shotten Eyes, Rheume or sore Eyes.

Take four spoonfuls of Rose water, of white Copperas as much as a pease, and of Allome and Sugar candied, of each as much as a pease all in powder, sometimes drop of this in the eye, and sometimes wash the eye with it, and lay Herbs to the wrists. Also Rosewater, Sugar, and Saffron is very good, Sugar candied is the best.

For a spot or itching in the Eyes.

Take Ground Ivy, Cellendine and Daisies, stamp them and strain out the juice, then put to it a little Sugar and Damask Rose water, and drop in the eye twice a day.

For sore eyes, or for any part inwardly disquieted by any Ache, Swelling, Wound or Stroke.

Take the leaves of Woodbind and Plantane, of each one handful, also three of four Dittony leaves, of Roach Allom well washed, the quantity of an egg, as much Verdigrease, three spoonfuls of pure honey, put all this into a vessel to be kept only for that purpose, put to it a pottle of fair running water, and after it hath boiled one quarter of an hour let it stand four of five hours; powre out the clear, and bury the grounds; if it be too sharp, put in some white Rose water. If the lids be sore with Rheume, or the eyes be red or burning, drop in, and wash the lids often with the white of an egge; if it be for a horse, put in more Verdigrease and Honey.

Another.

Take the Water of Roses, Saxifrage and Fennel, of each alike, and put to them a small quantity of Verdigrease, and boil it a little on the fire, and when if hath setled, take the clear, and see you wash Auxungium Poecati seven or eight times, and of that put in to your eye a little when you go to bed.

For Eyes blasted or swoln.

Annoint them with rape Oyle, and lay to a Plaister of Flower, Cream Hogs grease, Rose water and violet leaves bruised small, and boil all to a Poultice, and lay it to warm, change it as waxeth dry. Capons grease washed, and Tutia prepared and mixed with it is very good to annoint sore eyes.

For Ache, Strain or pain in the Head by sore Eyes.

Take of Plantane, Wood Betony and Ragweed, of each a handful, put as much flower to it as will make it a paste, the Herbs being first beaten small, make it a Cake, and make it through warm on a Gridiron, and lay it to the nape of the neck, and let it lye twelve houres, and lay fresh as you see cause.

A Purge for Choller, when there is Pain in the Head, or Rheume in the Eyes.

Take of Cene and of Ginger sliced one ounce, two ounces of Cassia, and six ounces of Sugar, stamp them all together, and boil them in a pint of Rose water till half be consumed, then put in two ounces more of Sugar, beat it well, and keep it close: Take of this Confection a quarter of an ounce in the morning and fast three hours after putting it into a draught of White Wine warmed, strain it,and so drink it, and use it in the Spring and Fall once in ten days for two months or six weeks. If you make but for one, you need make but half this quantity. It purgeth very gently.

For Eys that be troubled with sorenesse and rednesse.

Colewort leaves boiled in White Wine and Plaisters made of them, and laid one the eyes, is good for sore eyes that water much.

To wash them with the Water of Plantane is very good.

Also skivers or pricks of any kind boiled in fair water with red Roses amongst them, save the fat and drop it in your eyes mornings and evening is very good.

To take away spots of Blood in the Eye.

Take red Roses and seeth them, and let them be set warm to your Eye, it taketh away the spots of blood; it is good also for all Diseases in the Eye; for redness in the eye that cometh with a blow or any other violence; you must lay to it by and by Towe wet in Rosewater and white of eggs, juice of Wood-betony and Egrimony, and after the pain is mitigated you must lay a Plaister upon it made of a raw egg, Barly flower and the juice of Mallowes. If that do not help it, take wheat flowers, the juice of Mallowes, Mints, Smallage and the Oyl of an egg, and make a Plaister thereof, and lay it to.

For hardnesse that hath been long in the Eye.

Take a Scruple of Alloes, and melt it in Water of Cellendine at the fire, then put of it in the eye.

Or take powder of Cummin mixt with Wax like a Plaister, and lay it upon the eye: Or take Roses, Sage, Rew and Cellendine, of each alike, mixt with a little salt, and distil it, and thereof put a drop or two evening and morning in your eye. In stead of that water, it is good to take the juice of Vervain, Rue, and a little Rose water.

For the Pin or Web.

Take tops and crops of Herb Christopher, stalks and leaves a good quantity in the beginning of May, stamp them very small,then take a good quantity of May Butter, and stamp them together in a vessel, and strain it out, and set it in the Sun, and put of these into your eyes, it must stand a month in the Sun.

For a hurt in the Eye, that cometh by a stroke.

Take Pimpernel, Cellendine and Plantane, and put thereto the white of an egg, and womans milk of a male child, and Oyle of Roses, and put it in your eye going to bed; use this three or four times in a day.

Or take Egrimony and bray it, and temper it with White Wine and an egg, and make a Plaister, and lay to the outside of the eye.

For a Pearl at the beginning.

Take a Race of good Ginger, pare it clean, and rub it on a Whetstone, and make powder of it, and put the same powder into some Gascoin Wine, then strain it through a fair cloth, and put it into a glasse or Viol, and after nine daies you may use it, when you go to bed, lying upright, and likewise in the morning: Do this six or seven times.

For eyes that are full of Rheume, and bleared.

Take the juice of Rue four spoonfuls, and two of honey, mix them together, and when you go to bed put some in your eye.

Or take two or three roots and leaves of red Fennel, a branch of Cellendine, and a good race of white Ginger pared and beaten; if one serve not, take two, put all these into half a pint of water, cover it; and put of it in your eye when you go to bed, and an hour before you rise, strayning it when you use it.

To preserve the sight long.

Take a crop of Rue, and another of Camomile, and eat them fasting with a Figg two or three dayes in a week.

To clear the sight.

Take the white of an egg made as clear as water, and a spoonful of clarified Honey, and some fine Sugar; and mix them together, and keep it in a close vessel seven of eight weeks, then take Cotton and dip it in the liquor, and rub the eye-lids therewith within and with out.

For sore Eyes, and Megrim in the Head.

Take the whites of new laid eggs, and beat them to Oyl, then take a spoonful of Rose water, as much fine Sugar, and as much strong Vineger made of Malmesey or White Wine, put them to the Oyl and beat them together; then take Flax as much as will make a Plaister, dip it in the Medicine, and bind on each Temple one with a cloth, but take heed the Medicine do not touch the eyes. Do this three or four nights, and every morning the eyes will cleave together with Gum.

For the Megrim in the eyes.

Take new milk, and seeth it, and put it into a bason, and cover it with a platter, and with the dew that cometh wash your eyes and browes.
Or take three drams of the juice of Rue, and put in your eyes and ears, and stop your ears, and lye down on that side.

For a Pearl and Web.

Take Veinfrage, Ivie, Daisies, Sickwort, red Fennel, Seagreene, Pimpernel, May butter, bruise them in a Mortar, and let them lye in the froth five dayes, then make an easie fire, and set it over till it be melted, then strain it through a fair cloth, and put it into a Vial, and put thereof into your eye the quantity of a wheat corn. It will destroy the Web, and when your eye cleaveth together, wash it with Rose water.

Another.

Take the leaves of Sage, Hysop oculus Christi pulled downward, drink the juice of this with Monks pease otherwise called Wood-lice, stamped with the Herbs, and straine it in some Beer, and let the Patient drink it first and last three or four dayes together.

Or take the juice of Avens, Southernwood, and put this juice into Fennel water, and put it in your eye.

For Eyes that be fair to look on, and naught to see with.

Take Smallage, Fennel, Rue, Vervain Betony, Pimpernel, Eyebright, Sage and Cellendine, of each alike, wash them clean and stamp them, then take the powder of fifteen Pepper cornes, and a pint of good White Wine, three spoonfuls of good Honey, and fifteen spoonfuls of the Urine of a man child that is young; then put all these together, and let it boil over the fire a little, then strain it, and keep it in a vessel or glasse, and put of it into your Eyes; and if it dry up in the glasse, put to it a little White Wine. This is good for all kind of sore eyes, in fifteen daies it helpeth.

For the Small Pocks in the Eyes.

Take the strained juice of Pimpernel, and drop into your Eye morning and evening. This is good also for the Pin and Web, or Pearle in the eye.

For a Pin and Web.

Take Ivy leaves that groweth upon Ash trees, wipe them clean with a cloth, then stamp and strain them with womans milk, of a Girle for a man, of a boy for a woman; the sorer the eyes be, take the more juice, and the less milk. Drop this into your eye with a feather evening and morning, and twice in the afternoon.

For sore Eyes that cometh of a hot cause, as of a Rheume.

Take Elder leaves, and chafe them between your hands, and lay them to the nape of the neck.

For Bloodshotten Eyes.

Take a toast of leavened Bread, Houseleek and womans milk, a spoonful of Rosewater, the pap of an Apple roasted the yolk of a new laid egg, and boile them, take the toast, and lay it in red Wine not mingled, and let it lye halfe an hour, till it be soaked, then put into a fine cloth of two pieces, for each eye one, and the cloth must be between the eye and the toast and dresse it thus when you go to bed.

For Watering Eyes, and darknesse of sight.

Take May Butter and Honey, of each alike, and boil them together, and put in the white of an egge, and when it is cold, put it into your eye, and it will cleer up your sight.

Or take the leaves of red Roses, and temper it with the whites of eggs, and lay it to your eye when you go to bed.

For an excessive pain in the Eyes, when the
Flux of Humors be sharp in them.

Take milk hot as it cometh from the Cow, cover it with a Bason, then take the dew from the Bason with a feather, and put it in a glasse, and therewith dresse your Eyes.

For sore Eyes that be in the morning, full of
pain and water, so that they will not open
without great washing.

Take a new laid egg and roast it hard, then take a little white Copperas, and a little roach Allome, and a little Sandifer, then strain the juice, and drop thereof into your eye evening and morning, and wet a linnen cloth, and lay over your eyes.

For Eyes that have skins over them, or great pain in them.

Take black Snailes, and make an Oyl, and put thereto White Sugar candied, and Lapis Calaminaris, being first burned five or six times, and thus prepared, put in your eyes evening and morning with a feather.

Or take Daisie roots, Betony, flowers of Pimpernel, red Fennel, stamp and strain them with stale Ale, and drink thereof evening and morning; and lay outwardly to your eyes Rose water, womans milk, and the white of an egg, wet Tow or Flax therein, and lay it to your eyes; the Drink will be the better, if you put in the juice of Clestocks, a worm so called.

A Medicine that helped one that had a thrust in the Eye.

Take the right ground Ivy and Cellendine, and the green of a Goose turd, and womans milk, put them all together in a glasse, and when it is setled, put the clearest in your eyes.

An Oyle for burning of the Eyes.

Take the white of an egg well beaten together with the juice of Daisie roots and Houseleek, put them into an eggshell, and roast it hard, and thereof will come an Oyl, wherewith annoint the place pained.

Dr. Cademans Water for the Eyes.

Lapis Tutiae prepared half an ounce, white Vitriol half a scruple, red Rose water, Plantane water, or each one ounce, Egrimony water half an ounce, mingle them together, and let them boil gently, then clear it very well.

An excellent good Eye Salve.

Take a pound of May Butter, and set it in the Sun, to clarifie; and alwayes when it is melted powre the clear butter from the curds and whey that will be in the bottome; thus do this from day to day, until no more will come out, then put as much of the Herb Christopher, small chopt, as will be steeped in it, then set it again in the Sun in a glasse for the space of a month, in which time it will be rotten, then strain it through a fine linnen cloth, and so keep it in some Gally pot or Glasse that will not drink it up, and every evening as much as a small Wheat corne being put into the eye, will destroy any speck or Pin and Web, or and scale or thicknesse.

For, and of the Eyes in general.

In all causes of the eyes, observe the Nature of the person, his age, the time of the year, the sicknesse he hath had before, &c. It is alwayes good in all pains of the Eyes, that the Patient keep in a dark place, free from aire, lye high in bed, that the Rheume tarry not in the Eyes, but may fall down to the cheeks, seasonable sleep doth digest and congeal the matter; all vexation is to be avoided, as sorrow, anger, ill savors, &c. Also all vaporous meats. And this is a general rule, that so long as the pain lasteth, you shall lay upon the Eye the white of an egg, brayed with Oyl of Roses, for it stayeth the course of the humours, and asswageth all pain: or the white of an egge braied with womans milk, if the eye be red.

Of the Uthalmia of the Eyes.

This Disease is caused from the Flux of certain humours be they mixt or not, as from Choler, Phlegme, Blood or Melancholy, the signes whereof are these:

If it proceed of bloud, then are the Eyes and their veines puff'd up red, the Temples of the Head do beat, the uppermost Eye-lids do swell, the Eyes are moist, yet with little pain, but so moist, that in the sleep the Eyes do bake up.

If it proceed of Choler, then there is much pricking, burning with great pain and swelling, and not so red as the former, but moist and burning, that thereby sometimes the Apple of the eye is perished.

If it proceed of phlegme, then is there a compression and ponderosity in the Eyes with great pain, without heat or rednesse and by reason of the great moistness, some soreness and swelling.

If of Melancholy, then is there also great ponderosity with a sallow colour, with rednesse or compression: They do not bake together in their sleep, for that the Catarrhe or Rheum is too dry.

For the rednesse of the Eyes.

Take half an ounce of Tutia, make it glowing hot, and quench it fifteen times in Rose water, then bruise it small, and put into it a quarter of an ounce of Callamint stones, three cloves, and a half a pint of Malmesey, and mix them together.

This Collyria is for all redness of the Eyes.

Of Watry and running Eyes.

If the Cause be inward from any disease of the brain, and not through heat, you may perceive by this, viz. The Patient alwayes feels some heavy puffing up of the vains in the forehead and Temples of the head, and this reflux is for the most part augmented by neesing, falling both into the Eyes, and sharpnesse in the throat.

But if this humour be through heat, it bites the eyelids, and makes the hair to fall off; but if through cold, then contrary. In case it be through heat, the party must be purged with Pills of Cochia Aurea with Succo Rosartum, or with Pills of the five kinds of Mirabilans, and keep a good Diet.

If this grief come of a cold Cause its very convenient to eat a good deal of Fennel seed every morning, andn chew Rew and Valerian in the mouth, and annoint the eyes with the spittle.

Also if it proceed from the brains, this is excellent, Take prepared Bloodstone, one quarter of an ounce, Roses, burnt Ivory, red and white Curral, Amber, yellow Mirabilans, of each one dram, the juice of the Spirits of Frombois four ounces, temper then together, and keep them close stopped, put thereof daily into your eyes, and annoint your Eye-lids therewith. This dries the Rheume marvellously, and strengthneth the eyes from taking any moisture.

Also take the juice of Fennel and of Rue, of each one ounce, and of a childs Urine halfe an ounce, Alloes three drams, let it seeth a little, then strain it, and put a drop thereof into your eye. It cleanseth, drieth, and sharpneth the sight.

Also roast three Apples, take away the skin and cores, then temper them with the yolks of three new laid eggs, and lay it warm to the eyes.

Also if deflux cause much pain, take unwashed sheeps wool, burn it to ashes in a close stopped pot, bruise it as small as may be, and mix it with the white of an egge, and lay it on your forehead and temples. This asswageth the Catarrhe very quickly, and abateth the pain.

A Plaister for the Temples, or sore Eyes.

Take Alloes, Mirrhe, Mirtle leaves, Acatia, of each one dram, Mastick and Frankinsence, of each half a dram beaten small together, and make it to a Plaister with the white of an egg.

Likewise he ought to purge with Pills of Cochia, which be sharpened with the Trocisies of Alhandaly.

Also with the Confection of Hiers, and such like. Oyle of linnen being made thus, is very good for sore Eyes; viz. set it a fire with a candle, and lay the linnen upon an even piece of iron, tin or silver, and put it out quickly, and you shall find a drop of Oyle, the which take up with a feather. This healeth marvellously well the Imposthume of the eyes, taketh away the pain, and is good for a Fistula and Wounds in the Eyes.

FACE.

To take away the Scars, or Pockholes, or redness in the Face.

Take a good quantity of Lemmons, and slice them rinds and all, and distil them, laying them on fair sticks, that they touch not the bottom of the Still, and with the Water that cometh thereof, annoint the face, and it will soon take away the rednesse and scars of the face.

For a sawcie Face.

Take a pottle of White Wine and a quarter pound of Cinnamon cleane rubbed and winnowed, then seeth it in the White Wine, till it be half sodden away, then put it into a pot, and drink it evening and morning till the Patient be cured. Probatum.

An approved good Medicine to cool and repel the redness of the face that proceedeth of heat.

Take a quantity of running water, and a quantity of Brimstone, and as much Allome beaten small together, put them with the water into a glasse fast stopped, and so let it stand, & every morning and evening take a little out into a sawcer, and with a linnen rag wash your face therewith, and so let it dry in with wiping.

For Spots in the Face.

For a mans or a womans face that seemeth as they were drunken; take Watercresses, and cut them small, and put them in a small earthen pot, and put fair Spring water thereto, and let them boil together, and drink of that water morning and evening.

To make the Face fair.

Take the flowers of Beanes and distil them, and wash the face with the water.

Some say, that the Urine of the party grieved, is very good to wash the face, and to keep it from blemishing.

If the face be washed with the water that Rice is sodden in, it taketh away the Pimples, and cleanseth the face.

For heat in the face.

Seeth white Copperas in running water, and let it stand till it be cold, and then put in a little Camphire, and every morning and evening take a little of that water in a sawcer, and with a little cloth dipt in it, wash and bathe your face therewith, and let it dry in of it self.

A Drink for the Heat or Rednesse in the Face.

Take four handfuls of Wild Tansie, and boil it in two Gallons of small wort, let it stand until it be almost cold, then put to it a little Barme, and let it work, and when it is ripe, put it in a close vessel, and so let it stand three or four dayes; then you must drink of it every day twice, so long as you use it.

A excellent Water for the same.

Take twelve Lemmons, and pare them to the very juice, four new laid egges, shells, whites and yolks beaten all together, six spoonfuls of pure English Honey: Temper all together, and distil them with a very soft fire, and receive the water thereof in a glasse for your use, putting thereto a little Mercury to make it keep, and continue.

An excellent Lac Virginis to make the Face, Neck or any part of the Body fair and white.

Take of Alumen Plumosi half an ounce, of Camphire one ounce, of Roach Allome one ounce and dram, Sal gemmi half an ounce; white Frankinsence two ounces, Oyle of Tarter one ounce and a half; make all these into most fine powder and mix it with one quart of Rosewater, then set it in the Sun and let it stand there nine dayes, often stirring it, then take Littarge of Silver half a pound beat it fine, and searse it, then boil it in one pint of White Wine Vinegar, until one third part be consumed, ever stirring it with a stick while it boileth, then distil it by a Filter, or let it run through a thick Jelly bag, then keep it by itself in a glass Vial, and when you will use these Waters, take a drop of the one, and a drop of the other in your hand, and it will be like milk which is called Lac Virginis, wash your face or any part of your body therewith. It is most precious for the same. Probatum Dr. Walmesley.

For the Pimples in the Face.

Take Wheat-flower mingled with honey and vinegar, lay it upon them, and it cleanseth them.

To dry up any Pimples or heat in the Face.

Take Virgin Wax one ounce and a half, May Butter three ounces, melt them, then put to them Cerus half an ounce, Bole Armoniack a scruple, a little Rose water to wash it; after these are melted together, annoint the Pimples with it twice a day.

FELLON.

To ripen a Fellon or Boil.

Take Rue, Sage, and the fat of rusty Bacon, of each a like quantity, and stamp them all together, and lay it on a linnen cloth warm to the Grief.

Another.

Take an Onion roasted, put thereto Honey and Wheat flower, and so beat it all together, and lay it to the sore.

To kill a Fellon.

Take an egg and roast it hard, and take the yolk thereof, and take an Onion and roast it soft, and beat the yolk and the Onion together, and lay it to the sore, and it will kill the Fellon.

A Soveraign Salve to heal the Fellon.

Take the Soot of a house that is on the Beams, and break it to powder, and take the yolk of an egg, and bray them together, then lay it on a clean cloth, and lay it on the sore, and this will heal it.

An excellent Poultice to take away the anguish of a Fellon, and to break it speedily.

Take milk, and put therein crumbs of White Bread, and boil them together very tender to a Poultice, then take it from the fire, and put therein the yolk of an egg, and have ready some white Lilly roots, wrapped up in a brown paper, and roasted very tender, first bruise the roots into a pap, then mingle them well with the other things and so apply it warme to the griefe, and when it is broken use healing Salve.

For a Fellon.

Take Verjuice and crumbs of browne bread, and kernels of gray Soap and seeth all together till it be somewhat thick, then spread it upon a cloth, and lay it to the Fellon, and it will both kill the Fellon, and heal it.

For a Fellon in the Joint.

Take Bay salt, and beat it, then take the yolk of an Egg, and beat them together, and lay it to the joint.

Another for a Fellon.

Take twelve Snailes in the Garden, and beat them shels and all until they come to be a Salve; then lay them to the sore, and it will both kill, draw and heal. Also bruise Raisons, and lay them to the sore.

Another.

Take the biggest and fowlest Spider you can finde, and a quantity of black Soap, and one clove of Garlick, and bray them all together, and lay it to the Fellon as neer as you can, where you think it will break, and so let it lye four and twenty hours, then take it off, and heal it with some other Salve.

Also take Sage, Rue, Bay salt, Snailes and Bacon, and beat them together, and then lay it to the Fellon, and it will help.

Also make a Poultice of Bean flower of Wheat flower and honey, and apply it every morning and evening.

FISTULA.

Against a Fistula or hollow Ulcer.

First mingle the milk of Wortwort with fresh Hogs grease, and boil them together a little, and incorporate them, and put thereto powder of Mirrhe, and annoint a Tent therewith, and put it into the hole of the Ulcer.

For a Fistula.

Take the seeds of red Colewarts, the seeds of Tansie and Cabbage, of each a like quantity, and the great Madder, and make it into Pills and give thereof to the Patient thrice a day, and keep a Colewort leaf upon the Sore.

To heal a Fistula or Ulcer.

Take Figs and stamp then with Shoomakers Wax, and lay it to the sore on leather, and it will heal.

FLESH.

To kill dead flesh.

Take a pint of Malmesey, and a pint of Aquavitae, and flower, pound Parsley, and straine the juice into it, and drink it. And take Allome and Withy leaves, and boil them together in running water, and wash the wound therewith.

To try whether there be dead flesh in a Wound or no.

Take posset curd made of strong Ale, lay it to the wound; and if it look yellow, then there is dead flesh.

A Water to abate proud flesh, and to
clear a corrupted wound.

Take a quart of Ale or strong Beer, and a handful of Sage, and a piece of Allome, as much as a Walnut, and let it seeth till it come to a pint, and therewith wash the wound.

To clear a Sore or Wound of dead flesh.

Clarifie some Honey, and put it into the sore, and lay a Plaister over it, and in two or three dressings it will cleer the Sore, and take out the dead flesh.

To take out dead Flesh.

Take of Honey, of Oyl Olive, and of Wheat flower, of each a spoonful, and the yolk of an egg, and mix them well together, and spread it on a cloth, and so lay it on the sore; and it will draw and cleanse it.

FLUX.

For the white Flux.

Take the powder of the flowers of Pomegranats, and drink in red Wine.

For the red Flux.

Take Sperma Caeti and drink it, and truss up your self with a piece of black Cotton.

To stop the Flux.

Make a Caudle of Oatmeal, and put to it scraped chalk, brown Pepper finely beaten, then boil them together, and let the Patient drink thereof three of four times, and it will help.

For the Bloody Flux.

Take four or five eggs, and roast them hard until they be blue, then take a pint of Red Wine, and mix the yolks of the egges with it, then seeth it, and after it is sodden, put an ounce of Cinnamon into it, and let the Patient drink thereof two or three times in a day, and it will help.

Another.

Take Camock roots, make them in fine powder, and drink them in posset Ale, or put it into a Cake as you do Spice, and eat it.

Another.

Take linnen cloth, and make it like a Pill, and steep it in Aquavitae, and convey it into the Fundament, and in three or four dressings it helpeth.

For the Bloody Flux or Scouring.

Take a great Apple, and cut out the core, and put therein pure virgin Wax, then wet a paper, and lap it therein, then rake it up in the Embers, and let it roast till it be soft; then eat of it as your stomack will give leave.

PHLEGME.

To loose Phlegme.

Take an ounce of Ingibus Sirrup, one ounce of Sirrup of Violets, half an ounce of Sirrup of Roses, and half an ounce of Hisop.

A Drink to avoid Phlegme.

Take an Onion and core it, and put therein a little Mithridatum, and bruised Pepper, and then roast it soft, then take a pint of White Wine, and seeth it with a little white Sugar, and then straine it with the Onion, and give it the Patient to drink.

A Powder to break Phlegme.

Take of fine Ginger the weight of eight pence, of Elicampane roots, the weight of four groats, Anniseeds and Licoras, of each the weight of seven groats, and Sugar candied four ounces; make all these into powder, and eat it dry morning and evening.

FORGETFULNESSE.

Against Forgetfulnesse.

Apply Rue and red Mints with Oyl of Roses, and very strong Vineger to the nostrils, and it helpeth.

Also burn thine own hair and mingle it with Vineger, and a little pitch, and apply it to the nostrils.

GOUT.

For the Gout.

Take Snailes with shells on their backs, Barrel Soap, leaven, Baysalt and Honey, and pound them all together, and lay it to the grieved place.

Sundry Medicines for the Gout.

Take the grease of a fat Cat, of a Goose, of a Gray, Of a Fox, and the marrow of a Harts horn, Ivy, Sage, Rue, Virgins Wax, Frankinsence, the yolks of roasted eggs and Snailes, put them all in an earthen pot with a hole in the bottom for that purpose, and close it above with paste that no aire issue out, and put under the same pot another whole pot, and close them together, and put the neathermost in the ground, and compasse it about with fire, and there will distil a wonderful good Oyntment out of the uppermost pot, which will be good for the cold Gout.

Another Oyntment of great force for the Gout.

Take the juice of the wild Cowcumber roots, green Grapes and Pellitory, the leaves and Berries of Ivy, Juniper berries, Euforbium Castorium, the fat of a Graye, of a Goose, of a Heron, of a Fox, of a Beare, then take a fat Cat, and pull off her skin, and take out her guts, and fill her with the aforesaid things; and let it roast well upon a spit, and save the dripping, and resolve a little Wax therein, and use it.

Also a dog killed of thirty dayes old, and annoint the grief with the blood of the dog, it is very good.

Also take a fat Cat, and flea her, and pull the flesh from the bones, stamp it well, and put into the belly of a fat Goose, and put salt grease thereunto with Pepper and Mustard seed, of Pellitory, Dragon, Wormwood, Garlick, and Bears Suet, of each two ounces, of Wax two ounces, roast it, and keep the dripping.

Also mingle the ashes of Colewort leaves burnt, with fresh Hogs grease, and annoint the Gout therewith, and it will ease in three dayes.

For the Gout.

Take Tansie and Wormwood of each alike, Sheeps Suet according to your Herbs, fry them till they be green, and when you will use it, put a spoonful of Linseed therein; and if it be the hot Gout, lay it cold; if the cold Gout, lay it hot.

Another.

Take Tobacco leaves a good quantity, and put them into your own Urine, or milk, and set it on the fire till it be hot, then bathe the pained place throughly a good space, the lay some of the leaves thereon, and bind it up, and lye down.

For the Gout and the Palsie.

Take dead Horse bones, dryed in the field, and wash them clean, and seeth them long, and take the fat of them, that seethes aloft, and swims on the top, and therewith annoint any Gout and Palsie, of what cause so ever it come, and it will help.

For the Gout.

Take the juice of Broom flowers, and the juice also of Scala Coeli and Honey of each a like quantity, seethe them together, till it be of the thickness of Honey, and therewith annoint the place. One in London got much money by this Medicine.

For the Gout and Palsie.

Stamp Pellitory of Spain or Mastratia and seeth it in wine, and apply it, but if it be green then stamp it, and soak it eighteen dayes in Wine, and then boile it well, and put thereto Oyle and Wax, it is a special remedy.

GUMMES.

For Ulcers or any Infection of the Gums.

Take Labdanum, Frankinsence, Mastick and Curral, of each a like quantity, and make them into a powder, and lay them to the place infected, it confirmeth hardneth, and cleanseth the Gums and Jawes, and when the sore is well mundified, then it doth also incarnate and ingender flesh.

Also this is highly commended, Take Cipresse leaves or Mints halfe an ounce, a pint of well water, boiled to the one halfe, dip a cloth in it, and apply it to the griefe, and this defendeth the Gums from all bad Rheumes.

HEART.

For Faintnesse at the Heart.

Take the flowers of Centory, a good handful, clean picked from the green of Cene leaves clean picked from the stalks, a dram and a half, and of pure Cinnamon well bruised a quarter of an ounce, of White Wine a pint, and some Sugar as you list; put all these in a pot close covered, and set it in another pot of hot liquor for the space of an houre, then let it stand all night, and in the morning strain it into a faire pot, and put good store of Sugar to it, and let it simper til it come to a Sirrup, of this you may take two or three spoonfuls at a time in the morning fasting.

A very Soveraigne Medicine for one that
hath taken a cold at the Heart.

Take the Oyl of bitter Almonds and Wax, Capons grease and Rose-water, boil all together; then take black wool, newly plucked off the Sheeps neck, and wet it in the liquor, and put it in a quilted bag, and lay tt very hot to the stomack when you go to bed.

HEAD.

A Medicine for the Head ache.

Take Elder leaves, and a good quantity of Bay salt, and stamp them
together, and lay it to the nape of the neck, and by Gods help it shall take
away the pain.

For pain in the Head.

Take Camomile, Rosemary and Betony, of each a like quantity, and as
much leaven as Herbs, beat them together, then take a Nutmeg beaten very
small, and so much Wine Vineger, as will incorporate into a paste, which
you must apply warm unto the hinder part of the head, and to your
forehead, changing it evening and morning.

For Head Ache.

Take a piece of leaven, and the bignesse of an egge, and put to it
two spoonfuls of White Wine vinegar, and two spoonfuls of red Rose-
water, and a few red Rose leaves, mix them together, and warm them;
then take them, and spread them on two brown papers, then grate
Nutmeg upon it, and lay it upon a fire slice on the coals till it be very
hot, then take it, and lay it to the parties temples at night when he
goeth to bed.

For the Head Ache sundry Medicines.

The juice of Ground Ivy cast it into the nostrils purgeth the head and
taketh away the pain.
If the Rheume come of a cold cause, lay hòt Callamint or running time
bruised to the head.
Hisop boiled on embers, and laid to the head, stoppeth the Rheume.
The juice of Coleworts cast into the nostrils cleanseth and purgeth the
head.
The juice of onions cast into the nostrils, also doth the like.
This Plaister was proved for dizziness in the head, and is good for
any ache in the head: Take of Opium and of Saffron, of each one dram,
of Roses four drams, and thereof with Vinegar make a Plaister.
He that useth to take three Pills of Alloes, and the juice of Coleworts the
bignesse of a bean, shall never have the Head ache.

For the Head Ache.

Take an Herb called Alehoofe and fill a frying pan therewith, heat it hot
as you are able to endure it, and lay it to the aking place, and it will
remove the pain; then take more, and lay it to the place that aketh, and at
last it wil drive it clean away.

Another.

Take the whites of two new laid eggs, a little Aquavitae, and the juice of
Houseleeks, beat all together and therein wet some fine tow, and then lay
it upon the temples.

Of giddinesse in the Head.

This Disease is caused by much frequenting the Sun, and the head
being over heated, as also from the stomack, if it be overcharged with
any superfluity whereby the mouth of the stomack is hurt, and so
sendeth bad vapours to the head; but if it proceed from the blood,
which may be knowne by the redness of the eyes, the fulnesse of the
veines, then the party must have the veine opened behind the ear, and
bleed four ounces, and purge with seven drams of Reb steeped in
Whey all night.

Of the pain in the Head.

For the most part this pain of the Head proceedeth of the
intemperature of the four humours; namely, of Blood, Phlegme, Choler
and Melancholy.

If it proceed from Choler, the sign is evident, viz. belching or breaking
of wind upward with loathsomnesse and thirst, drynesse of the mouth,
tongue, and nostrils, the pain is pricking sharp, and rather in the right, then
in the left side of the head, heat over all the body, but especially in the
nostrels, no appetite, no sleep, the Pulses quick and lusty, the Urine
reddish, the face yellow; the surest notes are, if the time of the year be hot
and dry, the Patient young and hath used hot and dry things, to use cooling
Medicines, and a good cooling dyet.

Of heat in the Head through Melancholy.

It is described thus, It is not so great as the former, but with a
drynesse and sadnesse the heat is more evident in the left side of the

face, then in the right, it causeth disquietness and unnatural sleep, it causeth fearful faintheartedness, and carefulness, the colour of the face is red and blue, with a soure taste in the mouth, if the Patient be old, and if it be about Autumne, then the signes are more sure. Glisters are good in this case.

Of the paine in the Head caused by cold.

The signes are wearisomeness of all parts, as if the body were beaten and broken to pieces, the paine is not extreme without any swelling or thirst, sleepinesse, much spitting at the mouth and moisture of the nose, palenesse of colour, and somewhat sullen, the eyes run, and the mouth out of taste. In such cases use warm and dry Medicines, and purging, is very needful in this Infirmity.

Also this Wine following is excellent for this purpose. Take Rosemary two handfuls, Nutmegs one ounce, dryed Betony two ounces, Cloves two drams, being cut very small, put thereto eight quarts of good Rhenish Wine, let it stand three dayes; then for a weak stomack, drink a good draught at the beginning of meals, but for the Head ache at the latter end.

This Wine is very good for a cold, and moist braine, and hurtful for young folks and hot complexions.

The Dyet must be strong Wine, but very little, lest it disturb the Head, once in eight dayes, wash the head with the decoction of Camomile, Marjerome and Steches, and before meales, rub the head with warme cloaths, and after meales take a little Marmalade to hinder the vapour in ascending to the head. But because the Laxative Medicines, through their own power, do not expel all humours for which they be given, without such things as convey their operation towards some certain members which one desireth to purge, therefore take this Oximil following; and if you put thereto Nutmegs, Piony seeds or Cubebs, then doth it only purge the head, and no other part of the body; and if you put thereto Tamariscus and Caper roots, then it purgeth the Melt, and so for all the rest, but because we speak now only of the head, these are the Simples, or Herbs that do conduct the Medicines thereto; viz. Nutmegs, Cubebs and Piony, Penniroyal, Marjerom, Balsome wood and Seeds, Frankinsence, Beaver Codd, Labdanum, Mellilot, Squils, Spicknard, Hisop and Pepper.

Oximel, that is called at the Apothecaries Compositum, or Diareticum, take Fennel roots, and roots of Smallage, of each two ounces, the seeds of Parsley, of Butchers broom, Sparage, Smallage and Fennel, of each one ounce, take out the pith or core of the roots, chop them and seeth them in a quart of water till they be mellow, then strain them through a cloth, and add the Decoction of three ounces of sharp Vinegar, twelve ounces of Honey, let them seeth to a Sirrup; it doth attenuate all tough slimes, it driveth them out of the members, opens the obstructions of the Liver, Melt, and the Kidnies, and expelleth them.

A very good Medicine for Paine or Wind in the Head, which much hindreth the Hearing.

Take one Clove of Garlick, pill it and make three or four holes in it, then dip it in fine English Honey, and put it in your ear, and lye on the other side, and put in black wool after it, and continue this eight dayes, and it will expel the pain, expulse the Humour at the nose, and restore the Hearing.

For a White Scurf, or a Scabbed Head.

Take White wort, Cellendine, Ground Ivy, Mercury, Wormwood, and an Herb called Dead mens Bells, growing in Woods like Leek blades, of each of these alike, and stamp them, and mingle them with fresh grease.

And burne green Ash to ashes, and mix it with fresh grease, and annoint the place therewith.

To heal a Scald Head.

Take Lye that is made with the bark of an Ashen tree, and wash the head therewith, and annoint it with Quicksilver, killed in Barrowes grease, and fasting spittle.

Another.

Take yolks of eggs, and put thereunto as much Turpentine, then fry them in Swines grease, and stir them well together in the frying to a Salve, and so lay it to the sore head.

Another.

Take the roots of the small reeds that grow in ditches, burn them to ashes, and apply the ashes wet in Vinegar to the sore Head. This healeth the sore, and maketh the hair grow.

The bark of an Ashen tree being well boiled in water, with the Lye thereof, sometimes wash the Head to cleanse it, whiles the other Medicines be applyed to the same.

Another.

Take black Snailes, and stamp them very well, and in stamping them, there will be an Oyle come from them, and with the same Oyle, annoint the sore head.

For a sore Head.

First wash the head with pisse, and then annoint it with the dripping of a wild Duck, being roasted guts and all.

HOARSNESSE.

Against Hoarsnesse.

Put Sugar and the powder of Hisop in figs, and roast them on the coals, and eat them, and it will open the pipes.

JAUNDIES.

A good Medicine for the Black Jaundies.

Take the Berries of Ivy, that groweth upon the tree, and of the whole leaves of Ground Ivy and Mugwort, and put then in a woollen cloth, and then put it into an Oven when the Bread is drawne out; and when it is dry, make powder thereof, and take Saffron and powder of Gallingale, and use all these in pottage, and eat thereof.

Another for the Black Jaundies.

Take the gall of a Raven grated into powder, take some of it in a spoonful of Ale or Beer, temper it together, and drink it in the morning fasting.

A Medicine for the yellow Jaundies.

Take a little Athanatia, and eat it in the morning fasting, three mornings will be enough. It is much like Mithridatum.

Another.

Take a handful of red Nettle crops, and seeth them in a pint of Ale, and drink the same three or four daies together in the morning fasting.

IMPOSTHUMES.

For an Imposthume.

Take powder of Cene Alexandria one ounce, Ginger, Cinnamon, Mace, Coliander seeds, Anniseeds and Licoras, of each the weight of an eight pence, of Sugar two ounces, of Spurge seeds blanched twelve, beat them all smal to powder, and put them into a quart of Claret, and let it be brewed out of one pot into another, oftentimes in a day by the space of three dayes before you use it, then let it run through a Jelly bag, then take half a pint of the said Drink, and when you shall have need to use it, warm it by the fire, and drink it after your first sleep, and so ly still till it work, and offer to come; and then go to a close stool til it be clean come away, and then make a Plaister of red Mints, red Fennel, Wormwood and Sage, of each a handful, and a good handful of Cumin seed, and beat them small together, put thereto a good sawcer full of Wine Vineger, and set them all on the fire in a pan, and so stir them till they are almost dry, and then put them into a bag, and lay the same to your stomack, so that your stomack be not full of meat.

JULIP.

A most excellent Julip to refresh and cool any body distempered with heat or drougth in Agues or hot Diseases.

Take of Barley water a quart, and put it into a fair bottle of glasse, and let drop into the same some Oyl of Vitriol, or for the want of that, Oyl of Sulphur, and then shake it well all together to diperse the Oyl, and when you have perfectly tempered it, then take two very good

Pomgranats, and cut them in two, and squeece all the juice of them into it through some Colender or Strainer to keep out the kernels or husks; or for the want of Pomgranats, as much Sirrup of Violets, or Sirrup of Lemmons, as the juice of two Pomgranats may be; then take six penny worth of white Sugar candied, and beat it very small, and put it also in the Barley water, and let it dissolve therein, and drink thereof as need requires. It is the best Julip that was ever made by the Art of man.

ITCH.

To take away, or kill the hot Itch.

Take Brimstone, and as much Allom, with a spooneful of white lead, beat them small into powder, then take a quantity of Cream, and put the powder therein, and beat them well together, and therewith annoint the place that itches.

For an Itch.

Take a pint of Borus, two penny worth of Quicksilver, and four penny worth of Frankinsence, put these together, and stir them with your finger, and so annoint the hands and feet.

KIDNEYES.

Of the Kidneyes.

The Kidneyes are fastned very strongly to the Back bone, and that on the left side is right under the Melt, and that on the right side a little higher, so that sometimes it doth touch a great part of the liver, and they have sundry veins from the liver, whereby they draw blood with water, and also some part of the gall unto them, separating the same blood from the water, and keeping so much of the blood that sufficeth for sustenance, and vents through the Conduits, whereof each Kidney hath one by it self, descending into the bladder.

The Diseases of the Kidneyes are divers, as Imposthumes, Ulcers, &c. which appears by pissing of Blood, or like blood, as if flesh were washed in it, which Diseases arise either of heat, cold or gravel, &c.

The signes of cold Diseases are these, There is no great pain, nor heat, nor thirst, neither is the water high coloured, but much in quantity, because it is not wasted through the unnatural heat, which Agues, Winter and the Gravel augmenteth; for these Diseases a good Diet must be kept, all grosse and slimie meats being avoided, and likewise all cold Herbs; exercise presently after meat is very hurtful.

Pain of the Kidneyes through Wind, which spreadeth it self abroad, and the pain is more after one hath eaten then before, and is augmented through windy things, when the meat is half digested, therefore all windy things are to be avoided, and annoint the back with Oyl of Rue and Oyl of Lillies; likewise Conserve of Betony, and the confected roots of Pimpernel, Erinringo roots and Callamint is very good.

Pain in the Kidnyes through heat, is, when the Patient hath great thirst and a bad stomack, maketh very little Urine, and high coloured, and sometimes there is fat swimming upon it, and the rather in young, choleric, hot men, this is most dangerous, for through the heat which is mixed with a tough thick phlegmatick matter, the stone of the Kidney may grow; therefore the Liver Veine must be opened, and the Glisters administered whereby the guts may be cleansed, use cool Herbs, and purge with Manna and Succo Rosarum. Also use Saxifrage, Parslye, Cantharides, roots of Fennel, Butchers broom, &c. which are of a secret quality to convey the Medicine to the Kidnyes. Also Sirrups of Water Lillies and of Vinegar, and all things that cool the Liver and Spleen.

KNEES.

For pain in the Knees.

Take a Sheeps head newly killed, and slit it, and put into it a good handful of Plantane, as much Camomile, and so much Sage, and so much Rosemary, boil all well together until it be very tender, then take out the bones very clean, and chop all the flesh and herbs well together; then put in a handful of Oatmeal grets; and so boil it again until the Oatmeal be very tender, and so lay it to the Knees as hot as you may suffer it, and so use it as you see cause.

For ache in the Knees.

Take Rue and Lovage, of each alike, stamp them, and mix them with Honey, and fry the together, and lay a Plaister thereof warm to the sore.

For swelling in the Knees and Legs.

Take Lilly roots and red Cole, of each alike, seeth them in clean running water, and strain the Herbs, then take the milk of a Cow and Wheat meal, and temper it with the aforesaid Herbs, and set it over the fire, and stir it well till it be thick, and then lay it on with a cloth.

For Aches and Swelling in the Knees.

Take a quart of Malmsey, of Time one handful, and boil it together, and when it is half boiled, put in a piece of sweet butter, and let it boil together from a quart to a pint, and when you go to bed bathe your knees therewith, and let a cloth be wet therein four or fives times double, very warm, and lay it so warme to your knees six or seven times.

LAMENESSE.

For such as be stiff in their Limbs, or Lame.

Take five black Sheeps heads, a lapful of Arsemart, as much Mallows as much Balm, two good handfuls of Herb grace, four handfuls of Fetherfew as much Lavender Spike, two handfuls of Wormwood, two handfuls of Savage, one handful of Smallage, and two handfuls of Rosemary; all these will be as much as will fill a good sheet, put them all into a Lead, into running water a great deal, and pull off the stalks of the Herbs, and let them seeth a whole day; you must not skin the sheeps heads, but cleave them in sunder, and let the wool be on still, cutting off the hornes, and seeth the Heads until the bones fall asunder, then take out the bones, and skim off the fat, and keep it to annoint the Patient withal, and the Patient must sit in water up to the brests, and wash and bathe himself therein, and when he hath so done by the space of an hour, or as long as he can endure it, then lay him in a hot sheet into his bed, and there let him sweat, and so keep him close from aire two or three dayes.

A Soveraigne Medicine for Lamenesse in the Joints, to supple any sore, and to bring it into the Joint, which hath been long out; and for aches.

Take four or five young Swallowes out of the Nest being Flege, and put them into a stone Mortar, and stamp them feathers and all, then take

Lavender Cotton, Wild Strawberry leaves, Camomile and Setwal, of each a handful, stamp them all together very smal, then take a pint of more of May Butter, and half a pint of Neats foot Oyle, stirre them all together, and then put them into a Pipkin or liltle earthen pot with a cover; and close it well with Paste that no air issue out, then put that earthen pot into a brasse pot with water in it, and boil them two hours, then take them out, and set them as deep as you can in a muckhil two dayes, then take them up, and boil them two hours again, then take them out, and let them cool, and straine them through a linnen cloth, and when they be settled, powre out the watrish bloud from them, and keep them pure and clean, and lay them warm to the place grieved.

LEPROSIE.

For curing the Leprosie.

Take half a pint of English Honey, and a good handful of Herb-grace, beat it very smal, and put into the Honey, and boil them very well together till the one half be consumed, then strain it through a clean cloth, and with a feather annoint the sores therewith.

A Drink belonging to the same Medicine.

Take an ounce of Elicampane roots, one ounce of Fennel roots, when they be picked and pithed, one ounce or Burrage roots picked and pithed, one ounce of Niprial picked and pithed, then take a pottle of stream water, and boile all these roots till one half be consumed, then put in so much English Honey as will sweeten it to your taste, then straine it, and put it in a glasse bottle, then take a penny worth of Quicksilver, and kill it well with fasting spittle, and then put it into the Drink when it is through cold, and let the Patient drink thereof five spoonfuls in the morning fasting, and so much when he goeth to bed, and by Gods help it will cleanse him.

LASK.

For a Lask.

Take a good quantity of Wheat flower, and put it in a bag, seeth it very well, then take the same, and put it out of the bag, and so much as is soft, scrape away with a knife, the rest will be very hard, scrape it, and make pap with milk, and give it to the Patient twice or thrice a day, and it will help. Probatum.

To stay a Lask or Bloody Flux.

Take a few old Beanes, and parch them over the fire in a pan, and then beat them into a powder, then make an Aleberry of Sack or Ale, and put some of the powder therein, and seeth them well together, then let the Patient drink thereof warm, and with twice drinking, it will help.

Another.

Take milk somewhat hot, and put it in a dish, then take Red Wine, and put it in another dish, and let the Patient suck it out of both dishes with two quils or reeds both together, and in so doing it turneth into a curd, and stoppeth the Flux.

To stay a Scouring.

Take a handful of Rice, wash it in red Rose water, and dry it well, and beat it to powder, and make pap of it, and boil it with Cinnamon, and eat it.

Another.

Take Virgin Wax, and make it into Pills, and give it in the pap of an Apple, three at one time.

For a Lask or Flux.

Take the neather Jaw of a great Pike, and beat it into fine powder, and drink it in Beer or Ale, or in your pottage, and it will help.

To procure Looseness.

Seeth Mallowes and red nettles in fair water, and let the Patient sit over the hot fume thereof.

LIVER.

For cooling of the Liver.

Take French Barley, and boil it in a quart of fair water, when it is boiled, take it forth of that water, and put it in three pints of fresh water, then take of Violet leaves, Strawberry leaves, of each a handful, Succory, Buglos, Borage, of each half a handful, one good stick of Licoras, half a handful of Raisons of the Sun stoned, one spoonful of Anniseeds, let all these boil from three pints to a quart, then take the Liquor, and strain it, and put a handful of Almonds into it, and when you drink of it, take a spoonful of Rosewater and drink with it, and take two hours before you eat in the morning at the least, and likewise two houres before Supper.

For the heat of the Liver.

Infuse and steep Bread reasonably leavened in water, and a little Vineger, and eat thereof fasting an hour or two before other meats, and use Sallets of Succory roots sodden till they be tender.

Doctor Hills counsel for cooling the Liver.

Take Barley one handful, of Sorrel, Succory and Endive,of each one handful, a stick of Licoros bruised, Raisons of the Sun one handful, Anniseeds half a handful, seeth all these in a quart of faire water till halfe be wasted away, then strain it, and drink of it in the morning three times in a week at least.

A Drink to cleanse the Liver.

Take a quart of Rhenish Wine, and put thereto one ounce and a half of Cene, seeth it from a quart to a pint; then strain it, and put thereto three branches of white Mint, three penny worth of white Rose water, two Nutmegs sliced with a knife, six penny worth of white Sugar candied, and four penny worth of Angel Gold, and seeth it a little, and let the Patient take it morning and evening.

A good Medicine for the Liver.

Take Ivory, and burn it in a clean earthen vessel, and when it is burnt, take sweet Barly Wort, and put therein of the Ivory as you please, or put it into Ale, and drink it nine dayes together. Also drink the juice of Liverwort.

A Drink to mitigate all heat of the Liver and Spleen.

Take of Liverwort, Maidenhair, Endive, the flowers of Winter Gilliflowers picked clean from the stalks, great Comfrey, Tarragon, of each four ounces, of Spinage Water a pottle, of Licoras cleane scraped and thin sliced two ounces, of Ginger clean scraped and thin sliced, one ounce, boil all these together, stirring it now and then, and then put in fine Sugar candied one ounce and half, finely beaten to a powder, then let it boil half away, alwayes stirring it, and put it in some close glasse, and reserve it to your use: of this you must take a good draught every morning, and fast an hour after it.

A Broth to cool the heat of the Liver.

Take Violets, Time, Parsley, Watercresses, red Nettle Crops, and Clivers and red Fennel, of each alike, but somewhat less of the Water cresses, red Nettle crops and Fennel then the rest; shred all the Herbs, and make broth with Chicken, Capon or Mutton.

For the heat of the Liver.

Take three pints of Whey, Egrimony, Borage and Buglos, of each one handful, boil all together half an hour, then strain it through a fine linnen cloth; drink a good draught of this in the morning fasting, and at three of the clock: but before you drink thereof, take Smallage, and stamp it and strain it, and take two spoonfuls of the juice thereof, and put it into your drink before you drink it.

Against the stopping of the Liver, Lungs and Spleen,
and to comfort the Stomack.

Take two or three roots of Succory and Parsley, Sage of Jerusalem, Folefoot, Violet leaves, Scabious, Egrimony and Scurvigrasse, of each half a handful, Conserve of Red Roses one ounce, of Saffron one penny worth, and a Date or two sliced and the pill taken away, put all these into a Pullets belly ready drest, and sow up the open places, but put not in the roots, boil it in sufficient water till the flesh be sodden from the bones, and when it half sodden, put in the roots steeped before in Wine Vinegar, put in also three or four large Mace blades, of Raisons of the Sun one handful stoned, and a few Currans; and when it is sodden as aforesaid strain it, and drink every morning a good draught thereof fasting.

For all Griefs of the Liver.

Take the leaves, flowers and roots of Betony in Drink, Conserve, Electuary, Sirrup, or Potion, or Powder, is singular good for all Diseases of the stomack, Liver, Melt, Kidnies, Bladder, of Obstruction of the Matrix, the consumption of the Lungs, Coughs, Dropsies, continual Feavers, boile the leaves and flowers in Honey water, to have present Remedy.

Also seeth the Herbs and Flowers of Cammomile in Wine, and drink it to help the stopping of the Liver and Melt, to purge Choler, to expel Terms, to help the torments of the small guts, for the Griefes of the Kidnyes or Bladder, for difficulty of Breathing, Sighing, Wheezing, to warm a cold stomack, and to drive away any inward grief.

For the Liver, and to comfort the Stomack.

Take a branch or two of Ciprus, otherwise called French Wormwood, and a little Barme, and boile them in Ale and Drink it fasting.

LIPS.

For chopt Lips.

Take new Wax, Mastick and White Frankisence with Oyle of Roses, all made into an Oyntment, and annoint the lips, and it will cure them presently.

LUNGS.

A Preservation for the Lungs.

Take a pint of Wormwood Water and Liverwort almost a handful, and of Longwort a handful, Sugar one ounce; boile them all together till one part of the four be sodden away, and let the Patient drink thereof three spoonefulls in the morning fasting, and last at night, alwaies warmed. Probatum.

LEGGS.

For a sore Legge, or old ulcer.

Take Littarge of gold two pound, of Galbanum one ounce, Verdigrease foure ounces, Bdelium one ounce, Mastick one ounce and half, Opoponax and Aristologia of each one ounce, old Oyl Olive one pound and half. You must drie the gummes that they may be powdred, and frie them with your Oyle, then straine it and put thereto your Littarge, Verdigrease and Aristologia, one after another alwayes stirring it, lest the Littarge sink to the bottome, and so let it simber over the fire easily, then put to it three peniworth of turpentine, and of wax three ounces, and so make it up for your use in a Plaister.

It hath cured the Lord Wharton and divers others with two or three dressings when no Chirurgian could find a Cure for them.

For a sore Leg.

Take a stone lime, and slake it, and put it in running water, and put thereto of Quicksilver, white lead, and Bores grease of each one penny worth, mingle all together, and so annoint it.

To kill the Itch of the same, and to skin it.

Take a gallon of good Ale, and boil it to a pint, and then a linnen cloth, and wet it therein, and wash the sore withal.

Another.

Take of Ale, Allom, of each one half a penny worth, and boil it together, and melt a quantity of fresh Butter therein, and annoint it therewith.

A Plaister for festered Legs, being long sore.

Take March, and Wild Tansie, Plantane Morrel, Honey, and the white of an egg, and the milk of a Cow of one colour, and Barley flower, bray the Herbs in a Morter, and mingle all together, and lay it on the sore.

A Plaister for sore Eyes, broken or not.

Take a pint of Sallet Oyl, one pound of unwrought Wax, half a pound of white Lead, boile all these together in a brasse pan with a soft fire till it be as thick as pitch, stirring it with a stick, then dip in it a piece of Lockrum, and make thereof a Plaister.

MEGRIM.

For the Megrim.

Take a handful of Wormwood, and a handful of Betony, and a handful of Archangel, seeth them all together in a quart of good Ale, and a pint of White Wine Vinegar, the space of half an hour, and lay it to your forehead as hot as you may suffer it, and the longer you keep it thereto it is the better.

Another.

Take halfe a handful of the leaves of Rosemary, and seeth them in Vinegar till they be soure, then lay them upon a linnen cloth, and cast thereon a little Rosewater, and lay it to your forehead; as hot as you may suffer it.

A Plaister for the Megrim.

Take the Oyl of an egge, and some Cummin seed, and Frankinsence and wheaten flower, and two Nutmegs beaten all small and mingled with the Oyl of the egg, and make a Plaister thereof as big as a groat, and lay it to the temples of the head.

MOTHER.

For the Mother and green Sickness.

Take great Garden wormes, and slit them, and wash them clean, and then lay them in White Wine half an hour, then take them out, and lay them in an Oven to dry, and when they are throughly dryed, beat them into fine powder, and drink it in White Wine in the morning fasting, and fast two hours after it.

MOUTH.

For a sore Mouth.

Take the waters of the tops and leaves of red Brambles, Rosemary, Sage and Woodbind leaves, all severally distilled, of each a like quantity, and put them all together into a great glass, then put as much Allom small beaten into the same as will make it sharp, and so keep it to use as occasion serveth either for a Canker in the mouth, ranknesse of the Gums, or any other sorenesse.

Another.

Take Treakle, English Honey and burnt Allome, of each alke, then take tops of Rosemary, red Sage, Honey suckle leaves, Bramble leaves and Fennel of each a handful, stamp and strain the Herbs, and take the juice and boil with the other things til it be somewhat thick, then rub your mouth therewith.

For a sore Mouth or Throat.

Take Rue and red Sage, of each one handful, Groundsel and Sorrel, or each a little, cut them small, and then stamp them, then take as much Allome as a Walnut, and as much Copperas as a small Nut, and burn them to powder in a frying pan, then take a like quantity of each of them unburnt, and beat them small, then take a pint of running water, and put them all in it, and boil it halfe away, then take it from the fire, and strain it, then put to it three spoonful of English Honey, and so keep it in a glasse, and warm a little of it every time you use, dipping a cloth in it upon a little stick; and so wash the mouth twice a day, or more as you see occasion.

NOSE.

For stinking Nostrils.

Take the juice of lake Mints, and the juice of Rue, each a like quantity, and put it into the Nostrels when you go to bed, and it will help.

NAVEL.

For the Navel coming out.

Take beaten Mastick, and mix it with the white of an egg to a paste, and spread some it upon a cloth, then thrust downe the Navel, and apply it thereto, and when it is dry, renew it again.

NIPPLE.

For a chopt Nipple.

Take a white Lilly leaf out of his Oyl, and apply it, its very good.

OYLES.

To make Oyle of Mallowes for Imposthumes, and Ripenings, and to mitigate Aches.

Take of Garden Mallowes two handfuls, stamp them small, and put to them a quart of Oyle Olive, and let it stand nine dayes, then boil them till it wax green, then strain it, and keep it in a box for your use.

This keepeth open, draweth and asswageth the paines of Imposthumes, and mollifieth, it being laid hot with moist wool, then take a fine linnen cloth, and dip it in the oyntment, and lay it warme to the sore, and bind it fast.

Also Mallowes made in a Plaister ripeneth greatly, and mitigath the pain of Imposthumes, and especially in ripening of womens breasts.

To make Oyle of Poplar buds.

Take of Poplar buds half a pound clean picked, and stamp them small, and weigh them, and look what they weigh put the like weight of pure Hogs grease, and half the weight more, then stamp it together in a stone Mortar to one substance, and then put them in an earthen pot, and cover it close that no air come to it, and let it stand so six dayes till it be hoary, then take it forth, and put it in a clean pan, and let it boil on a soft fire, always stirring it till the Herbs be parcht, then strain it, and keep it for your use. It will allay all the heat about a mans body, and procure sleep.

In like manner make Oyl of Marsh Mallowes.

To make Saint Johns Oyle.

Take the flowers of Saint Johns wort, and pick away the green husks very clean, and take a quart of the purest Sallet Oyl, and put it in an earthen pipkin, and put in it as many of the flowers as will make it thick, then set it on hot embers and there let it boil very softly, and when you think the strength is boiled out, strain out the flowers very hard, and if they be boiled enough they wil be as harsh as herbs fied in a frying pan with butter, and when you have strained out all very clean, put in as many fresh flowers as you did before, and let them boil in the like manner, and so shift it till your Oyl looks as red as a Ruby, then strain out all the flowers, and put it in a glasse, and keep it close stopped.

This Oyl is very good for any greene Wound or any bruise in any part of a mans body; you must take heed you do not over boil it, and it is good for any ache.

A very good Oyle or Balsom for any green Wound.

Take a quart of White Wine, four pound of Oyle Olive, two pound of Turpentine, the leavs and flowers, or seeds of Saint Johns wort two great handfuls, and bruise them, and put them with the other things into a great double glasse, and set in the Sun eight or ten dayes, then boil the same glasse in a kettle of water with some straw in the bottom, which done, strain the liquor from the Herbs, then put into the liquor the like quantity of Herbs, flowers and seeds, as you did before, but no more Wine nor Oyl, use it as you did before, and then you have a great Secret.

To make Oyl of Hypericon.

Take of the best Oyle Olive three pound, of the best Turpentine three pound, white Frankinsence half a pound, Wheat sweet and clean picked, Hiperico and Saint Johns wort, of each halfe a pound, Valerian four ounces, Carduus Benedictus four ounces, of White Wine or Sack a quart, take the Herbs and cut them small, then put them into a tinned pot that hath as narrow mouth as may be, then powre in the Wine, and let them stand and steep six hours, then powre in your Oyl, and stop up your pot very close that no aire can get forth, set the same on a soft fire of coales without smoak or flame, let it boil very softly, stirring it now and then with a wooden slice, and having stirred it, stop it up again, and so let it boil till the Wine be consumed,which you shall know in this manner, by dropping the Oyl into the hot coales, the which Wine being not consumed, will hisse in dropping on the coals and being consumed it will not hisse but burn very clear. And so the Wine being consumed, take it from the fire, and straine the liquor through a thick canvas cloth: Then make clean your pot, and put the liquor (that ran through the canvass) therein, and set it on the fire again, then put in your Turpentine and Frankinsence, the Frankinsence must be beaten and searsed, and let them boil very softly, stirring it with your slice the space of a quarter of an hour, then take it from the fire, and strain it through another strainer. This Oyle must be put in a Glasse bottle, and the mouth stopt very close.

How to cure with this Oyl.

First you must wet a fine linnen cloth in White Wine, and wash the wound with the Wine being warme, and the bloud and corruption being cleansed, fill the wound with the Oyl, as warm as the Patient can suffer it, then lay a linnen cloth wet in the Oyle upon the Wound, and upon that another cloth wet in the White Wine, and so dresse it morning and evening. If the Wound be deep, take a Sirenge, and spurt in the Wine to cleanse it. And thus may you cure deep wounds without any Tent. The Wound being come to a Plaister, to skin it, take of the said Oyl one ounce, of Turpentine one ounce, of Virgins Wax one ounce, boil them together till the Turpentine and Wax be melted, and thereof make a

Plaister to skin the Wound, and keep it in a pot very close stopped for your future use.

To make Oyle of Adderstongue.

Take a quantity of Adderstongue, chop it smal, and in the chopping of it, sprinkle on it some White Wine, then put the Adderstongue into a quantity of Sallet Oyle, according to the quantity of your Adderstongue, and boile it very well, then strain out the Herbs, and put in fresh Herbs so prepared as aforesaid, and boil it again. Thus do several times, and keep it for your use.

OYNTMEMTS.

An Oyntment for a Bruise.

Take a gallon of sweet Butter unsalted, well washed in the month of May, and a handful of Broom flowers, and bruise them in a Mortar, set the Butter and them over the fire, and boil them well, and strain them into a Galley pot. This is good for a woman in her Child-bed, and it is good for a sore Brest, before it be broken.

A very good Oyntment.

Take Rosasolis, Sallet Oyl and Neats Foot Oyl, and boil them alltogether over the fire.

To make the green Oyntment.

Take one pound of Sheeps suet, and melt it, and skim it, and put thereto one ounce of Verdigrease, and half an ounce of Salgemmi in fine powder, and stir it well together, then take it from the fire, and put into a clean box, and keep it, for it may be kept many years. It is good for Cankers, and to heal old Wounds, and to fret away dead flesh, and it will keep a Wound from festering. It is good for Morphew and for Scabs, and there is no Oyntment that worketh so strongly as this doth. Probatum.

To make another green Oyntment.

Take of Sage, Rue, of each a pound; of Wormewood, Bay leaves, of each half a pound, of Mellilot Herbs, and flowers, of Camomile flowers, of Spike,

Rosemary, red Rose leaves, Saint Johns wort and Dill, of each one good
handful, of Marsh Mallowes two handfuls, chop these Herbs and Flowers as
small as may be, and stamp them and weigh them, and put thereto the
weight of pure sheeps suet, chop it small, and mince your Herbs and it
together, and stamp it in a stone Mortar to one substance, that there be no
suet seen, but all green, put it in some fair pot or pan, and put thereto a pottle
and a pint of Oyl Olive, and work all these together in the pan with your
hand to one substance, and cover it close with some clay or paste about the
edges that no air come in nor out, and let it stand so seven daies, then undo it
and take it forth, and put it in a clean pan, and set it on a soft fire, always
stirring it till the Herbs begin to wax parched, and then strain it into some
fair pan, and then put into it these Oyls following, Oyle of Roses, Oyl of
Camomile, Oyl of White Lillies, Oyl of Spike, and Oyl of Violets, of each
one ounce, stir them all together, and reserve them to your use.

   The infirmities that this Oyntment is good for, are these; for Stiches,
Bruises' Aches, Palsies, shrinking of Sinewes, Gouts, and Sciaticaes, the
Ache of the Back, Lamenesse, Plurisies, the Cough, the soles of the feet
being annointed; for extreme pain in the head, make a cap for the crown of
the Head of linnen cloth, and lay in it the wooll of a quick Sheep, plucked
from the flanks and cods, pick out all the moates, and make it cleane and
card it, then straine it with this Oyntment, and baste it, and lay it some what
warm to your Head. It is good for the Cholick, and for the Spleen, and for
the cold Dropsie of the Liver. If you will have it to be more pleasant of sent,
and more nourishing, add thereunto of the Gums of Labdanum one ounce
and a half bruised fine to powder, of the Gum called Storax Cremitie three
quarters of an ounce beaten well to fine powder, mingle the other stuffe and
this together, and strain it, and keep it to your use.

An Oyntment for the heat of the Raines,
or elsewhere in the Body.

   Take Oyl of Roses six ounces, of clear white Wax, two ounces scraped as
fine as may be, dissolve these together on the fire, and skim them as clean as
may be, then have a dishful of Rose water, and three spoonfuls of Rose
vineger mixt together, strain your other stuff into it, and labour it a long time
in the liquor, and last of all have ready Camphire a dram in fine powder, and
work it till it be cold. This is a good Oyntment for the back, head or eyes.

An Oyntment for a Bruise or Ach[e].

   Take of Dill, Vervaine, Mugwort, Henbane, the tops of Camomile,
Lavender, of every one a like quantity, then take May butter, and shred the

Herbs small, and put them in the May Butter and stamp it well in the Butter, then let it stand a fortnight, and then fry it well, but take heed you burne it not, and then strain it, and keep it to your use.

A very good Oyntment for all Aches and shrinking of Sinewes, for blasting of the Face, and for greene Wounds.

Take of Mellilot, white Dothet, Adderstongue, Valerian, of each three handfuls, May butter well clarified in the Sun four pound, your Herbs must be shred small, and then stamped very wel by themselves, and after stamped againe with your clarified butter, and so let it stand six or seven dayes, then boil it over a temperate fire until the Butter be green, stirring it alwayes till it be taken from the fire, then strain it, and keep it for your use.

The white Dothet doth grow in moorish grounds where Rosasolis growes, and groweth very neer the ground like a Plantane, but a more yellowish greene leaf, it beareth a blue flower on a tall stem and smal; no Herbal maketh mention of this Dothet.

An Oyntment for any Swelling or Sore. It is good for many things.

Take three good handfuls of Rosemary, and as much of Hisop stripped, Rosen as much as a Walnut, and one pound of fresh May butter, boil them all together until it be green, then strain it into pots.

A very good Oyntment for any Ache.

Take two pound of fresh new butter, and clarifie it till it be clear, then take a handful of the youngest Bay leaves, of Camomile, red Sage and Herb grace, of each two handfuls, chop the Herbs, then boil them in the clarified butter a pretty while till it be green, then straine it, and keep it for your use, and when you use it, let the place pained be well chafed therewith against the fire. You must also put in it with the rest a handful of Smallage.

An Oyntment for a Wrench or Strain.

Take the white of an egg and a spoonful of Honey, and beat it to an Oyle, the boil Bove wort with Sallet Oyl or Butter to an Oyl, and mingle it together.

An excellent green Oyntment for a strain or Bruise.

Take a handful of Camomile, of Bay leaves four handfuls, of Smallage foure handfuls and a half, of red Sage four handfuls, of Herb grace three handfuls, chop the Herbs and stamp them, then take five pound of fresh Ewes Butter, and boil it, and when it riseth, take it from the fire, and let it stand, then take off the skum cleane, and then put in the Herbs together, keeping it stirring, and when it is well boiled take it off, and let it stand till it be cold, then strain it into an earthen pot well glaz'd, and keep it to your use, it will continue a year or two.

An Oyntment for Legs that itch with heat,
or to cool or heal any Sore running of a hot humour.

Take a handful of Houseleek, stamp it very small, and mingle it with thick Cream, and annoint the sore therewith.

A Soveraign Oyntment to strengthen Sinewes,
and good for Lameness.

Take half a pound of Swines grease, half a pint of Sack, Camomile and Betony, of each a handful, as much Sage, half a handful or Bay leaves, halfe an ounce of Cloves, chop the Herbs small, and beat the Spice small, and let it boil all night on the Embers, then strain it out, and use it.

An Oyntment for all Aches, Lamenesse of Sinewes,
Stiches, Bruises, Plurisies, or Gout.

Take Sage and Rue cleane picked of each a pound, of Bay leaves and Wormwood of each half a pound, of Rosemary three handfuls, Camomile flowers one good handful, Dill and Spike of each a handful, of sheeps Suet, the skin picked off, three pound, of sweet Sallet Oyl three pints and a half, the Herbs must be chopt smal, and the Suet minced as fine as may be, then beat the Herbs and Suet together into one substance, put into as earthen pan, and put thereto your Sallet Oyl, and work it with your hands until it be well mingled together, then cover it with a dish, and close it with paste, and so let it stand six or seven dayes, then take it forth, and put it into a broad pan, and put thereto one ounce of Mace smal beaten, then boil it with a soft fire, and stir it well till the leaves be parched, put into it three ounces of Oyl of Licoras, two ounces of Oyl of Spike, then strain it, and put it into a glasse for your use.

An Oyntment for any Ache or Bruise.

Take the leg bones of a male Deer, and break them, so as the marrow may be taken out, and put it into a Posnet, then put to it a pretty quantity of Daisie roots, and the like of Elder buds or leaves, as much Camomile and a little Balm, all clean picked, then put in the marrow, and let them boil a pretty while, then strain it, and keep it for your use.

An Oyntment for a Strain.

Take a pound of Rosemary leaves and flowers, one pound of running Mallows leaves and flowers, and a good handful of Camomile, but wash them not, gather them when the dew is off the ground, chop them very small, and stamp them with a wooden pestle, put to them a quart of May butter well clarified in the Sun, stamp them all together til they be wel mingled, then put them in an earthen pot and stop it close, and let it stand nine dayes, and then seeth it on the fire, and stir it wel for burning, and when it is greene, strain it through a Canvasse cloth, and keep it for your use.

A greene Oyntment to be made in May, an approved good one for diversthings.

Take young Bay leaves and Wormwood, of each halfe a pound, red Sage and Rue, of each a pound, all must be gathered in the heat of the day, pick them clean, but wash them not, beat them very small in a great Mortar like greene sawce, then take three pound of new Sheeps suet, clean picked and shred smal, beat all these together til they be wel incorporated, then put to them a pottle of the best Oyl Olive, work it wel with your hands til it become all one substance and colour, put it into a new earthen pan, and let it stand there close covered in some cool place eight dayes, then boil it on small coals almost a whole day stirring it wel, and after it hath boiled four hours or more, put to it four ounces of the best Oyl of Spike; and to know when it is throughly boiled, then take a drop thereof in a sawcer, and if it be a fair green colour, take it off, and strain it through a new piece of course canvass, and put it up in Gally pots, it will last seven years.

It cureth all Straines, Swellings, Aches, Kibes, Cramps, Scaldings, Burnings of all sorts, all outward pain or griefs, easeth Sciatica and Gout, and all kinds of swellings in the face or throat.

An Oyntment for any Ache.

Take Camomile, Bayes, Marygold, Dill and Mallow leaves of each a like, chop them, and boil them in fresh butter or Sallet Oyle, and so strain it forth, and when you use it, warm it, and so annoint the place.

To make Flos Unguentorum, the flower of all other Oyntments.

Take of Rosen and Perosen, Virgin Wax and Frankinsence, of each a quarter of a pound, of Mastick one ounce, Harts Tallow or Deers suet one ounce, of Camphire two drams, Olibanum four ounces, the Rosen, Perosen, Frankinsence, Mastick and Olibanum must be beat apart in a Mortar into very fine powder, and searsed, then melt your Wax and Deers Suet, being first cut in small pieces together, stirring them very well with a clean stick for fear of burning to, then put in your powder of Rosen when they be throughly melted, shaking it in by little and little, and likewise your powder of Perosen, Frankinsence and Mastick, one after another, stirring it continually together till all the Powder be melted, in no wise suffering it to boil, but so soon as you perceive it to be throughly melted, take it off and strain it through a strong course cloth into a pottle of White Wine boiled seething hot, so long as any thing may bee gotten through the cloth, and so stir it till it be no warmer then bloud warm, then put thereunto a quarter of a pound of Turpentine and your Camphire, stil stirring it, and when it is cold, make it up into rolls of a reasonable size, and put it up in parchment to keep, and so you may keep it a long time, if you keep it dry; if you find any knots in it in the rolling of it up, by reason of the negligent stirring of it, take them out. And for a Fistula, put therein four ounces of Mirrhe. In the Mortar before you do grind the Camphire, you must grind three or four Almonds, and take them out with a feather, and stamp your Camphire therein, and grind it very small, and take it out with a feather, &c.

The Effects of this Oyntment.

It is good for old and new Wounds, for amongst all others it is most cleansing and wil ingender good flesh, and it healeth more in a night, then any other in a month, and suffereth no corruption in a wound, nor any ill flesh to be ingendred. It is good for a Festure and Canker. It draweth all manner of ache out of the Liver, Spleen and Reins of the back. It breaks Imposthumes, it is good for the Headach & for the singing in the brain, and for all manner of Imposthumes in the head or body, for blowing in the ears, and for sinews that be strained of shrunk. It draweth out any thorne or broken bone, or any evil thing that is in a wound; it is good for the stinging or biting of any venemous beast; it rotteth all manner of Botches, and healeth the same without fear; it is good for the [ ] of the space Members, the Flux, the Menstrous, if it be laid to a womans Navil; it helpeth the Emrods, and is very good to make Cerecloth for the Gout, all Aches and Pestilent Botches. If you lay this Plaister to a little Sore or Wound, one Plaister wil serve twice, if it be clean wiped; also if you lay it to any place where the skin is not broken, you may let it lye thereunto til by the moisture that it draweth from the sore place it falleth off; and so from time to time you must do it til you find release of pain, and being driven thin upon a cloth you must lay it that it may cover all the sore.

PALSIE.

For the Palsie.

Take half a pound of sweet butter, a pint of new Cow-dung, and boil them both together till it come to a Salve, then lay half of it upon a woolen cloth, and lay it to the nape of the neck, and when it is cold apply the other half warm.

Another.

Take White Wine and Sider, and take a good deal of red Sage, and boil them well to the one half, and wash the Patient where he shaketh, and if his Head shaketh, wash the neck as hot as may be suffered, and keep his neck warm and his joints at all times.

Against the Palsie.

Take a handful of Sage, of Southern. wood, Spike of Lavender, of each alike, boile these in a gallon of running water, and strain it into a stone pot when it is boiled away to a pint and half, then every morning take three or four spoonfuls thereof luke warm, and gargarise therewith, and put it forth again. Also take some of the same water warm, and chafe the place with a spunge.

Of the Palsie.

This shaking is a continual strife of natural powers, which are raised with out ceasing. It hapneth; first by looking from a great height, by sudden fear or sudden joy, or much cold or great heat, or much bleeding; for remedy, use three leaved grasse, Cummin and Steches, by Glister or otherwise; of Oyls, use Oyl of wild Cowcumbers, Oyl of Dil, of Clivers Artico, which Herb is very good against the shaking Palsie.

PLAGUE *or* PESTILENCE.

For the Pestilence.

Take half a handful of Rue, as much of Fetherfew, and one handful of Marigolds, a handful of Burnet, a handful of Sorrel, a quantity of Dragons, either the root or the crop, as the time of the year requireth; then take a pottle of running water, and let them boil over the fire till half the water be consumed, then take it from the fire and let it cool, and when it is almost cold, straine it through a fair linnen cloth, and then let the sick body drink thereof, and if it be too bitter, put thereto a quantity of loaf Sugar, of else powder of Licoras.

This hath been proved of a certain by great men, and hath holpen almost an hundred Persons in divers places; and where there were three persons in one house sick, two of them drunk thereof, and the third would not, and he dyed, and the two that took it lived, and this was proved of a certain. This Medicine must be given betimes before the Purples do appear, and it will cease by the grace of God.

A Medicine against the Plague.

Take a handful of Sage vertue, a handful of Hens grease, a handful of Elder leaves, a handful of red Bramble leaves, and stamp them all together, and strain them with a fair cloth in to a quart of White Wine, and then take a quantity of Ginger, and mingle them all together, and drink thereof a spoonful every day fasting for ten dayes together, and for the first spoonful you shall be safe for four and twenty hours, and after the ninth spoonful you shall be safe for all the yeare after. And if it shall happen that any be strucken with the Plague before this Medicine be taken, then take water of Scabious and water of Betony, and a quantity of fine Treakle, and put them together, and drink it, and it will put out all the Venom, and if the Sore do appear, then take leaves of Elder, and make a Plaister thereof with Mustard seed stamped together, and lay it to the Sore, and it will draw out all the Venome, and (by Gods grace) recover the party.

A precious Water good against all Poisons and Pestilences.

Take Turmentile, Scabious, Dittony, Pimpernel, of each a like quantity, distil them all together, and drink of it.

An approved Medicine for the Plague.

It taketh one like the Ague, with cold: as soon as it taketh them and complain of it, take five, seven or nine leaves of Garden Spurge, nine is the most, stamp them small in a dish, and put to it warm milk or Posset Ale, and let the sick body drink it, and presently go to bed and sweat; then take a great Onion and take out the core, and put into it Mithridatum, then lay on the top again, and rost it very soft, then beat it very small in a dish, and put to it three spoonfuls of White Wine Vinegar, as much Sugar as will make it pleasant to take, and as soon as the stomack is purged, give him of the Onion as much as you can, for that will draw out the Sore in four and twenty hours (by Gods grace) and keep the Patient very hot and warm, and give him hot Broths and Drinks, and keep him in a sweat four and twenty hours, and after keep him very hot, and when the Sore is come out, roast an Onion with Treakle and Vinegar, and lay it to the Sore to draw it out, and have a Chirurgion to launce it.

For the rest of your houshold, give them every day Mithridatum and Treakle, and take Centory and Madder, and boil it in Beer, and let them drink now and then thereof.

An excellent Drink against the Plague, Small Pox or Meazels, and for the cure and prevention thereof.

Take a pint of Dragon water, three pints of the best Malmsesey or Muskadine, boil therein of Rue and Sage, of each a handful, and let it boil till one pint be boiled away, then strain it, and afterwards set it on the fire again, and put thereto long Pepper, Ginger and Nutmegs beaten to powder, of each one ounce, boil all these a little more, and then take it from the fire, and put therein of the best Mithridate one ounce, of London Treakle two ounces, and a quarter of a pint of the best Angelica Water, and use it as followeth. If you think your self to be infected, take one spoonful of this at a time morning and evening luke-warm, but if not infected, take it but once or twice a week at the most, half a spoonful at a time, in any Plague time; and when they that are infected take this, let them lye down and sweat two or three houres in the bed; and when they be well dryed, and warm kept, let them drink none but warme Drinks or Caudles, and so by Gods assistance they shall be well. This Drink will keep good half a year if it be close kept.

A good Drink against the Plague.

Take of White Wine one quart, and put therein the juice of these Herbs following, of Elder leaves, Rue leaves, Wormewood and Scabious, and put in a spoonful of good Treakle, and the powder of a good Race of Ginger, stir all together, and drink three spoonfuls of this every morning for the space of nine dayes together: This preserves you from the Plague, and if you be infected, it wil expel it; and if it come to a Botch, stamp the leaves of red Brambles with Mustard and Honey, and make a Plaister, and lay it to the Sore. Probatum.

An excellent thing to defend the Plague.

Take twenty leaves of Rue, two Walnuts, and two figs, and a graine of Salt in the morning fasting with a little Wine.

A good Preservation against the Plague.

Take of the best Hungaria or Roman Vitriol, with a little Amber, and dissolve it in Vineger of the best, then take a litle Rosewater, and mingle therewith, and every morning take half a spoonful thereof, and cast it on a brick made hot in the fire, and let the chamber where any abide be perfumed every day, and t will take away all corruption and poison out of the Chamber, so that the Spiders will nor endure; of all outward Medicines, there is none better then this, by the advice of Doctor Matthias a Germane, and Doctor Butler of Cambridg.

A Water for the Plague.

Take Turmentile, Scabious, Betony, of each a like quantity, distil them together, and they will make the best water for a Surfet or any manner of poisonous Disease, if you drink it in the morning fasting.

A Water to be made in May, good against the Plague or Surfet.

Take Cellendine, Rosemary,Rue, Pellitory of Spain, Scabious, Angelica, Pimpernel, Wormwood, Mugwort, Betony, Egrimony, Balme, Dragon, and Turmentile, of each half a pound, shred them somewhat smal, and put them to five quarts of White Wine, stop it close, and let it stand three daies and nights, stirring it morning and evening, then take the Herbs from the Wine, and distil them in an ordinary Still, and when you have distilled the Herbs, distil the Wine also, wherein is vertue for a weak stomack. Take of either of these three or four spoonfuls in the morning or any other time, as occasion serveth, walking after it till you shall feel your selfe inclining to sweat, then go to bed, or betake your self otherwise to rest.

An approved Medicine for the Plague.

Take a root or smal handful of Saxifrage or Meadow Parsley, one good spoonful of Sassafrass wood smal beaten, one half root of Tormentile or Setwal, Elder berries one good spoonful, or a handful of the leaves of Rue, red Sage, and red young Bramble leaves, of each a handful, two spoonfuls of old black Ivy berries, Harts horne scraped very small as much, eight Figs dryed, eight Races of white Ginger, and two Oranges, stamp them all together in a Mortar, steep them all at least twelve hours in a quart of White Wine, and half a pint of White Wine Vinegar, then strain them through a fine cloth, and drink every morning a spoonful fasting, and take nothing in two hours after, and as much at night; if you be to go abroad into any infectious place, carry in your mouth one half root of Tormentile, taking the wind as much as you can of all infectious persons and places. This is to be done before you be infected, and when you are infected, you must keep your self warm and out of the ayre for twelve dayes, drinking this as before; and if there be any great danger, you may drink a spoonful every three or six hours, and it will with Gods blessing bring the Infection out in Sores, which being done, the worst is past; only take heed of cold to drive in the Sores again, and use warm Poultices which may draw them to a head, ripen, and so break them.

A Preservative against the Plague.

Take of Sage, Rue, Elder leaves and red Bramble leaves, of each a handful, stamp them all together, and strain them through a cloth with a quart of White Wine, then take a quantity of Ginger, and mingle it together, and drink thereof morning and evening a spoonful nine dayes together.

For the Party Infected.

If you be infected before you have drunk the aforesaid Medicine, then take a spoonful of Scabious Water, as much of Betony, and a quantity of fine Treakle, put it together, and drink it, and it will expel the Venom.

To break the Botch.

Take Bramble leaves, Elder leaves and Mustard seed, and stamp them all together, then make a Plaister thereof, and lay it to the Sore.

A Medicine for the Plague.

Take three slips of Herb grace, and six spoonfuls of Vinegar, and beat them together, then strain them, and put thereto one ounce of Treakle, and one ounce of Sugar, and stir them together, and set it on the fire and make a Sirrup thereof, then take a Sage leafe, and every morning take as much as a bean upon the same leaf and eat it.

A Drink against the Plague.

Take one ounce of Sorrel Water, as much Dragon water, and a dram of Treakle, and put thereto a dram and a halfe of Powder Imperial, and give it to the Patient in Ale within four and twenty hours after he is infected.

Another.

Take a handful of Savory, and boil it in a quart of Wine Vinegar with a spoonful of graines beaten being put therein, and drink it every morning with Sugar fasting.

Another.

Take in the morning fasting one dry Figge, one Walnut, and four or five leaves of Rue chopt all together, and eat it, and after drink a cup of Wine.

PILES.

A good Medicine for the Piles or Emrods.

Take a very old and hard white Dogs turd, which will be on the top of Molehills, and seeth it in Sallet Oyl very thick and so put up the Piles therewith, and it will help very quickly.

A Plaister to mitigate the pains of the Piles and Emrods.

Take the pap of an Apple, and put thereunto the yolk of a new laid egge, work them well together, then put in nine cleaves of Saffron small ground, of Linseed twenty cornes finely ground, these boil all together on the Embers alwayes stirring it, of this make a Plaister and lay it to your grief.

A Medicine for the Piles.

Take a good handful of Mullet leaves, and a good handful of Elder leaves, and stamp them very smal in a Mortar, and boil them in fresh butter very well, so that it may be very strong of the leaves, then strain it, and keep it for your use.

For the Piles.

Take a fair great Pippin or Apple, and cut off the top, and take out the core, then fill the same with Capons grease and the powder of Saffron, and roast the apple in the Embers till it be soft, then stamp it, and make thereof a Salve, and spread the same upon a piece of leather, and lay it to the Sore being well warmed.

Another.

Take a pint of Sallet Oyl, Rosemary tops, Sowthernwood, Hisop, Lavender, Camomile and Costmary, of each almost a handful, and a good handful of red Rose buds, stamp all these herbs in a stone Mortar, then put them into the Oyl, and let it stand nine dayes, then boil it half an hour, and when it is almost boiled, put into a quarter of a pint of Aquavitae, and so keep it for your use.

Another.

When they come forth and swel much, bathe them (with the water that Mallowes Fenicrick and Onions have boiled in) very warm, and after the bathing, apply unto it this Plaister following, Take the finest and inner part of a roasted Onion, beat it in a wooden dish with May Butter, and a little powder of Saffron, and annoint the Sore.

To heal the Piles and Emrods.

Take the leaves of green Elder, and boil them in a pint of water, and four spoonfuls of White Wine, then take a piece of cloth three fingers broad, and take the leaves so boiled as hot as you can suffer them, and so apply it a good while, then rub it with a little May butter. Probatum.

For the Piles or Emrods. Mrs. Wing.

Take Oystershels, as thick as you can get them, and the newest, and burn them in the fire till they be red hot, then take the inner white of those shels, and beat them in a Mortar very smal, then sift them through a piece of Lawne, then take some Linseed Oyl in a sawcer, and warm it, and annoint the Piles first with that Oyle, then strew the powder thick upon the Piles, then take a cleane rag and dip it in the Oyl, and lay it upon the Piles, and dresse it so twice every day, this is a sure and approved Medicine, and faileth not to help. Probatum.

PLAISTER.

To make the Black Plaister.

Take a pint of Oyl Olive, and halfe a pound or red Lead, and boil them together, and stir them with a slice of wood continually until it be black, then take it from the fire, and put in a pennyworth of red [ ], and a quarter of a pound of Rosen and set it on the fire againe, the fire may not blaze, and stir it, then powre a little of it on the side of a dish, and if it stick to the dish it is enough, then let it stand until it be cold, and then make it up in rolls for your use. It is good for any ache, new wound that bleedeth, or an old Sore, and to stanch blood.

An excellent Plaister.

Take Harts suet four ounces, Rosen and Perosen, of each half a pound, white Wax and Frankinsence, of each foure ounces, first melt the Suet and Wax together, then powder the Gums, and put thereunto, and when they have relented together, strain them through a canvass cloth into another vessel, and put thereunto a pottle of White Wine, and set it on the fire again, and boile them to the consuming of the Wine clean away, stirring it with a staff, then take it from the fire, and when it is almost cold, put to it four ounces of Turpentine well washed in White Wine, two drams of Camphire well powdered, then make up your Rolls, and lap them in Parchment. This Plaister is good for Wounds both new and old, for Bruises and for Aches; and it doth mundifie Ulcers and old Sores without pain, and comforteth the members that it lyeth on. It is good both for Fistulaes and Cankers that are ulcerate.

A drying Plaister.

Take Oyl of Roses eight ounces, white and red Lead, of three ounces, Cerus six drams, Littarge of Gold, Sanguis Draconis and Bole Armoniack, of each one ounce. Camphire one dram, make all these into a fine powder, and mixt it with the Oyle, and set it on a soft fire alwayes stirring it, and let it boil til it be Plaister like. This Plaister is good to dry the Sores in the legs.

An excellent Plaister for any Sore old or new.

Take the yolk of an egg, as much ordinary Turpentine, and as much Herb grace chopt and stamped, mingle all these well together, and spread them on a cloth and lay them to the Sore.

A Plaister for all manner of Swellings in any place.

Take Parsley, Herb Christopher, and crumbs of sowre bread, beat then small together, and boil them in White Wine, and make thereof a Plaister, and lay it to warm.

To make a Parracelsus Plaister.

Take Gum, Galbanum and Opoponax, of each one ounce, Amoniacum and Bdelium, of each two ounces, beat them smal, and put them in an earthen Pipkin glazed, and powre on them as much White Wine Vinegar as will serve to steep the Gums in, so let them stand one day and one night, the next morning boil them in the same Vinegar on the gentle fire of coals, and when they be throughly melted, pour them out hot into a bag, and wring them well, and cast away that which remaines in the bag, then take the liquor so strained, and let it boil in a pot till the Vinegar be consumed clean away, and in boiling you must stir it continually lest the Gums burn to the bottom. Then take Oyl Olive one quart, new Wax halfe a pound, put them into an earthen pot glazed, such a one as is of sufficient bigness, and set it over a fire of Coals, and let it melt softly, then put into it one pound of Littargy finely beaten into powder, stirring them continually with a wooden slice, and when they be all well mixed together, and of the colour of tawny, then take it from the fire, then take of the aforesaid Gums that were first boiled, the quantity of a nut, and put thereto, and so by little and little put in all the Gums, and being well mixed together, then set it over the fire again, take heed withal, lest the matter be over heated and run into the fire, for it is very hot of it self; then put into it these things following, Take of the two kinds of Astrology rotunda, Calaminaris, Mirrh and Frankinsence, of each of then one ounce, beat them into powder, then put them into the said matter, and powre upon the same one ounce of Oyle of Bayes, and last of all put into it four ounces of the best Turpentine, then boil all together, and stir it continually; and when you would know whether if be sodden enough or no, put a little thereof into cold water, if it be not soft that it will not cleave unto your fingers it is enough; but if it cleave it is not enough, but let it boil until it is enough, then take it from the fire, and pour into a Bason of cold water, then annoint your hands with Oyl of Roses, and work it well with your hands two or three hours, and make it into Rolls and keep it.

It is good for old and new Sores, it draweth and cleanseth, it wil not suffer any Sore to putrifie, but if there be dead flesh in the Sore before it be laid on, it will not take it away. It is good for sinewes cut or pricked with thornes, it will draw out of Wounds, Iron, Wood or Lead, and it is good for the biting of venemous Beasts, it is also good for Biles, Fistulaes, Cankers, Shingles, and for Saint Anthonies fire. Sir Thomas Porter hath found by often experience a speedy help for bones out of Joint, so that laying on two or three of these Plaisters, hath healed in fifteen dayes Armes out of joint; when you do lay up this Salve, keep it in an Oyly paper.

PLURISIE.

A good Medicine to ripen a Plurisie.

Take a fair Costard, and cut off the crowne, and pick out the core, but make no hole through, and then put in all these powders, of Bores tooth the weight of four pence, of the Powder of Rubarb grated as fine as may be, the weight of a three pence, of Cinamon the weight of a penny, of the powder of white Sugar candied the weight of two pence, put all these into the Apple, and cover him again, and lay him on a tile on the Embers, and roast him till he be soft as may be, then cut it in sunder, and give the sick party in the morning half of it to eat, and fast two hours after it, then eat some good broth, and take the other part of the Apple the next day, so that both the dayes are good to take a Medicine on.

An approved Medicine for the Plurisie.

Take a quantity of Horse dung which is kept in the Stable, strain it with Ale, then put to it a good quantity of Treakle and some Ginger, and let the Patient drink thereof morning and evening lukewarm as much as he can endure.

A Plaister for the same. Probatum.

Take a good handful of Brooklime, and shred it very smal, and boil it in fair water till it be very tender, then take a quantity of Sheeps suet and wheaten bran, and boil them together till it be thick, and so lay it to his side where the pain is, as hot as may be endured.

For the Plurisie.

Take a quart of White Wine, put to it two handfuls of Cummin, as much Oaten bran newly bolted, bruise the Cummin, and boil all to a Poultice, and put it in two bags hot, lay one to the side pained, and when it cooleth, lay to the other, and so continue changing them three or four hours.

Or take Earth-wormes and fry them in Vinegar, and spread them, and lay them to the side pained.

Another.

The Plurisie cometh of cold humours, therefore beware you take not much cold or any cold thing. Malmesey sod with Camomile is very good.

A sweet Apple roasted, and eaten with powder of Licoras and Sugar candied, is good eaten in the morning and at night. A sweet Apple also is best with Olibanum. Also a Plaister of Pitch is very good laid to the side.

Another.

Annoint the place where the paine is with the Oyl of Linseed.

For the Plurisie.

Take four Spanish Balls newly gathered from a Horse, stamp them and strain them with a pint of White Wine, and as much beer, & put to that a penny worth or Treakle being first melted, and give the party to drink thereof twice a day, and not to eat or drink one hour before nor after: if you be sure it is the Plurisie, let him blood within three dayes, but if he be longer before he be let blood, be sure you let him blood on that arm on that side where the pain is. Also if when after blood letting he fall worse again, this Drink is a very good Medicine for that Sicknesse taken by overmuch labour or lying on the ground.

There must be laid also to the side that the stitch is on, for the Plurisie, this following:

Take a pint of new milk, make batter of it with wheaten flower, as thick as you do Fritters, put to it three spoonful of Honey, and a groats worth of Saffron, boil it to a Poultice, and spread half, and then grate it over with Nutmegs, and lay it warm to the side, and when it hath been on twelve hours, then lay to the other half, and make more if you see cause.

Also if you boil a piece of leaven, as big as a good Apple, in Vinegar, the quantity of four spoonfuls, and as much Rose water, and a few Rose leaves to a Poultice, spread it, and grate it thrice over with Nutmegs, and lay to the pained side: It is also very good for the Plurisie, or for any pain in the side.

If you take two handfuls of Horse-dung, two Races of Ginger powdered, boil them in a quart of White Wine being bound in a cloth, boil it to the one half, then drink a good draught morning and evening, and after you have drunk it, cover your self warm and sweat; this way is also very good. If the party be costive, give him gentle Purgations, as Cassia Fistula, or use Suppositories or Glisters.

For this Sicknesse Tessers are good, and the water of Mallowes, Violets, Borage or Bugloss, Sugar candied also.

Take also of the Water of Broom flowers, Scabious and Carduus Benedictus, of each three spoonfuls, put in Sugar candied, and let the party drink so much morning and evening, and annoint the side with Oyl of Broom flowers.

To know whether one have the Plurisie or no.

Hold in thy breath as long as possibly thou canst do, and then if thou canst not let thy breath pass from thee without coughing, assuredly thou either hast it, or art in danger of having it forth with.

For the cure of the Plurisie,

Thou must be let blood forthwith, then take the quantity of a Walnut of Carduus Balsom, and eat it upon a knifes point, and take again presently the like quantity of the same Balsom, and melt it in a sawcer at the fire, and with a soft clean linnen cloth dipped in the Balsom, wash and bathe thy left side well, as hot as thou art able to suffer it, then warme the said cloth, and lay it double over the place pained, and bind it on, and ly down to rest, and by Gods blessing thou shalt fine it a present Cure.

For a hot Plurisie.

When any get a pricking pain about the ribs with a cough and an Ague, then use this Glister, Take sixteen ounces of Broth wherein a Lambs head or Calvs feet have been sodden, put therein one ounce of Sugar, the yolk of one egg, two ounces of Sallet Oyle, salt one dram and halfe, temper them well together and use it.

PRICKING.

For the pricking of a thorn, Swelling or Ancomb.

Take Birdlime and spread it on a piece of Glovers leather on the Allome side, and lay it on as far as the swelling goeth, and let it lye four and twenty hours, and then renew it again.

Another for the pricking of a thorn or needle in any joint.

Take fine boulted flower, and temper it with White Wine, and boil it together till it be thick, then lay it on the Sore as hot as may be suffered, and it will open the hole, and draw out the anguish, help the aking, and heal it: for want of White Wine take Ale or Beer. It is good to heal a Boil of Whitlow.

POULTICE.

To make a Poultice for Wounds or Swellings.

Take a good quantity of Marsh Mallowes, or of other, if you cannot get them, and boil them in clean water, then cut them small, and take White Wine dregs, and of good Ale as much more, your Mallowes being shred, put it into your dregs, and put in some Deers Suet and Sheeps Tallow melted, and crumbs of brown bread, boil all these together till it be thick, always stirring it to keep it from burning, then lay it warm every dressing upon a woollen cloth, it dissolveth hardnesse and swelling. The Lady Farnehams Poultice.

Another Poultice to mollifie and dissolve.

Take the crumbs of white bread, seeth them in milk, and put to it Oyl of Camomile and a little Saffron, then take it from the fire, then put to it the yolks of two new laid egges, and so make of it a Poultice, and lay it to the sore.

An approved good Poultice to lay to an Ache or Pain.

Take a good handful of Mallowes, another of Smallage, a handful of Linseed, as much of Oatmeal grets pounded together, a pottle of well water, halfe a pint of milk, and Deeres Suet as much as an egge, or else so much of Sheeps Tallow, then boil all these together till it be thick, then lay it to the Patient where the pain is, being spread upon a linnen cloth.

A very good Poultice for Wind gotten into joints.

Take Wormwood and Dill dryed and beaten to fine powder, of each one handful, of Sheeps dung three handfuls, of Camomile flowers half a handful, of Cummin seeds two ounces, seeth them all in Lye, and let it boil together until it be very thick, then spread it upon leather, and lay it upon the place grieved warm: but first annoint it with Oyle of Rue. Mr. Smart.

A Poultice for a Bruise or Strain.

Take Claret Wine, Balme and Rose-leaves, boil them together till they be thick, then lay them to the Sore as hot as the Patient can suffer it.

A Water to wash the place before you apply the Poultice.

Take Mallowes and Smallage, of each a handful, boil them in a quart of Vineger to a pint, then wash the place pained as hot as you can suffer it.

An excellent Poultice for the Ague in a Womans brest or Legs.

Take Houseleek, Smallage and Mallowes, of each two handfuls, shred them small, then take a handful of Linseed, and bruise it finely in a Mortar, take also a handful of Oatmeal or wheaten bran, some Roses of a Rose cake, every leaf pulled from another, Sheeps Tallow one pound, shred it well, then put all these into a gallon of running water, and boil them together till they become thick, then put thereto a quart of Cowes milk, and let it boil still till it be as thick as a Plaister, stirring it often, then when the legg or brest is washed with the water aforesaid, spread the Poultice on a cloth all abroad, and lay it to the leg or brest as hot as may be suffered, and let it lye so till it be dry and hard, and then renew it, but if the leg or brest be not very hot and red it shall not need.

A Poultice for any Swelling.

Take of Violet leaves and Groundsel, of each a handful, of Mallowes and Chick weed, of each halfe a handful; shred them smal, and let them seeth wel in running water, and thicken it with Barly meal being finely sifted, and spread it on a cloth, and so lay it on the place pained, and bind it fast, and shift it twice a day till it be cured.

PURGE.

The Manna Purge.

Take half an ounce of the best Cene, lay it in soak in a pint and half of Posset Ale on the Embers in a close covered pot two hours, then put it into a posnet, and put to it a Parsley root or two, one Fennel root, two spoonfuls of Anniseeds, a stick or two of Licoras scraped and bruised, a few Raisons stoned, boil all together to half, then strain it, and put into it one ounce of Manna, and four penny weight of Rubarb being grated and put in a clout, and laid in soak in the aforesaid liquor with the Manna one hour, when the Manna is melted wring the rubarb, strain it, and put to it three spoonfuls of Sirrup of Roses, and drink it blood warm in the morning, and eat a mess of Mutton pottage after it.

To Purge, the Moon being in Scorpio, Cancer or Pisces.

Michocanum two drams, which is two six penny weights, grate it with a Grater, and pound it smal, steep it in a penny pot of White Wine all night, and in the morning about six of the Clock, warm it milk warm, and drink it off, and half an hour after take eight or ten spoonfuls of Mutton broth, with a few Raisons or Currans in it, and it will work downewards, and purge away moist humours causing Phlegme to breed in the body.

Of Catapusia being small seeds, you must take two and twenty or four and twenty of them in quantity, and take off the outer hulls, and beat the inner graines small in a Mortar or pewter dish, then mingle it with a little Ale or White Wine which is best, warm it a little, and take it as abovesaid, and it wil void as the other.

And if you should at any time have any continuing Lask by occasion of Medicine or otherwise, seeth a little Rice without any salt or butter, and eat it with a little Cinnamon, and it shall presently stop it.

Another to purge Phlegme.

Take a handful of Groundsel, wash it clean, and boil it in a pint of Ale, skim it, then put in half a handful of Raisons or Currans, and boil two ounces of Sugar candied, boil all together again to half a pint or lesse, then strain it, and drink it milk warme fasting at six a Clock, and fast till eleven, then take some Mutton broth.

Another.

Take Elicampane roots, and make Conserves of it, use it in this manner, first wash the roots clean, then slice them in pieces as big as your little finger, seeth them in fair water until they be tender, then take them up, and pound them, and strain them through a haire sieve, then set them over the fire, and put to them the double or trebble weight of Sugar, and when it is perfectly incorporated or mingled, take it off, and keep it in a Gally pot. The time to gather the roots is when the leafe falleth away.

A Dyet Drink to Purge withal.

Take Anniseeds, Licoras, Cene, Hermodactilus, of each one ounce, of Sassaparilla five ounces, scrape away the outside of it, and bruise it a little, and cut it the length of an inch, then bruise your Licoras, and put your Anniseeds to it, and put them in a pot to steep in two gallons of Conduit or running water four and twenty hours, the boil them until a third part be consumed, then put in your Cene, and half an hour after put in your Hermodactilus, the outside being pared away, and slice them as you do a Race of Ginger, and within an hour take it from the fire, and let it rest in the pot two hours, then strain it in a bag as you strain Hypocras, so let your first draught in the morning be luke-warm fasting, and at Dinner and at Supper what you think good, for you must drink no other Drink till that be spent.

A Purging Ale.

Take the juice of Scurvigrass foure pound, of Watercresses two pound, of Brooklime one pound, of Water Mints half a pound, of dry Wormwood four handfuls, of the roots of Madder four ounces, of the roots of Monks Rhubarb three ounces, roots of Horse Rhadish one ounce and a half, the roots of Saxifrage one ounce, of Cene four ounces, of Juniper berries half an ounce, of Anniseeds, Coriander seeds and Ginger, of each six drams.

Another.

Take a pint of the Whey of Goats milk, of Cene half an ounce, of Ginger clean scraped and thin sliced, Anniseeds and sweet Fennel seeds well dusted and lightly bruised, of each the weight of four pence, let them stand one hour, or one hour and a half on warm embers in infu[ ]g; the next morning to a draught hereof put a spoonful of Sirrup of Roses, and as this agreeth with you, so take it three or four dayes together, or every other day.

Another.

Take a pottle of the same Whey, boile therein Betony, Colts foot and Hisop, of each one handful, and drink thereof as you have occasion.

A very easie Purgation.

Take halfe a pint of Malmesey, or somewhat more, and half a quarter of an ounce of Cene, and two Races of Ginger sliced, then put them both into the Malmesey, and stir it well and let it stand all night, and then strain it, and drink it, and keep your Chamber, and you shall have four or five stools.

Another.

Take clarified Whey, and put into it a handful of Violet leaves, and half a handful of Polipodium of the Oak called Oak fernes, and drink a good draught of it luke-warm, and wash after it.

To procure Looseness.

Seeth Mallows and red Nettles in fair water, and let the party sit over the hot fumes thereof.

A Purge.

Take Aron or Wakerobbin, one dram of the powder thereof with two drams of Sugar, is good to cut gross humours, to purge the stomack of Phlegme and Melancholy.

Or else the root either green or dry, one dram thereof being taken in drink with as much Treakle, is a very special good Purgation.

To purge Phlegme and Melancholy.

Fetherfew dryed into fine powder, and two drams thereof taken with Honey or sweet Wine purgeth by stool Phlegm Melancholy, and Sadness.

Also take Peniroyal with Honey and Aloes to purge Melancholy, and for the Cramp.

To cleanse the Stomack from rotten Phlegm and Melancholy.

Drink the Seeds of Hollioaks.

Also Cene the cods and leaves in powder one dram, doth purge Phlegm and Melancholy.

To purge Phlegme and Choler.

The great Garden Dock leaves drunk in Wine, purgeth Phlegme, Choler and Water.

A Purging Drink.

Take two gallons of new small Ale, and put unto it a good handful of English Madder, a handful of Dock roots bruised, two handfuls of Scurvigrasse, a handful of Scabious, two ounces of Cene, two ounces of Anniseeds, two of three sticks of Licoras finely scraped, and all those things bruised, then put them into the new ale, and let them work therein, so let it stand two or three dayes and then drink thereof morning and evening.

PAINE.

For pain in the Joints.

Take a pennoworth of Aquavitae, Oyl of Exeter, three ounces of Sage, of Herb grace, Clerk Robert, of each a handful, stamp them small in a Mortar, then take your Aquavitae, and straine them together a good while, then take a spoonful thereof, and annoint the Sore place against the fire.

For the pain under the side.

Take the toast of a Wheaten loaf, and butter it, and toast it again, and butter it twice more, then toast it againe and butter it with Soap, and hold it against the fire till it lather, then lay it to the side where the pain is.

For paine in the side that cometh of Wind.

Take one handful of Cummin seeds, as much of Anniseeds, two handfuls of Rue, seeth these together in running water from a pottle to a quart, put to it half a pint of White Wine Vinegar before it be cold, dip a Spunge in it, and wring some of the liquor out of it, and lay it to the Patients side as hot as may be suffered, and when it beginneth to wax cold take a new.

POISON.

For the Poison of a Toad, or other Poison.

Take a handful of Plantane, and a handful of Parsley, and stamp and strain them into a little raw Cream, and mingle it well together, and annoint the place grieved therewith.

PISSING.

For pissing a bed.

Take a Boares pisle, and dry it, and make powder of it, and drink it in Ale or Beer.

POCKS.

A Medicine for the Small Pox.

Take two handfuls of Salt, and put it into a pint and a halfe of water, and stir it well together, then set it upon the fire and let it boil well, and in the boiling you must skim it, so that there be not any skum seen, and when the Small Pox are come well forth, and that the Swelling doth asswage, you must take a fine cloth, and bath them with this Brine, being warme, three times a day: And when they begin to grow brown, use this Oyntment, take a piece of Bacon, and roast it on a spit, and set a dish of fair water under it, putting thereto some Rose water, and let the Bacon drop into it as it doth roast, and when it is roasted, take the dripping and the water and work it well together, and it will be a very good Oyntment, then put it into a Gally pot, and twice a day annoint the places with a feather, but in case lay not on too much, for that will make them moist, and make them stay longer.

Another to take away the Redness.

Take fair water in a Posnet, and put thereto half a pound of Butter, then set it on the fire, and let it boil softly, and skim off all the froth very clean, then take it off the fire, and let it stand till it be throughly cold, then powre the water from it, and put it in clean water, and set it upon the fire again skimming it very clean, and do this nine times together, put every time your butter must be cold before you put it into a new water, and the last time being very cold, take it clean away from the water, and put

Rosewater to it, and work them very well together, and put it up in to a Gally pot, and with a feather twice or thrice a day annoint the rednesse of the face; and if these Medicines be used as they should be, it will take away the rednesse, and make the face not to have any holes in it.

For the Small Pocks in the Eyes.

Take red Rose water, white Sugar candied beaten very fine, and brest milk, and temper these very well together, and with a feather dresse the eyes and it will keep them from the Small Pocks. If it be for a man, you must take the milk of a Girle; if for a woman the milk of a boy.

For the Small Pox or the Meazels.

When the Pocks are white at the first coming out, let a woman (that gives suck) milk some of her milk upon them, and apply a paper thereupon and do this every day, and they will not pit. Also take a new laid egge, and [ ] it in fresh butter, and then poure it into cold water, and being cold put it into a pot, and put Rosewater thereunto, and stir it so long till it become like an Oyntment, and with it annoint the face, and the eyes especially, and it will preserve the sight from the Pocks; and when as any one hath Pockholes, annoint them with Barrowes grease betimes, and it will help.

Also for them that have the Small Pocks falne into the eyes, let them take Pimpernel and stamp it, and strain it, and take the juice thereof and drop it into the eyes where the Small Pocks are with a feather morning and evening, this is a special good Medicine for a Pin and Web or Pearle in the eyes.

Also for the Small Pocks or Meazels take Dragon Root, it purgeth all the inner parts, or the distilled water given to drink with Treakle is very good to drive them out.

Also Figs eaten before a meat, provoke sweat, and thereby expel all stinking humors, and therefore are good for the Meazels or Smal Pocks, and to be given to Children to bring them out speedily.

Also an excellent Medicine to drive them out, seeth Fumetory in Rue water, and drink it.

Also to heal the Pocks or any Scabs, seeth Houndstongue in Red Wine, and drink thereof, and also apply it to the Sores.

Also to drive out the Smal Pocks, drink a spoonful of Sallet Oyl with three spoonfuls of Malmesey, and the quantity of a Hasel nut of Treakle in it.

Also to take the print of the Small Pocks out of the Sore, take one ounce of Sperma Ceti, and as much Deers Suet, and melt them together, and when the Small Pocks are ripe, annoint the face therewith with a feather, and if the Pocks be in the Throat, then give the Patient a little Sirrup of Blackberries, such as grow upon Briars, but take them when they are red, and pound them, and strain them, and put as much Sugar thereunto as there is of the juice, and seeth them together till they boiled away to the one halfe, then give the Patient a little in a spoon three or four times in a day, and that by Gods help will cure them; and the very like may be done with Gooseberries before they be too ripe, and these may be taken and made into Sirrup, and kept seven yeares if you will.

A Drink to put out the Small Pocks.

Make a Posset with Ale and milk, and take away the curd, then take a red Fennel spout, and boil it well together, then strain it, and put thereto a quantity of Nutmegs and Treakle, and English Saffron mingled warme together.

QUINZIE.

For the Quinzy.

Take milk and a flint stone, and make it red hot, and quench it twice in the milk, and take Vervain and Collombine leaves, and seeth it in the milk, and fine Honey, and so give it to the Patient to drink.

Another.

Take the paring of the threshold and Sallet Oyl, and fry them together, and lay it warm to the Patients throat.

RAINS.

An excellent Medicine for the running of the Rains.

Take a handful of the inner rind or bark of the Sloe-bush, the outermost black skin or rind being cut or scraped away; then put the same into a quart of the purest and strongest Ale you can get, and let the same boil well from a quart to a pint, when it is so boiled, take the rind out of the

Ale, and let it stand until it be cold, then divide it into two parts, and drink it two mornings together, and fast after it every morning two or three hours. Probatum.

For the Raines of the Back.

Take half an ounce of Venice Turpentine, and let it be wel washed in Plantane Water or Rose water, and then mix it with fine white Sugar, and make thereof four or five balls, of which you must eat three in a morning fasting, and drink White Wine or Rhenish Wine immediately after.

RHEUME.

A good Medicine for the Rheume distilling down the throat, and causing pain in the Teeth.

Take two handfuls of Hisop, strip it from the stalks, rowle it in a brown paper somewhat wet, then lay it to roast under embers until it be roasted very soft but not burned, then take it off, and lay it upon a linnen cloth, and so lay it upon the mould of the Head as hot as may be suffered, and so put it fresh three or four times, letting it lye from the evening to the morning.

For the Rheume distilling into the Eyes or Lungs.

Take of Rosemary, red Sage, sweet Marjerom, of each a handful, of Betony half a handful, seeth them in a quart of Balme Water until it cometh to a pint, then strain it, and make up the Decoction with Sugar; and for the Lungs you must put in some Hysop, and a few Anniseeds and Licoras before you boil it.

An approved Receipt to be Drunk first and last for a Months Space, good for Rheums and Aches.

Take of Licoras one ounce, of Cassia in the Cane, and Cene Alexandrina of each four ounces, sweet Fennel seeds one ounce, Madder roots two ounces, of large Mace ten pence in weight, of Cinnamon fourteen pence in weight, Hermodactilus three ounces, of Polipodium three ounces, of Coriander seeds three ounces prepared, two or three yellow Dock roots, use the rind; a good handful of Scabious, a handful of Egrimony; All these are to be used thus, the Polipodium scraped, the Licoras scraped and bruised,

the Madder roots scraped and sliced, the Hermodactilus sliced, Mace
bruised in a Mortar with the Cinnamon and Licoras.

Then put all these Simples together in a bag, with a pound weight to
cause it to sink, but let it not touch the bottom, then tun four gallons of
good Ale, and about a week after you have tunned it, drink there of first
and last and continue it a Month or six weeks together.

For a Rheume in the Head.

Take the roots of white Beats stamped and strained, and put the juice of
them into a glass, and snuff up thereof into your nose with a quill every
morning twice in a Month, and it will help.

Of Rheume.

Rheume is nothing else but a defluxion that falls from the head into the
throat or brest, which doth otherwhiles so stop the pipes of the Lights and
throat that its ready to choak, also these Rheumes fall into the nose, and
cause the pawse.

These Rheums are caused divers waies; as from gross meats which
cause vapours, or of cold, or from a sharp North wind which bloweth
suddenly after a South wind.

The cold Rheumes are knowne by these signes following, as
wearinesse, heavinesse of the whole body, sleepiness, heavinesse of the
head and forehead, palenesse with full vaines, stuffing of the head or nose,
swelling of the eyes, pain in the throat, motion to vomit, swelling of the
Almonds; the Remedy, is to use dry and warm Herbs, as Sage, Fennel,
Mints, Rosemary, Marjerom, Time, &c. and after meat use something to
close the stomack, as prepared Coriander, toasted Bread, &c. and walk in a
morning fasting.

Hot Rheume, the signes thereof are these, viz. the face is red, mixt with
a pale or black colour, great heat in the nose with itchings, when the
mouth and the throat is full of bitterness and sharpnesse, and if the head be
hot in feeling, its thus to be cured, he must be let blood, and use this
Gargarism.

Take Sirrup of Jaunbes, of Violets and Poppy seeds, of each alike
temper them with Barley water; Or take Jaunbes, Sebestians, Violets,
white Poppy seeds and Quince kernels decocted in Barley water, use it in
the evening after meat, it is passing good.

Also take Sirrup of Poppy seeds Sirrup of Mulberries, of Roses, and
well water of each three ounces, of Wine of Pomgranats one ounce, make
it warm, and gargle therewith.

RICKETS.

For the Rickets in Children.

Cut the middle gristle of both the ears, and with the blood annoint the belly and the Navel with a little Cotton wool, then boil Harstongue and Liverwort in Milk or Broth for their usual Dyet.

Another.

Take Bay berries bruised and sweet Marjerom, of each a handful, and boil it in Beer, with three or four blades of Mace, and so drink it often.

Another.

When the former will not help, take Fennel seeds and Dill seeds, of each alike, but most of Dill, boile them in Beer and strain it, and sweeten it with Sugar and drink often.

RUPTURE.

A Plaister to keep up the Rupture.

Take Knotgrass and Shepherds Purse, of each one handful, of Comfrey and Solomons seale, of each half a handful, beat them into an Oyl, and thereof make your Plaister. This Oyl will be preserved all the year in a Gally pot.

A Drink for the Rupture.

Take long Plantane, Yarrow and Knotgrass of the redest colour, of each a great handful, Daisie roots, Dove f[]ot, Mousear and Borage, of each a small handful, wash them very clean, and shred them grosse,then take three quarts of milk, and two quarts of White Wine, set the milk on the fire, and when it doth seeth put in the Wine, and as the Curd ariseth take it away, and being clean, put in the Herbs, and let them boil gently a quarter of an hour, then take it off and straine it; and preserve it in Glasses, and let the Patient drink thereof in the morning fasting, and so in the evening almost a pint at a draught, and do so one week.

Another.

Take Comfrey roots, Daisie roots, and Pollipodium of the Oak, make them into a fine powder, and drink thereof every morning the weight of six pence the space of a fortnight, fasting an houre after it.

For the Rupture in Children.

Take Frankinsence half an ounce, Aloes a quarter of an ounce, beat it small and mixt it with the white of an egg unto an Oyntment, and therewith annoint the child upon his Rupture morning and evening.

Also take the root of Aron halfe a pound in powder, and give thereof unto the child every day for nine dayes together, one dram with water of Parfoliata, and tye the Rupture with a Boulster close upon it, and unto it.

RESTORATIVE.

A Restorative.

Take Treakle, Sallet Oyl, Sugar candied, Cinamon, powder made with Licoras and Sugar, of each a penny worth, mingle all these together, and take a quantity thereof as much as a Nut both morning and evening.

Another.

Take a quantity of Ale or Beer, and put therein over night three of four sprigs of Rew, and drink thereof evening and morning for a good space, and it will keep your stomack in good order.

A restoring Medicine for any decay of the inner parts.

Take Live Honey, and put thereto tops of Balme, Cowslip flowers, Borage flowers, Bugloss flowers, and tops of the Gilly flowers, and let this remain in the Honey the space of a Month, stopping the pot very close that no aire come in, let it stand all the said time in some warm place, either in the Sun or by the fire side, then distil it in a glass Still, with a little water, and drink thereof every morning a good draught.

A Restorative made of an Herb called Rosasolis.

This Herb groweth in the Meadows in low Marish grounds, and in no other places; it is of Horseflesh colour, and groweth very long and flat to the ground with a main long stalk growing in the midst of six branches springing out of the roots round about the stalk with a hoar colour, and a main breadth and length; and I do warn you in any wise not to touch this Herb when you gather it, with your hands, for then the vertue is gone: you must gather it by the stalk, and so pluck it out of the ground, and put it in a glasse or pewter pot; the leaves of this Herb are full of strength and vertue. Take of this Herb as much as will fill a pottle pot, but wash it not in any wise, then take a pottle of Aqua vitae, and put them both together in a large vessel, and let it stand (being chopped) just three dayes and three nights, and on the fourth day strain it through a clean cloth into a glasse or pewter pot, and put to it half a pound of Licoras beaten to fine powder, and half a pound of Dates, take out the stones of them, and cut them into fine slices, and mingle all these together, and stop the glass of pewter pot close that no Aire come into it, and drink of it at night to bedward half a spoonful with Ale, and as much in the morning fasting, for there is not the weakest man or body in the world that wanteth nature or strength, or that is cast into any Consumption, but it will restore them again, and cause them to be strong and lusty, and have a marvellous hungry stomack, and that very shortly; for he that useth this Medicine three times shal find a great change, and comfort in it, and as he feeleth himself, so he may use it.

It cured one Mr. Stubbs who dwelt in Westminster, and was in a great Consumption, and very neer unto death, being sick continually for eighteen weeks, and all the Physicians in London had forsaken him; these things were sent him to drink from an outlandish man, and in three times drinking of it he walked upon his feet.

RULES for Health.

A very good Rule for Mans Health, to be used in every
Month of the Year, written 1607.

In January use no Physick but warme clothing, eat warm meats, and drink White Wine fasting, it is wholsom.

In February forbear Physick and letting of blood, take no cold for fear of Agues, which are easily gotten.

In March forbear grosse feeding, purge by Potions, Bathing or Blood-letting.

In April Physick is good upon occasion, except Nature wil remedy of it self.

In May rise early and walk in the fields with a light breakfast, and use Physick upon occasion.

In June, if Physick, take it early in the morning with small dyet; clarified whey with cold Herbs is very good.

In July use cold herbs, cold meats, no Physick, no extreme exercises, use Rivers rather then Bathes.

In August use moderate Dyet, beware of surfetting or cold after heat for fear of Plurisies, sleep not in the day.

In September use Physick if need require, and bathe or bleed, and use fruits if they be sound and ripe.

In October use hot meats and drinks to nourish blood, and beware of cold for fear of Agues.

In November use hot meats and drinks and wholsome Wine, provide warm clothing, and go dry foot.

In December use none but Kitchen Physick and warm clothing, use merry company, and good Hospitality.

SALVE.

To make an especial good Salve.

Take Sallet Oyl one ounce, fresh and unwasht Butter one ounce, Sheeps Suet one ounce, Virgin Wax one ounce, Rosen beaten to very fine powder four ounces; Mastick four drams beaten very fine, Olibanum one ounce beaten to very fine powder, honey half an ounce, boil them all together till they come to six ounces, and then put it into a Gally pot, and put thereto some reasonable quantity of Venice Turpentine.

To make a very good Balsom.

Take half a pint of the best Aqua vitae, a quart of the best Wine Vineger foure, ounces of Storax, Mirrh one ounce, Galbanum one ounce, Gum Dragon one pound, eight graines of Musk, as much as Ambergreece, three pound of the best Sallet Oyle old and sweet, half a pound of Oyle of Lawrel of the best, Öyl of Spike one ounce, Oyle of Hypericon and Oyl of Juniper berris, of each two ounces, Oyl of Peter one ounce, half a pound of Virgin Wax, four ounces of red Saunders, and a quarter of an ounce of Saffron.

An approved Salve for any Greene Wound.

Take a pound of Butter, half a pound of Sheeps Suet, a penny worth of Rosen of Frankinsence and Turpentine, of each two penny worth, boil all together a good while except the Turpentine, for that must be put in afterwards, and boil but little, then strain it into a Bason of fair water, and then strain it out for your use.

A white Salve to heal a cut or green Wound.

Take a quantity of Mutton Suet, and almost half as much Rosen, shred the Suet very small, and melt it on a soft fire, and when it is well melted, beat the Rosen, and put it in, and let it boil together, stirring it continually till it be cold.

To make an excellent Salve.

Take the roots of Marsh Mallowes, wash and pick them clean, then slit them and take out the inner part of the pith, and cast it away, and take the outer part that is faire and white, and cut them into small pieces, bruise them in a Mortar, and take of them half a pound, and put it in a new earthen pan, and then thereto Linseed and Fenicreek of each two ounces a little bruised in a Mortar, then take Malmesey and White Wine of each a pint, and stir all these together, and let them infuse two or three dayes, then set them on a soft fire, and stir it well till it wax thick and like a skum, then take it off, and straine it through a new canvass, and thus have you ready the Mustellage for Plaister; Then take fine Oyle of Roses a quart, and wash it well with White Wine and Rose water, then take the Oyl clean from the water and Wine, and set it on the fire in a brasse pan alwayes stirring it, and put thereto Littarge of Gold and Silver, of each eight ounces, Cerus six ounces, red Coral, Bole Armoniack, and Sanguis Draconis, of each two ounces, and let them be finely powdered and searsed, then put them into the Oyl over the fire alwayes stirring it, and let not the fire be too big for burning of the stuff, and when it begins to wax thick, put in ten ounces of the aforesaid Mustellage by a little at ounce, or else it will boil over the pan, and when it is boiled enough you shall perceive by the hardnesse or softnesse of it, dropping a little of it on a sawcer or cold stone; then take it off, and when it is cold, make them in Rolls, and lap them in parchment, and keep them for your use. This Plaister resolveth humors in swolne legs.

To make a Salve for all manner of Wounds.

Take the juice of Smallage and Plantane, of each alike, honey and the white of an egge alike, put Wheat flower to them, and stir them till they be thick, and let it come to no fire at all, and so lay it to the Sore, and by Gods grace it will heal it.

A good Salve for greene Wounds or old Sores.

Take half a pound of Sheeps Suet, as much Barrowes grease, as much Wax, as much Rosen, and a pint of Sallet Oyl, set them all on a soft fire, and when they be melted, put in the Rosen finely beaten, boil them all together and skim them, then put in two pennyworth of Verdigrease, and last of all two ounces of Turpentine, and so let them boil a walm or two more, then take it up and keep it for your use; if it be an old Sore, put four pennyworth of Verdigrease, and three ounces of Turpentine.

SCIATICA.

For the Sciatica.

First take as fat a Goose as you can get, and when she is ready drest, then take a couple of the fattest young sucking Cats you can get, and flea them, and cut them into gobbets, and put them in the belly of the Goose, and so roast it as long as it will drop, then take the liquor and annoint the place pained with it, and bathe it before the fire as hot as you can suffer it, and dip a brown paper therein, and lay it hot to the place with warme cloathes to keep it fast to all night. Do this for the space of three or four nights together.

For the cold Sciatica or benumnesse of the Thighs or Legs.

Take a pint of aqua vitae, a pint of Wine Vinegar, a quarter of a pound of Oyl of Bayes, the juice of four or five handfuls of Sage, a Sawcer full of good Mustard, the Gall of an Ox bladder, and chafe them in the bladder, an hour or more, that the Oyl may be well mingled with the rest, and annoint the place therewith against a good fire, and let the Patient go warm into bed and sweat. Probatum.

A Soveraigne Medicine for the Sciatica.

Take half a pint of Aqua vitae, halfe a pint of White Wine Vinegar, and one Oxe Gall, almost a handful of Bay salt, and a handful of the tops of

Rosemary, and shred them small, and put them in a little Pipkin all together, and let it be ready to boil up, and then take it off, and chafe the place pained with it, with your hand so long as the Patient shall be able to endure it, and do it very warm against the fire, and then take Nerve Oyle, and annoint it, and then take a Scarlet cloth, and bind it up or cover it warm, and this do morning and evening.

CERECLOTH.

To make a Cerecloth.

Take Virgin Wax, Deers Suet, Rosen, Pitch, and Barrowes grease, of each a like, and boil them together until they be half consumed, then do it abroad upon a linnen cloth somewhat thin, and lay it to the place grieved as hot as may be suffered.

A singular Cerecloth for all Bruises, Aches and Wounds whatsoever.

Take a pint of Sallet Oyle of the best you can get, and half a pound of red Lead, and as much Rosen as a Walnut, boil all together upon a soft fire till it be somewhat black, stirring it continually, and when it is cold rowle it up, and keep it for your use. You may keep it seven years, and it will be exceeding good if you keep it from the heat of the fire. Probatum.

To make a Cerecloth for an Ache.

Take Olibanum and Sallet Oyle with Wax, Rosen and Stone Pitch, and boil them together.

A Cerecloth for all Members that be out of Joint or any consuming member and grieved with cold moistness that consumeth, it bringeth the Member again to his natural place.

Take six ounces of Wax, three ounces of Rosen, two ounces of Mastick, Armoniacum, Galbanum and Olibanum of each one ounce, of Fenicreek, Wormwood, Camomile and Cummin, of each of these in powder one ounce, Oyl of Crastorum and Oyle of Camomile flower: of each one ounce, of Vinegar five ounces; melt the Rosen, and Wax, and the Oyles together, and then put in the Galbanum and Armoniack steeped in Vineger and strained, and so put in the powder last of all, stirring it together, and thereof make your Cerecloth.

To make a good Cerecloth.

Take one pound of Galbanum finely beaten to powder and searsed, as much fine Rosen beaten and searsed, as much Pitch, of Sheeps Suet four ounces, of Cummin two ounces, Labdanum one ounce, of Cloves one ounces, of Mace one ounce, of Saffron half an ounce.

SORE.

For a new cut or Sore.

Take Brimstone and scrape it fine and mingle it with May butter, and annoint a Tent or a little lint throughly, and put it into the Sore or Cut, and it helpeth.

To dry up and to heal a Sore.

Take the burned Ashes of a Rhadish and strew it upon the Sore, and it will dry up and heal.

To break a Sore that is swoln.

Take Spurge and shred it small, and boil it in Whey, and thicken it with Oatmeal, and lay it warme to the Sore, it is also good for a womans brest.

Also for the breaking of a Sore or Boil, take Coriander seeds made into fine powder, and mix it with Honey, and this being implaistered upon a Boil or a Carbunkle will in a short time destroy it. Or take a little of a Calves curd.

STONE.

A Water for the Stone.

Take Ashen Keyes, Stichwort, Saxifrage, Mother-time, Broom flowers, Hawes, Hips, Bramble leaves, Pollipodium of the Oak, Pellitory on the wall, put all these together of each alike, and Still them, then to every pottle of water put half a pound of Anniseeds, and so let then stand four and twenty hours, then put them in the Still again, and still them all together, then drink of it as you need, and if it happen that the gravel come too fast and will not avoid, then stil Ivy berries and Parsley, and drink two spoonfuls of it, and it will avoid the stone if it be never so great.

A present Remedy to avoid the Stone.

Take a handful of Pellitory on the wall, a handful of Parsley, and a handful of Parsley seeds a little bruised, boil these things in a quart of White Wine until a third part be wasted, then strain it , and wring into it the juice of a Lemmon or two, then with this Wine and some milk make a Posset as clear as you can, and drink thereof a good draught twice or thrice a day, but not with meat, nor when the stomack is empty from meat.

> When the Stone is avoided and the pain ceased,
> to preserve you from the like again, make a Broth,
> and break fast three dayes every week thus.

Take a Chicken or a piece of Veal, three young Mallowes, Marsh Mallows are the best if you know them, one handful of Violet leaves, or of Mercury, or of Pellitory of the wall, one handful of Apothecary Barley scalded, half a handful of great Raisons stoned, boil these in water until the meat be enough, then take of this broth, without thickning or seasoning, with a little Sugar, three hours before dinner.

For the Stone, and to provoke Urine.

Take a quantity of Normandy glasse being clean without rust of canker, burn it in the fire a good space, then beat it in a Mortar, then take an old Cambrick cloth, and sift it very fine, and give the Patient a spoonful or two of the same powder to drink in Malmesey, being pained, and it will help by Gods grace. Probatum.

An approved Medicine for the Stone.

Take a gallon of new milk from the Cow that is all red, and thereinto put one handful of Pellitory of the wall, wild Time, Saxifrage and Parsley, of each a handful, two or three Rhadish roots sliced, steep all these in milk one night together, and in the morning distil them with a moderate fire, then take of that Water six spoonfuls, and six spoonfuls of Rhenish or White Wine, and a little Sugar, and some slices of Nutmegs, make it luke-warm, and drink it fasting, and fast after it three hours, using temperate exercises. Take this two or three dayes together every fortnight or oftener if need require. The best time to distil this Water is towards the end of May.

For the Stone.

Take two or three unset Leeks, and stamp them, and strain them, and drink it in Malmesey in the morning, strain as much as the Patient will drink at twice; after this, to bedward take some Sack and Sallet Oyle, and beat it, and drink it hot, that will make the Stone slide.

A present Remedy for the Stone in the back or Bladder.

Take Saxifrage, Philippendula, Peniroyal and Parsley seeds, and stamp them together, and strain them into a cleane Vessel, and let the Patient drink thereof with racked Rhenish Wine. Probatum.

A Medicine for the Stone.

Take Ivy berries, and stamp them wel, and put it in White Wine, and give the Patient to drink thereof, and let the Patient make Water through a cloth, and you shall see the avoiding of Stones and Gravel.

For the Stone.

Take Foxes bloud and Hares blood of both alike quantity, and dry them in an Oven, then beat it to powder, and seeth it in a little White Wine, and drink it as warm as you can suffer it.

To make a Glister for the Stone.

Take a good handful of Mallowes, as much of Camomile, and as much Pellitory of the wall, three or four crops of Herb-grace, a quantity of Beets, and a quantity Mercury, one ounce of Coriander seeds, one ounce of Cummin seeds, bruise the seeds and seeth them and the Herbs all together in a pottle of running water, and let it seeth till halfe be consumed, then strain it, and take three spoonfuls of Sallet Oyl, and three spoonfuls of Honey, and half a handful of Bay salt bruised, so put it into a Glister pipe and use it.

For the Stone.

Take the inner bark of Elder, and seeth it in Beer or Ale til it have a good strength of the Elder, then strain it, and drink it morning and evening, and it will break the Stone.

A very good drink for the Stone.

Take a pint of White Wine, and half a pint of Ale, and make thereof with milk a pottle of posset drink, and take away the curd very clean, and boil in it two or three roots of Mallowes, Marsh Mallowes are the best, and some Licoras till a quarter be boiled away, then drink half in the morning, and the rest at night.

For the Stone or strongurion.

Take half an ounce of Anniseeds, a quarter of an ounce of Licoras, Calamus Aromaticus, French Gallingal, Mirrh, Gum Arebeck, Gum Traganthum, Diatria Papira, or Piperion, Pine Apple kernels, white Orris roots, Storax, Benjamin, Cipresse and Labdanum, of each a small quantity, then beat them all together, take also half an ounce of large Mace, white Archangel, Mead Parsley and Garden Parsley, Camomile, Mallowes, Fennel and Spiere Mint, of each halfe a handful, then take three quarts of White Wine, and put them together in a brasse pot or a Posnet, and boil them a pretty while, then take it off, and strain it through a cloth, and put it in earthen vessels, and keep it cool it will drink the better, and take six spoonfuls morning and evening for three dayes together when you find your self ill, and do not foreslow the taking of it. Porbatum.

A Plaister to apply to the side for the Stone.

Take Mallowes, Herb grace, Pellitory of the wall, the green tops of Fennel and Camomile, of each two handfuls, seeth them in water till they be tender, then presse out the water from them, then stamp them very small, and put in Oyle of Lilies, Oyl of Camomile, Oyl of Dill, Oyl of sweet Almonds, and Oyle of Scorpions, of each one ounce, let them boil on a Chafingdish and coals a good while, then put to it as much wheat flower as wil make it thick like a Plaister, spread it between two cloths, and apply it to the Patients side as hot as may be endured.

For the Stone.

Take the weight of a French Crown of Pulvis Hollandi, drink it in a quantity of White Wine, stirring it well in the cup that it may not curd, drink it in the morning betimes, or at what time the Patient pleaseth keeping himself warme in his chamber all that day, for it will give him three or four stooles, and drink some warm broth after it, and use this once a Month.

More belonging to the former Medicine.

Take once a week after the former, eight spoonfuls of Deal Wine, and eight spoonfuls distilled from the berry of the Hawes, make it sweet with Sugar, and slice half a Lemmon into it, and some sliced Ginger.

For the Stone in the Kidneyes.

There is great pain in the raines of the back, which draweth downwards; stirring encreaseth the pain, they are much inclined to vomiting, the body is bound, Urine raw and watrish, often provoking to pisse, but not without pain, the Urine avoids with gravel, sand and slime, yea sometimes mixt with blood.

To know it from the Chollick, first its not so sharp as the paine of the Chollick.

Secondly, The Chollick doth appear beneath on the right side, and stretcheth from thence upwards toward the left side, but the pain of the Kidneyes begins above, and stretcheth downwards, and a little more towards the back.

Thirdly, the pain is most of the Kidneyes fasting, the Chollick otherwise.

All Saxifrage and other things good for the Stone, are good for the Kidneyes, but not for the Chollick.

Lastly, there is found in the Urine gravel or sand, and not in the Cholick or pain of the guts.

To restrain the growing of the Stone or Gravel.

Take Turbith one dram and an half, Hermodactilus one dram, Diagridy six graines, Salt of India two grains, Ginger half a scruple, Annis and Mastick, of each three grains, Sugar Pellets one ounce, white Sugar half an ounce, steep them together in three ounces of Water of Smallage or Maidenhair all night, and wring it out well, and drink it; if the matter be in the stomack, then take a Vomit that it run not towards the Rains. This Vomit may be made of reddish Orange seeds, the middlemost rind of Elder and Nux Vomica.

SIRRUP.

To make a Sirrup for one that is short winded.

Take a good handful of Hisop, a handful of Horehound, and seeth them in a quart of running water to a pint, then strain it through a fair cloth, and put in Sugar to make it pleasant. Use this morning and evening with a Licoras stick some three spoonfuls at a time.

To make Sirrup of Roses.

Your liquor must be ready to seeth, then put therein as many Roses as will be well steeped in the same water, and cover it close, and when the Roses be throughly white, then strain it, and set it on the fire again, and so you must use it thirteen times, and to every pint of your water or liquor you must put into it a pound of Sugar, and let it stand together for the space of one night steeping and skim it clean, and seeth it over a quick fire a quarter of an hour, then take whites of egges, and beat them well together, then take the pot off the fire, and put into it the whites of your egges, and then set it on the fire again, and let it seeth a good space, then let it run through a Jelly bag, till it will stand upon your nayl.

To make a comfortable Sirrup.

Take a handful of Egrimony, and seeth it in a pint of Water till half be consumed, then take out the Egrimony,and put in a good handfuls of Currans, & seeth them til they be ready to break, then strain them, and make a Sirrup of them, then set it on a chafingdish and coales,and put thereto a little white Saunders, and drink it either hot or cold.

Sirrup of Sugar candied.

Take Sugar candied, and put it into a clear bladder, and tye it, but so as it may have some vent, then put it into a bason of water, so that the water come not over the top of the bladder, and cover it with a pewter dish, and let it stand all night, and in the morning take of it with a Licoras stick.

Doctor Deodates Scorbuttical Sirrup.

Take the juice of Garden Scurvigrass, Brooklimes and Watercresses, of each six ounces, and after it hath stood till it be clear, take sixteene ounces of the clearest, and of the juice of Oranges and Lemmons, of each four ounces, make it to a clear Sirrup with so much fine Sugar as will serve the turne.

STRAINE.

For a Strain.

Take of Elland leaves, Sage, Fennel, Fetherfew and Mallowes, of each a handful, and seeth them in thick milk till the milk be almost consumed, and then lay it to the place very warm.

SUPPOSITORY.

To make Suppositories for such as be bound and costive.

Take English Honey, white Soap and some salt mixt together, and fryed, then make a roul or peg thereof, and put it in the Fundament, it will make the Patient go to stool within an hour and a half, for so long or until it work, he must keep it in his body.

Another.

Take a long piece of Coperas, being white, and smooth it, and annoint it with some butter, and so minister it to the Patient, and let him keep it in his body an hour and half, if it work not before, and he shall find great ease and help: These kind of Suppositories will serve twice or thrice at the least.

SINEWES.

A good Medicine for the Sinewes that be shortned or shrunk.

Take the head of a black Sheep, Camomile, Barly, leaves of Sage, of each one handful, and bray them together in a Mortar, and then boil them all together till they be well sodden, then let it stand to cool, and then draw it through a Strainer, and lay it on the place grieved, and by Gods grace it shall soone amend.

For shrinking of the Sinewes.

Take Hogs dung and half a pound of Oyle of Roses, seeth it in a new earthen pot, and apply it as hot as you can endure it.

The Composition of a Cerot to mollifie Sinewes and Joints that have been long displaced.

Take the leaves of Mallowes cleane picked from the stalks eight handfuls, of Gentian three handfuls, of Archangel one handful, then take of Oyl Olive a pint, of Oyl of Roses, Oyl of Camomile and Oyl of Dill, of each half a pint, boil all together, and in boiling of them, strow on one ounce of Anniseeds, and one ounce of graines beaten into fine powder, and when they be made well sodden, beat them in a Mortar with the yolks of eggs.

For a Sinew that is strained.

Take Groundsel, Brooklime, Fitch, Bruisewort, Nepe, Petty Morral and Hemlock of each alike, stamp them, and boil them in a pan over the fire, and lay it to the Sore as hot as the Patient may suffer it, and it will ease the aking and swelling, and heal it in a little space.

For Sinewes that be shrunken or grown together.

Take the water of shell Snailes and Shoomakers Oyl, of each alike, and temper them wel together, then take new Snailes and seeth them in running water, and gather off the Oyle and put it to the other Oyle; and temper them well together.

STOMACK.

For the pain in the Stomack.

Take Mackerel Mints two handfuls, and of sowr leaven one handful and an half, stamp them very small, and put to it a good quantity of Mace beaten to fine powder, and so much Wine Vinegar as shall incorporate all into a liquid paste, which you must spread upon a linnen cloth; apply it warm to the Stomack twice a day.

For heat in the Stomack.

Take a pint of stale Ale, and half a pint of Endive Water, and put thereto as much Sugar as will make it sweet, then set it on the fire, and skim it clean, then take a piece of white loaf as much as an apple, the crust taken away, and three or four whole Mace, then let it seeth one walm after, and then take and drink it luke warm (the bread taken away) whenever you feel the heat in your stomack.

To make one have a stomack to his meat.

Seeth Centory in fair water, and let the Patient drink it luke-warme fasting, three dayes, each day three spoonfuls, it purifieth the stomack and brest also.

A good Powder to digest well.

Take Centory and Pellitory of Spain, Anniseeds, Licoras, Grains of Paradise, Ginger and Cinnamon, of each alike, beaten and searsed into fine powder, and drink thereof morning and evening half a spoonful in Wine or Ale.

To make Hiporcras for a weak Stomack.

Take a pint of Aqua vitae and put it in a glass, then take two ounces of Cinnamon, and one ounce of Ginger, of Cloves and of Graines, of each two Penny worth, of Nutmegs one Penny worth, beat them all together, into grosse powder, and put them all into the glasse to the Aqua vitae, and shake it very often for nine dayes together, and then drink it with Wine or Ale, half a spoonful or a quarter with halfe a pint of Ale.

To cleanse the Stomack from rotten Flegm and Melancholy.

Drink the seeds of Hollioaks.
Also the cods and leaves of Cene in powder, one dram taken with broth of a Chicken or Mutton, doth purge phlegm and Melancholy.

For a cold and stopping in the Stomack.

Take one handful of sweet Marjerom, a few Marigold flowers, a penny worth of Caraway Comfits, a penny worth of Parsley seeds, two penny worth of Dates, a half penny worth of Raisons of the Sun, boil all these in a quart of White Wine till halfe be boiled away, then put in two ounces of brown Sugar candied, and a little Mithridate.

SHINGLES.

For the Shingles.

Take the green leaf of Colts foot stamped and mingled with Hony and apply it, and it will help.

SPOTS.

To cleanse the skin from all scars and spots.

Make balls of a little bignesse of the juice of the inner parts of a Pumpkin and bean flower, dry them in the shadow and wash therewith before the fire.

SWELLING.

For a Swelling.

Take two handfuls of Wheaten meal, and a pint of Cow milk, and a handful of Rue, and shred it small with a spoonful of fresh grease, and boil them all together till they be thick, then lay it on the swelling.

For Swelling in the Legs.

Take a handful of Archangel, a handful of red Fennel, and two handfuls of Mallowes, and a handful of Brooklimes, then seeth all these Herbs together in a gallon of running water to a pottle, then bathe the leggs with the water hot, and lay the Herbs on.

For all Swellings and Wrenchings, &c.

Take a pint of Milk, Oatmeal, dryed Rose leaves, Mellilot flowers, of each a handful, and a little Deers Suet, and seeth it till it be as thick as pap, then lay it to the hurt as hot as may be suffered:

For Swelling in the Legs.

Take Wormwood, Parsly, Camomile, Cumin and Ash rods, of every one a handful, and seeth them in the Patients Urine, and make a plaister, and apyly it.

For Swelling of Sinewes.

Take Smallage, Lovage, Groundsel, Brooklime, Sengreen and Bruisewort, stamp them, and put thereto a little wheaten bran, Sheeps Tallow, and some Barrowes grease, fry them well together and make a Plaister thereof, and lay it to the place grieved.

For Swellings or Bruises.

Take milk, wheaten meal, red Roses and Camomile, of each a handful, seeth all these together until they until they be thick, then spread it on a cloth, and lay it to till it heal the Patient.

For Swelling in the Joints.

Take Groundsel, Daisies, Booklime, Chickweed, Petty Moral, Herb Bennet, take of each of these alike, and fry them with Sheeps Suet, and put thereto crumbs of soure wheat bread, and so bind it to with a cloth warm.

For any Swelling that looketh red, or for the Ague fallen into any part of the body.

Take Houndstongue, Camomile, Daisie leaves and roots, Plantane leaves and roots, and Adderstongue, of each a handful, pick them clean, but wash them not, chop them small and stamp them, then take a pound of fresh butter, of Sheeps Suet half a pound, set them over the fire, and so let them boil until it look green, then strain it out, and keep it in an earthen vessel to use all the yeare.

For a Swelling.

Take three handfuls of Mallowes, and a pottle of running water, and boil the water and Mallowes together, then bath the swelling therewith a good while, then take a good quantity of Suet of the Kidney of a fat Sheep chopt, and so boile that together with the Herbs againe, and being hot, lay it on a red piece of cloth all night, and the next morning renew it, and so from time to time till it be asswaged.

Another.

Take two quarts of Barley, and two gallons of running water, a pound of Boars grease, four new laid eggs, a handful of Bay salt, of the tops of

Rue, Sage, Camomile, Rosemary, of each a handful, a quart of new Barm, chop all the Herbs together, then let it boil to two quarts, and when it boiled sufficiently, then stop it close until it be good case to lay to the place pained on a piece of new red cloth, and renew it as occasion shall require.

It is called by the name of the Jewes Bath, and it is an excellent thing for this purpose.

For a White Swelling.

Take Woodbind flowers, Water, and Wheat flower, and make thereof a thin paste, first annoint the Swelling with Oyl of Linseed, then lay on a plaister of paste.

FALLING SICKNES.

Divers and sundry Remedies for the Falling Sicknesse.

Take powder of Hawthorne, and drink it with Wine, it healeth the Falling Evil.

The braines of a Fox unto Infants, cureth this Disease.

Also Powder made of Opoponax, Castorum, Antimonium and Dragons is a most Soveraign Medicine.

The like vertue hath Antimonium alone with Castorum.

Or Antimonium alone received with water.

The ashes of a dead mans skull drunk is wonderful good.

Five leaved grasse drunk three and thirty times together, doth perfectly heal this Disease.

The red stone found in a Swallow healeth the falling Evil.

It hath been proved that Mistletow drunk healeth this Disease.

Piony tied about the Patients neck keepeth him from falling.

Also cut a Frog through the midst of the back with a knife, and take the liver, and fold it in a Colewort leaf, and burn it in a new earthen pot wel stopped, and give the ashes thereof unto the Patient in his sickness to drink with good Wine, and if he be not healed at once, do so by another Frog or more, and without all doubt it wil heal him.

A Rhadish stampt and bound to the braines will heal one of this Disease.

The bloud or gall of a Lamb drunk with Wine cureth it.

The stone that is found in a Harts head stamped and given to the sick party doth the like.

The braines of a Camel mixt with Oyl of Roses, wherewith annoint the Patient before and behind over all his body doth heal it, which is a wonderful experiment, and true.

The dung of a Peacock taken in drink doth the same also.

Take Mares piss new made, and heat it, and let the party grieved drink thereof as warm as he may, this will help by Gods grace with three or four time taking. Probatum.

A good Medicine for the Falling Sicknesse.

Take young Ravens when they be fledged before they touch any ground, flea the skin and feathers off clean, and pull out all the guts and entrels, and wipe it very clean, and then put it into an Oven, and dry it that you make powder thereof, then beat flesh and bones together very fine, and searse it, and take a quantity as you think good, and let the Patient drink it with Ale or Wine when the Fit begins, and by Gods grace it will help. Probatum.

STITCH.

For the Stitch in the side.

Take Camomile, Spieremint, Wormwood and Southernwood, of each a hand ful, then put a few cold ashes in the bottom of a pewter dish, and upon them hot embers, then clap the dish, Herbs and all over with a linnen cloth, and lay to the side somewhat higher then the paine is, and it will drive away the pain downwards.

For the Stitch of the Stomack or Heart.

Take young Broom of one yeares growth, distil it, and drink it, and it will help the Stitch; and if it be in such time of the year that you cannot get the water, then take Broome and make powder thereof, and drink it in Ale or Beer.

For all manner of Stitches in any part of the Body.

Take Mousear and Shee Holm, Stitchwort and Spierement, of each alike, and dry them upon a tile, and make powder of them, and drink it with Ale or Beer.

Another.

Take some wool, and baste it on a piece of linnen cloth, then take Oyle of Camomile, and warm it, and sprinkle it thereon, and lay to the pained place, being first annointed with the Oyl.

SWEAT.

To cool a Sweat withal.

Take a Chicken and boil it in fair running water, then take Burnet, Burrage, Marigold leaves, Parsley and Sorrel, of each a handful, then boil all these together with a little salt, then take the yolk of a new laid egge, and put to halfe a pint of the broth, and drink it hot.

To abate too much sweating.

Take Balm, Burrage and Rosemary, of each alike, and steep it four and twenty hours or more in Ale or Beer, and drink thereof evening and morning.

Also the water of the Decoction of Strawberries is good to be drunk for overmuch heat or sweating.

SLEEP.

To make one sleep.

Take a handful of Betony, a handful of Rosemary, and a handful of red Rose leaves, brown bread crumbs, two spoonfuls of womans milk, two spoonfuls of Rosewater, a spoonful of Vinegar, and boil all them together, and lay it to the temples of the Head.

Another.

Take an Onion and roast it soft, and take Camomile and shred it, and lay it upon the Onion, and so bind it upon the nape of the neck.

A good Medicine to make one sleep.

Take a pint of Milk and seeth it, and let it cool, then take Cream thereof and the white of an egge, and a little womans milk, and a little Rosewater, beat them all together, and spread them on a cloth, and so lay it to the forehead.

A Medicine of Doctor Cranmers to bring sleep.

Take twenty or thirty Almonds or more, and beat them with a spoonful of Poppy seed that is white, then take two handfuls of white Poppy leaves, and as much of Lettice leaves, and seeth them from a quart to a pint, and with that water strain the Almonds to make Almond milk to drink, and let them that cannot sleep, drink of it last to bedward.

For one that cannot sleep in sicknesse, but raves.

Take the juice of Houseleek, a good quantity, as much womans milk, and as much Rose vinegar or else Rose-water and vineger, and mix them well together, and then wet flax in it milk warm, and bind it to the temples of the Patient, and also wet flax therein, and make round together like a ball, and bind it in the palmes of the hands, and it wil give great ease.

Another to make one sleep.

Take the white of a new laid egg, and beat it with a spoon until it cometh to an Oyl, then let it stand a while, and take the froth of it from the Oyl, and put thereto Rose-water, Vineger, and womans milk, and lay it to the Patients forehead in a linnen cloth, and when it is dry lay on more. Probatum.

Another for one that cannot sleep.

Take the Oyl of Roses, and put thereto a little good Vineger, and heat them wel together, and put it on a Cloth, and bind it to the forehead, it is a comfortable Remedy.

TASTE.

Losse of Taste.

The signes of the Humour that causeth this Infirmity; viz. The Blood yeildeth a sweet taste: Phlegme also somewhat sweetish with much spettle, humidity of the head, of the tongue, and the whole body.

Choller causeth bitternesse, saltnesse, and a salt phlegme; if no taste, then is the mouth of the stomack troubled with many superfluous humours; If Melancholy, then is the taste tart. There may be also be sure signs taken from the tongue; if it be white, its not only a sign of cold, but also that the stomack, head and liver are full of phlegme; if red, then the malady is of blood and hot Rheumes; yellownesse is a sign that the choller is the cause of all; if a blackish lead colour, it signifies Melancholy, unless in hot Feavers, then must the Patient be dyeted according to the grief.

TEETH.

For Tooth ache.

Take running water, and put into it a Rosemary branch, a branch of Sage, and a branch of Rue, and let it lye three of four hours, and then wash your mouth with the water.

For a swelling in the cheek or Tooth ache, and good for the Stomack.

Take a handful of Bay salt, a quantity of Cloves, Mace and Nutmegs, and put it in a bag and warme it good and hot, and lay it to the place grieved.

A Powder to keep Teeth clean and without Ache.

Take dry Sage, Allom, Pepper and Bay Salt, of each a like weight, and make all these in powder, and preserve it in a box, and take a Sage leaf with the Powder, and rub your gums with it when you please.

A Medicine for the Tooth ache.

Take Fetherfew, and stamp it, and strain it, and drop a drop or two into the contrary ear to the pain, and then lye still a half hour after.

To make a Tooth fall out.

Take the roots of Marigolds, and put it in thy mouth on that Tooth that aketh.

For any Swelling that cometh by Tooth ache.

Take a quantity of Sage and Woodbind leaves, and seeth them very tender in White Wine and a little Honey, then wash the inside of your mouth with the water thereof, and lay the Herbs to the outside of the grief very warm.

For the Tooth ache.

Take every night a little salt, and let it melt in your mouth, and when it is melted, gargarise it well in your mouth, then spit out, then take five leaves of Rosemary, and chew it wel, and hold it to your teeth.

A hollow Tooth cured for ever.

Lint shaved and dipped in Oyl of Camphire, then roll it in Bole Armoniack and burnt Allom, being beat very small, and make it into balls like paste and stop the hollow tooth, and lay lint thereon, and let it remain in the Tooth four our five houres, then take it out, and wash the Tooth: cured for ever.

To keep Teeth from rotting.

Take white salt, and in the morning fasting hold it under your tongue till it do turn to water, and with that water wash your Teeth.

To make the Teeth white.

Take one drop of the Oyl of Vitriol, and wet the Teeth with it, and rub them afterwards with a course cloth, although this Medicine be strange, yet feare it not.

Of the Teeth.

Some men heave thirty two Teeth, some eight and twenty, and some have thirty.

The Physicians write, that the foremost Teeth are engendred of pure and superfluous moisture of the Scull, the middest of a reasonable good humor, and the hindmost of a grosse humidity.

All Imposthumes or Corruption of the Gums or Teeth, if there be much blood and moisture with it, then that part is to be purged with yellow Marabus and sowre Dates according to his ability, and wash the mouth with this water, viz. Take blossomes or pills of Pomgranats, Acorn cups and Roses, of each one ounce, and boil them in water, and wash the mouth with Vinegar and Allome.

For loose Teeth.

The cause is blowes, thrusts, defluctions that fall out of the head into the Teeth, which loosen their roots, or of great drowth after long sicknesse, the corruption of the mouth and teeth may be also cause the same.

The Remedy is, Take half an ounce of Allome, Rose buds half an ounce, Bedegar Red Wine one pint, boil them unto the one half, and take this into your mouth warm often, and hold it a good while therein, for it is very good.

Also to wash the mouth often with Rosemary and Wine is very good.

TYMPANY.

For the Tympany in a Woman.

Take a handful of blossoms of the Marygold that is yellow, stamp it and strain it, and give the juice thereof to the sick in a draught of Ale, and drink the same fasting.

An Oyntment for the same.

Take the herbs, stalks and leaves of the said Marigolds chopt small, and fry them in Goose grease, take the liquor that cometh of the frying of the herbs, and annoint the Patient all over the belly, and in a short time the Disease will vanish away.

A Plaister for the same.

Then take the Herbs so fryed, and lay on a Plaister of Black wool, and bind it over all the belly, which will help likewise.

The like for a Man.

Take the Marigold that hath black grounds, and use them for a man, as the other in all respects.

TETTER.

A good Medicine to kill a Tetter.

Take Lemmons and distil them rinds and all, and with the water thereof wash the Tetter, and sometimes annoint it with the juice of Ribwort.

TONGUE.

For a sore Tongue.

Seeth five leaved grass in Vinegar, and gargarise therewith to help a sore mouth, tongue or throat.

Of the Tongue.

The swelling of the Tongue is of blood or phlegme that falleth out of the head:

If it be of cold phlegme, the tongue and the face is alwayes white, and the mouth full of moisture, then rub the tongue with Sirrup or Wine of Pomgranats, and Dates boiled in sweet Wine, of each alike, and purge the Head, and use Barley water boiled with Pruines, Barberries, Cinamon, use this as a cooler. Also preserved Raspices, or anything made of them is to be used.

THIRST.

To abate excessive thirst.

Take a pottle of fair water, Endive, Succory, Violet leaves and Borage, of each a handful, Lillies half a handful, two Fennel roots, two Parsley roots, and seeth them from a pottle to a quart, and put a little Sugar to it, and drink it as you shall see cause.

Also seeth the leaves of Rosemary in well water, and drink it cold with a little of a Pomgranat.

Also hold Purslain under the tongue.

VEYNES.

To knit Veines.

Take Frankinsence one pound, Mastick one ounce, Bole Armoniak two ounces, beat all into fine powder, and mingle it with the white of an egge, then spread it on a linnen cloth, and apply it.

To mollifie Veines that be dry and stiff.

Take Oyl of Camomile, and Oyle of Linseed, and mingle it with Capons grease finely tried, mix them together, and this wil open the Veynes.

For straining of a Vein.

Take half an ounce of Coral and beat it fine, and drink it in red Wine morning and evening.

For a broken Vaine in the Stomack to knit it, or for any inward bleeding and casting of bloud, &c.

Take the leaves of Plantane, Shepherds Pouch, of each one handful, of Hartshorn half a handful, of Nettles and Mints, of each of them as much as you can hold betwixt two fingers of Barley, (the outer skin taken off,) three spoonfuls, of Yarrow half a handful, and one quarter of an ounce of Cinamon, boil all these in two quarts of fair water till half be consumed, then strain it, and put to the liquor strained as much Sugar as wil make it sweet: let it boil a little againe, then put thereto as much White Wine Vineger as wil make it sharp, and let the Patient take three or four spoonfuls ever in time of thirst; boil an equal quantity with a black Hen drawne and washed, but not pulled, and then put an equal quantity of the broth and the juice of Mutton half roasted, and boil them between two dishes, until there remain no taste of rawness. And if the Patient cast any more, presently take two spoonfuls of the juice of Mints, one spoonful of White Wine Vineger, and as much soure leaven as two Walnuts, boil them to the consumption of the juices; and make thereof a flat cake, and strow upon it fine powder of Nutmegs, and apply it hot to the brest, and give the Patient two spoonfuls of the Cordial following about three of the Clock, and between nine and ten at night, and at eight in the morning, and fast one hour and an half before, and two houres after at the least. And give a Suppository made with two Positives of Honey, and one of salt, every day, if the Patient cannot go to stool.

Diacatholicon half an ounce, Confectionum de Hameck halfe an ounce, comixt in a penny pot of White Wine.

Lotian water good for a heat.

A little Cinamon and Ginger and Venice Turpentine made into Pils, and take three every morning.

Ising-glasse and Saffron boiled in a red Cowes milk, and drunk three times for the same.

Church yard wormes washed and sliced, dried and drunk in Beer five several times or mornings, is good for a sore throat, as the Kings Evil, & c.

VOMIT.

A Vomit for the green sicknesse.

Take one handful of Goundsel, and one ounce of Currans, boil them in a quart of Ale, until it come to the quantity of a draught, the strain it, and drink it blood-warm, and fast two hours after it, and when the Patient hath once vomited, drink Posset Ale between every Vomit until it cease.

To stay Vomiting.

Take Mint Water and Carduus Benedictus, of each a pint, bruise two Nutmegs, and let them boil to a pint, and make it sweet with Sugar, and drink it first and last.

Another.

Take Cloves, and boil them in faire water or beer, and put Sugar thereto, and drink it.

A Vomit.

Take an ounce of Green Ginger, as much of Treakle, and as much of Malmsey, put these together, and drink them bloud warm.

UFULA.

For falling of the Ufula.

Roast an egge hard, then cut it long wayes, and take out the yolk, and fill the place full of Cummin seed fine beaten, and lay it to the nape of the neck as hot as may be endured, then take a good quantity of Sage, and boil it in milk, and so drink it warm as can be suffered keeping the head warm.

For a child that is Jaw fallen and Roof fallen. See before in Children,

A Water for a sore Mouth, or the falling of the Ufula.

Take Bramble tops, Ivy berries, green Rose leaves, and some Allome, seeth all these in drink, and make thereof a Lotian, and gagarise therewith.

For the falling of the Palate of the Mouth.

Take of Cummin in powder two great handfuls, of white salt four, of the powder of Camomile flowers three, and the powder of three Nutmegs, mingle these together, and put them into a bag of linnen cloth cut round, and then quilt it, and use to lay it on the mould of your head all the day and night, if need so require.

URINE.

To make a mans or womans Water run strong from them.

Take of Gromel seed half an ounce, of Cene cleane picked from the stalks, a quarter of an ounce, of Ginger scraped and sliced thin, of Cinnamon scraped and bruised of each of them one dram, of Damask Pruines the stones taken out seven, of White Wine a pint, put all in the Wine, and cover it close, and stop it with paste, and set that in another pot of hot liquor for the space of one hour or more, that the pot may be hot, then take it forth, and when it is cold strain it, and after put in Sugar to make it toothsome, and then drink it.

For one that cannot hold his Water.

Drink Nepe a little before Supper, and also for pissing a bed in a cold cause, drink three drams of the powder of Frankinsence in Ale.

An excellent approved Medicine for the hard and slow passage of in man or woman.

Take two quarts of good Wort, and boil it in a skillet by it self without any Hops, till it come to a pint and a half, then when it is cold take it and put Barm to it till it be ripe drink, and ready to cleanse, then take drink, barme and all, and boil it againe, and boil in it the quantity of two Nutmegs of Civil Soap, then skim it very clean, and drink thereof at night when you go to bed, and in the morning when you rise; when it is done make more.

To cleanse the Ureters or Conduits of Urine, and to open them. See before in Stone.

WATER.

A Water to cure all manner of Wounds and Sores be they never
so stinking; and all manner of Cankers in the nose,
mouth, throat or elsewhere.

Take a handful of red Sage, a handful of Cellendine, and as much
Woodbind leaves, take a gallon of running water, and put the Herbs into it,
and let it boil to a pottle, then strain it, and take the liquor and set it over
the fire again, then put thereto a pint of English Honey, and a good
handful of Roach Allome finely beaten, a penny worth of graines grosly
bruised, and let them boil all together three or four walmes, and then skim
it off with a feather, and when it is cold, put it in an earthen pot or bottle,
so as it may be kept close: and for a green wound take of the thinnest of
the water, and for an old wound the thickest, the Water first being well
shaken together, and after you have well cleansed the old sore with White-
Wine, then take fine lint and wet it in the water, and oft times bathe the
wound, and with the lint cover the wound, and if there be any holes in the
wound, fill them with lint made like a Tent, and so cover the wound with a
piece of bladder, the more better to continue your lint with moisture, and
dresse your wound twice a day.

To make Barley Water.

Take a penny worth of Barley, a penny worth of Raisons of the Sun, a
penny worth of Anniseeds, a half penny worth of Licoras, two quarts or
more of water, boil all together till halfe be consumed, then strain it, and
when it is cold, drink it, your Licoras must be sliced into small pieces.

To make Doctor Stephens Water.

Take a gallon of good Gascoigne Wine, then take Ginger, Gallingal,
Cinnamon, Nutmegs, Graines, Cloves, Mace, Anniseeds, Fennel seeds,
Carraway seeds, of each a dram, then take red Mints, red Rose leaves,
Garden Time, Pellitory of the wall, Smal Marjerom, Rosemary, Peniroyal,
Sage, Wild Time, Camomile, Lavender, Avens, of each one handful, then
bruise them all in a Mortar, and beat your Spices small, then put your
Spices and Herbs into your Wine, and let it stand twelve hours, stirring it
oftentimes, and then still it in a Limbeck. The first pint is the best, the
second is good.

The Vertue of this Water.

It comforteth the spirits, and preserveth greatly the youth of man, it helpeth the inward Diseases coming of cold, it helpeth the shaking of the Palsie, it cureth the distraction of the Sinewes, and helpeth the Tooth ache; it comforteth the stomack very much, it cureth the Raines of the back, the Canker and cold Dropsie; it helpeth forth the Stone in the bladder, also it helpeth a stinking breath, and the Conception of a woman that is barren; a spoonful of this Water to some is sufficient, to others two or three once in ten dayes sufficeth.

A Water for a green Wound.

Take a gallon of fair running water, a pottle of White Wine, of Wormwood, Motherwort, Bramble buds, Hawthorn buds, Basil, Mints, Avens, Egrimony, Bovewort, Wood Bugloss, Woodbind, Plantane, Ribwort, Daisie roots, Betony, Wild Angelica, Sanicle, White Bottles, Scabious and Dandillion, of each one handful, and put them into the Wine and water, and let them boil together till the half be consumed, then strain out all the Herbs, and boil the liquor with a quart of English Honey very softly till it be clean skimmed, then take it from the fire, and when it is cold put it into a glass, and keep it for to wash any green wound, which it will cure, although never so dangerous, drinking also at a time three spoonfuls of it.

A Water to heal a Wound.

Take Woodbind leaves and Sage, of each a handful, boil them well together in a little water, and put in a piece of Allome and a little Honey, and wash the wound therewith, laying a little lint to it, and it wil heal it.

An excellent Water to wash any Sore withal,
and will be a means to gather skin.
Doctor Wheads Water.

Take brown Sage, brown Fennel, Rosemary, Violet leaves, Liverwort, Hartstongue, Bryar leaves, Plantane leaves, Woodbind leaves, five leaved grasse, Egrimony, Wild Tansie, of each one handful; take all these Herbs, and boile them in an earthen pot with a pint of White Wine, and three pints of running water till it comes to a quart, then take the Herbs and strain them in a bason, then take as much Allome as three Walnuts, and put it in the water, and let it boil up, then take it, and put it in a bason till it be almost cold, then put in a quarter of a pint of live Honey, and presently put it in bottles, and stop it very close.

To make a cordial Water.

Take of the tender leaves of green Angelica four handfuls, of the like leaves of Carduus Benedictus two handfuls, of the like leaves of Balm and Sage,of each one handful and an halfe; let all be shred small, Licoras bruised five ounces, the seeds of Angelica two ounces, the seeds of sweet Fennel three ounces, let both be bruised well, the Spices of Aromaticum Rosarum, & Diamoschum Dulce, of each half an ounce, infuse them all in six quarts of good Sack four and twenty hours, then distil them in a Limbeck with a soft fire according to Art, and draw forth of the best water a pottle: whereunto after two dayes put half a pound of the finest Sugar, dissolved in half a pint of good red Rose water in a fair pipkin on the fire, when the Rosewater is hot with the Sugar, then put in your hot water, and let it stand over the fire till it be throughly hot, then take it off, and put it in glasses, and keep it as excellent to comfort the spirits, and against infection, you may draw forth of good smaller water a quart.

A very precious Water made of Cinnamon.

Take one pound of good Cinnamon, and bruise it a little, and lay it a soaking four and twenty hours in four pints or four pound of Rosewater, a pint and half of Muskadine or white Wine, then put it into a Limbeck glass to distil upon hot ashes, or else in a pot of hot water.

This Water is good against the pain of the Spleen, the pain in the head, the Mother, to provoke Urine, to stay vomiting, to expel all venemous colds. You may take four pints of White Wine, putting to it half a pound of Cinnamon, and use it as aforesaid.

WEN.

A Medicine to put away a Wen or Curnel.

Take black Soap, mixed with unflaked Lime made into powder, lay it to the Wen of Curnel, and by Gods grace it will help.

A Medicine for an unbroken Wen.

Take the crumbs of Barley bread, the bignesse of an egge, and as much White Wine Vinegar as will make it into a soft paste, and spread it upon a cloth, then take an old wooden ladle, and set it against the fire and it will sweat, then take a feather and wipe the sweat off the ladle, and annoint the Wen therewith, then take a plaister of the paste and lay it on the Wen, and dresse it three times a day after the Sun is risen, and before the going down the same, every time fresh paste, and divers times the ladles sweat. Probatum.

For the drawing and healing of a Wen when it is broken,

Take a handful of Marigolds blowne, of them that have black in the midst, and half a handful of Rosemary leaves stripped downward, and half a handful of Pellamountain, half a handful of Hysop, half a handful of Valerian, all stripped downward as before, and all these Herbs must be boiled in six ounces of unwasht Butter over a soft fire till the one half be consumed, then strain the Oyntment through a clean cloth, then put the Oyntment over the fire, and put in an ounce of Bee Wax, and boil it again dozen turnes, then put it into a fair pot, and keep it for your use.

WOMAN.

To make a Woman to be soon delivered,
the child being dead or alive.

Take a good quantity of the best Amber, and beat it exceedingly small to powder, then searse it through a fine piece of Lawne, and so drink it in some broth or caudle, and it will by Gods grace presently help the Patient to be delivered.

To make a Womans Disease to come to its right course.

Take young Southernwood, Betony, Caunapitum, Centory, the roots of Cellendine, St Johns wort, with the flowers, of each of these as big as your thumb, yet put but in one root of Cellendine, of White Wine a pint and an half, of Raisons of the Sun (the stones taken out) half a handful cut in pieces, these boil until a third part be wasted, then strain it, and put to it three and forty blades of Saffron made to powder, of Graines the weight of two pence beaten, then boil it a little again; and of this drink a draught in the morning fasting, with as much Treakle as a Hasel Nut, and at night a draught without Treakle.

For the green Sickness.

Take fasting every morning of one Cowes milk, one pint hot from the Cow with a few Mints bruised in it, and let the party stirre about after it.

An approved Medicine for the green Sickness or the yellow Jaundies.

Take seven or nine Lice out of a cleane bodies head, and put them into bread and Butter, or Conserves of Roses, or into Ale or Beer, or any other thing you shall think fit, so that the party grieved may eat them all alive, and know not of it for loathing the Medicine.

A Medicine for the Green Sickensse, and also to scowre the body.

Take three sticks of a fig tree, and three sticks of a Walnut tree, and a handful red Sage, and a good handful of Peniroyal, a pound of Raisons of the Sun, stones and all, three Cap Dates, stones and all, bruise them all together, and put them all in a pottle of White Wine, and seeth it from a pottle to a quart, then strain it, and put into the drink one ounce of the best Sugar candied, and drink thereof morning and evening: it is good. Probatum.

A Medicine for a woman that is in travel.

Take seven or nine leaves of Dittony, a pretty quantity of Germander, a branch or two of Peniroyal, three Marigolds, a branch or two of Hisop; take all these and boil them together in a pint of White Wine, or a pint of Ale, and after it is boiled, put into it Sugar and Saffron, and boil a quarter of an hour or more, and give it the Patient to drink warm.

For the after Burthen.

Take one little branch of Motherwort and six blades of Saffron, pound them together, and then put to it six spoonfuls of Ale, and then drink it blood warme all at one draught, and fast after it half an hour.

A good Medicine to provoke the Termes in a Woman.

Take Wormwood and Rue, of each one handful, five or six Pepper Cornes, seeth them all together in a quart of White Wine of Malmsey, strain it, and drink thereof.

Mallows sod in Wine, and drunk is very good.

Also take Sage half an handful, of Cloves, Mace and Saffron, of each half a scruple, stamp them all together, and bind it in a fine cloth, and hang it a night and a day in a pint of good Wine, wringing it oftentimes out into the Wine, then divide it into three parts, and take one part five hours before meat, the second part in the afternoon, and the other part after supper; but this is to be done in the wane of the Moon, and eat very little.

A Medicine for the Green Sickness.

Take the weight of a French Crowne of Rubarb, of French Wormwood and Egrimony, of each half a handful, steep them over night in a quart of Ale, and slice a Nutmeg and put therein, and so take it three several mornings at three draughts; and this being done, you must make more, and use it in that sort six mornings more. See before amongst the Vomits for a Vomit for the Greene Sicknesse, which is to be taken before this Medicine.

To procure the red Menstrues.

Take of Clary leaves and of Hisop, of each one handful, of Parsley half a handful, stamp them and straine them, and put part of the juice thereof into an empty eggshel, and put thereto the yolk of an egg only with a little Sugar candied in powder, then stir it, and set it on embers, and when it is through hot, sup it up, and fast after it two hours, and this do three mornings together in the beginning of the Moon, within five dayes of the Change.

To stop the White Menstrues.

Take a pottle of running water, of pure Cinnamon half an ounce, halfe a Pomgranat Pill, of Knotgrasse halfe an handful, boil these together till the water come to a pint, and thereof make a caudle for three mornings.

Also take Sassaparilla six ounces, Pollipodium of the Oak, Cene and Fennel, of each four ounces, of Caraway seeds one ounce, of Licoras scraped and bruised two ounces, Egrimony and Maidenhair of each two handfuls, Liverwort one handful, Scurvigrasse two handfuls, new Beer or Ale three gallons; these particulars must be stamped to powder, and all put into a bag together with the Scurvigrasse stamped, then hang the bag in the vessel of Ale or Beer, the yeest being first taken away, and so stopped very close that no aire get in, then drink thereof the quantity of a pint two hours before dinner, and so at Supper. It purgeth all humours in the body; it will not suffer the bloud to putrifie, nor phlegme to have Dominion, nor Melancholy to have exaltation; it purgeth the wind, it defendeth the stomack, it nourisheth, profiteth and preserveth the Heart, it ingendreth a good colour, it comforteth the sight, it nourisheth the mind, and is good against the Stone.

To stop the red Menstrues.

Take a good handful of Lavender tops and boile them in a quart of Posset drink, till it come to a pint, and drink it off hot with some Sugar, if you please.

For the Green Sicknesse.

Take half an ounce of the powder of steel, as you have at the Steel-makers, but the Needle makers have the best; wash it in three or four waters, and dry it, one ounce of Cremer Tartary, two Nutmegs, Licoras the weight of six pence, make all into fine powder, and mix them; take every morning the weight of six pence in broth, and fast two hours after, and after this Receipt hath been taken, let the party be purged once or twice.

WOUNDS.

For great Wounds in the head.

Take dry Wormwood or green (green is the best) and a new laid egge, shell and all, and beat them together very fine, and make a Salve thereof, and lay it to the place hurt very thick, and let it lye four and twenty houres; and if the party be much pained, change it, if but a little pained, let it lye four and twenty hours more, and then dresse it with other Salve as need requireth.

A Medicine for any Cut, Wound or Sore.

Take of Rosen and Perrosen of each half a pound, of Olibanum four ounces, of Harts Suet four ounces, of Mastick two ounces, of Mirrh one ounce, of Comfry half an ounce, of White Wax four onnces, let your Rosen, Perrosen, Olibanum, Mastick and Mirrhe be made into fine powder and searsed each by themselves, then take your Suet, and Wax, and dissolve them upon a soft fire, when they be melted, put in all your searsed powders, always stirring them till they be all melted, then have ready a pottle of White Wine hot in a faire pan, and straine all your stuff through a Canvas cloth into it, then put in two ounces of good Turpentine, and then

your comfry beaten to fine powder, alwayes stirring it till it be cold, and
then make it up in rolls, and keep it for your use. This Oyntment is very
good for new Wounds and for the Bloody Flux, and the Wind Cholick,
being spread upon a cloth, and laid to the Navel. It is called, Flos
Unguentorum, The flower of Oyntments, of which see more at large in
Oyntments.

WIND.

To make one long winded.

Take half a pound of Almonds, and lay them in cold water till they
blanch of themselves, then beat them very smal in a Motar, Licoras three
ounces, scrape off the bark or rind, and beat it fine in a Mortar, and take as
muck Anniseeds, two ounces of Sugar, and beat them small as before, and
work them together and use it.

For the avoiding of Wind.

Take the juice of red Fennel, and make a posset of Ale therewith, and
drink thereof.

Another to expel Wind.

Take of pure Sugar four ounces, of Rose water as much as will
moisten your Sugar, put it in a possnet, then have ready these Spices
following, White Pepper, Black Pepper, of each half a dram, pure
Gallingale sliced and finely minced, Ginger pared and minced fine, of
each of these one scruple and a half, pure Turbit white and gummy clean
scraped, thin sliced and minced very fine two scruples, skim your
Rosewater and Sugar clean as may be, and let them boil on a soft fire,
then put in all your Spices, and stir them wel, then take it from the fire,
and stir it till it be cold and thick, then put it into a gally pot, and reserve
it to your use: of this you may take at a time the quantity of a
pennyworth or two pence.

For the Wind of the Stomack.

Take a handful of Tansie, and a handful of Sorrel, and beat them
together, and strain them, and make a posset of White Wine, and put in
it the juice of the Herbs, and drink it in the morning, and fast after it a
while.

VVORMES.

For a Ring-worm.

Take a Dog berry, and with the juice thereof rub the Ring-worm, and it will help it.

For the running Worm that eateth the flesh.

Take a handful of Wormwood, and a handful of Herb grace, a handful of Fetherfew, a handful of Vervain, a handful of Herb Robert, a handful of Wild Bugloss, boil these Herbs in half a pound of unwashed butter, then strain it through a clean cloth and annoint the place with a feather, and lay upon the wound Oak leaves with the smoothest side next the wound, the leaves must be withered, and so bind up your sores with linnen clothes, dressing it twice a day after the same manner, but remember your herbs be stamped before you boil them in your butter.

To kill the Canker and Worm that eateth the Teeth.

Take an egg that is layed on a thursday, and empty it, and fil it with salt, and so set it on the fire, until it may be made in powder, and rub the Cankered teeth therewith, and it both kills the Canker, and destroys the worms that eat the Teeth. Probatum.

For Wormes in a Child, to rid them away, if they be almost past Remedy.

Take of Wormwood and of Walnut leaves, of Rue and unset Leeks, of each one handful, and put to an Ox gall, and fry them all over the fire, and lay them on a cloth, and lay them on the childs navel all night; and that wil help them: and on the morrow, take half a pint of Malmsey, and put into it four or five spoonfuls of Wormwood water, and as much Mint water, and warm then together, and drink it one or two dayes, and this will help without doubt. Probatum.

For the Ring-worm.

Take a handful of Violet leaves, an handful of Columbine leaves, and a handful of Rosemary leaves, stamp all these together, and boil it in a quarter of a pound of unwasht butter, and a little Deer Suet, and when it is half boiled away, strain it, and put it over the fire again, and let it boil two or three turnes, then put it up for your use, and strike a Plaister therewith, and lay it on the Ring-worm, dressing it twice a day, and washing it every two dayes with White Wine.

For the Wormes.

Take Curraline in powder as much as will lye on a groat in new Milk three mornings, three dayes before the Full or New of the Moon. It will help old folks and sucking children; it is a groat an ounce.

For the Ring-worm.

Take black Soap, and almost as much Ginger in powder, and mix them well together, and annoint the place therewith four or five dayes together, and this will cure any Tetter or Ring-worm.

WHITES.

For the Whites.

Take a quarter of a pound of Ising-glasse, and boile it in a pottle of milk to a pint and half, then put to it Nutmeg, Cinnamon and Sugar and red Rose water, and so make it to a Gelly.

WOOD BETONY.

The Vertues of Wood Betony.

It saveth mens bodies by the vertue it hath in it, and by Gods help, for who so beareth this Herb about him, preserveth him from Evil Spirits, and this Herb must be gathered in the Harvest time, early in the morning before Sun rising.

Also he that drinketh of the juice of Betony, it will break the stone, and cast it with the Urine.

Also if it be drunk with hony, it is good against the Dropsie.

Also it is good against the outrage of wicked blood.

Also the juice of Betony mingled with Rose-water put in the ear, amendeth the hearing.

Also the powder of Betony sodden with hony, helpeth them that have the bloody Egestions, and marvellously comforteth the stomack.

Also the leave of Betony mingled with salt, and make a Plaister thereof, is a great help to green Wounds being laid thereto.

And the leaves of Betony with Rue evenly proportioned, sodden together is good for akings in the eys, and the blood of the Egestions, it putteth away that which annoyeth the Eyes.

Also it draweth away all venom in the body of man.

Also take four handfuls of Betony, and three cupfuls of Red Wine, and seventeen Pepper cornes, and break them smal, and seeth it, and drink it, it purgeth the veins.

Also take an ounce of Betony, and an ounce of Plantane, and drink it with warm water, and it will destroy the Quotidian Feaver.

Also take powder of the root of Betony, and drink it with luke-warm water, it will purge the phlegme.

Also take the weight of a Bean of the powder of Betony mingled with honey, it will comfort the stomack, and the digestion.

Also make a Garland of Betony, and lay it about an Adder, and he will kill himself within it.

Also take Betony well warmed by the fire, and then bound to the forehead, it provoketh sleep, and putteth away wicked blood, and destroyeth the heat of the eyes.

Also Betony sodden in Wine, and held in the mouth, helpeth the Tooth ache.

Also Betony sodden in Wine, purgeth the veines, the spleen, and the stomack.

And the juice of Betony mingled with salt, and put into the nostrils purgeth the Evil savor of the nose.

THE KNOWLEDGE AND ORDERING OF WINES.

A true Receipt to fine any piece of Wine
Spanish or French.

Take Isinglass half a pound, and steep it in as much of the hardest French White Wine, let the Wine cover it, and let it stand four and twenty hours then pull the Isinglasse in pieces, then put a little of the same Wine to it, then let it lye, three or foure times a day squeeze and break it with your hands till it come to a cleer Jelly, and as it thickens, put more of the same Wine to it, then when it is come to a perfect cleer Jelly, take a pint or a quart to a Hogshead, and so according to that quantity as you have occasion, over draw the same piece of Wine that you beat up, three or four gallons, then put in the same quantity of Isinglass into the Can of Wine you overdraw, then stir the Isinglass, and break it very well together into the Wine, then put it up into the same piece of Wine, and beat it with a staffe exceeding well together, then fill it up top full, and so let it lye. And for the French Wine Bung it up very tite and full. Spanish Wine you may bung up or open as you please.

To fine any piece of Browne Wine that is quailish and brown, be it Spanish or French.

Take a pint of the same Jelly of Ising-glass, and a quantity of milk, as you shall find the piece of Wine in brownesse, and so put the Ising-glasse and the milk together, and stir it very well, then overdraw the piece of Wine eight gallons, then with a parting staff, stir it two or three blowes, then suddenly put in both milk and Ising-glass into the Butt or Hogshead, then beat it up extraordinary well, fill it up very full, and this will fine in a day or two.

For French wine that comes over upon the Lees, that is brown and faint.

Take one pound of Alablaster dust sifted, and overdraw the Hogshead three or four gallons, then put this dry dust into the bung of it as it is upon the Lee, then take a staff, and give six good strokes, then fill it up top full, the more you stir it, the better it will be upon the Lee, and nothing will be seen, but grow perfect good, the longer it lyes the better it is, and when you see good you may Rack it.

How to make any piece of quailish Spanish Wine fine.

Take halfe a quarter of a pound of White Stirch, and about a quart of small writing sand, and a pint of Ising-glasse, and one handful of Bay salt, and the whites of two eggs, and beat them with a little Brush very well, then overdraw the Wine, and put it in all together, and so beat it up all together extraordinary well and fill it up, and this will make it perfect fine.

To make Wine sweet that stinketh or is unsavory or Musty.

If the fault be in the Cask, you must draw it out into a fresh Cask and Lees, and let none of the old Lees come out of it, therefore draw it not too neer: then thus use him, Take twelve eggs, both whites and yolks, and beat them short, then take of Ginger, Cloves, Oras, Graines, of each two pennyworth, and one pennyworth of long Pepper, put the eggs into a quart of Damask Rose water well mingled together, and put it into the Wine, then beat the Butt half an hour; let all the Spices be grosly beaten, then take two grains of Musk, and bruise it well in four spoonfuls of Damask Rose water with the back of a spoon and put that into the Butt, then beat the Butt again gently a quarter of an hour, then take Ambergreece, Manus Christi, of each two graines, and beat them well, and put them among the Spices, and put all into a bag, and tye it fast to the Bung, and let it hang almost to the bottom two dayes; then draw it up softly to the middle, and there let it hang two dayes; then draw it almost to the top, and let it hang one day; then take it out, and roll the Butt a little, and in two dayes broach it, and it will be very sweet.

If Claret or Red Wine be faint.

First draw him out into fresh Lees, and put into him four or five gallons of the best Allengant, then turne him over twice in the Lees, and let him lye with the Bung upright a week before you broach him, and it shall have both a good colour and taste.

For Wine of any sort that groweth long.

Take two pennyworth of Roach Allom in powder, and draw your Hogshead four or five gallons, then strew in our powders, and shake it well half an hour, then fill it up, and broach it with in three dayes, being well and close and stopped.

If White Wine and Sack hath lost its colour.

Take four gallons of skimmed milk, over draw the Hogshead six gallons, then take the yolks of four eggs, beat them, and put them into the milk, and after beat them together, then put them into the wine, and beat the Wine well, then stop it close, and in five dayes you may broach it.

To keep Wine fresh and sound all the year.

You must fill your Vessels once a month or six weeks, fill your Red and Claret with the best Red Wine, for Red doth preserve the Clarret, as White doth the Malmsey and Bastard, and fil White with White. And so all other Wines with the same; and those you intend to preserve, give them their Lees all in one day, then at night, lay them all upright,and be careful to keep them right. If they lack vent in any place, they will be faint and spoil. July and August are the most dangerous to keep the said Wines sweet.

For Sack that hath Flying Lees in it.

Draw it out into a fresh Butt with fresh Lees, and make a good Parel with the whites of eight egges, and beat them with a handful of Bay salt, and put it into the Sack, and if it be any whit tawny, put thereto two gallons of new milk, and beat the Wine wel, then lay it upright, stop it close, and in two dayes broach it.

A Note of all kind of Wines that prick,
with their perfect remedies.

Imprimis. For every Pipe take half a pound of Whiting to flavour your Wine, Long Pepper one ounce, Cinnamon half an ounce, the eighth part of an ounce of Orras, as much Cloves, a little Anniseeds the which must be beaten to powder, and put them into a bag, and hang it in the Wine with a piece of Lead to sink it, two dayes, and then take it out, and see, if it do not change let it hang one day longer, then put four of five gallons of Bastard Sirrup, which must be well beaten into it.

How to make Sack white, being otherwise coloured.

Take two pounds of white starch, and two gallons of milk boiled together the space of two hours, then take it from the fire, & let it be cold, and staff it, and put it into a Butt that is clean and sweet, then beat the Starch and milk together with two handfuls of white Salt, and put into the butt, and beat it with a staff, and it will fine and white.

To help Claret that is tawny.

Rack it, and take halfe a pound of Turnsil, two gallons of Red Wine, one of Allegant, two ounces of Red-wood small ground, mingle them together, and put them into the Hogshead, and stop it close, and in three dayes it shall have a most perfect colour.

For Sack that beginneth to be long.

Take three pennyworth of Roach Allome, burn it, then beat it small, then take a pint of Burrage water, and wring into it the juice of four Lemmons, then beat the Allom and liquor together, till it be short, and put it into the Sack and beat the Butt well, and stop it close and in three dayes it shall be perfect.

For Malaga that pricketh.

Overdraw the Pipe two Gallons, then put in the Pipe half a peck of Limestones, and chalk, and three pennyworth of Roach Allome, burn it, and strew it in the Pipe with a handful of white Salt, and beat that gently, and this only shall help it.

To give your Muskadine, Malmsey, Sack or Bastard
a pleasant sweet taste, and sent,
although it be very faulty.

Take a quarter of a pound of Coriander seed, Cloves, Nutmegs, of each half an ounce, two pennyworth of Orras, one pennyworth of Callamus, Musk, Manus Christi, of each one grain, beat them all well, and put them into a bag, then put a pint of Rosewater into a dish, upon a Chafingdish of coals, and when it is hot, let the outside of the bag drink it up, then first put in to the Butt or Pipe, one gallon of Spanish Cute, and roll it well, then hang the bag into the Pipe, neer to the bottom one day and night, then draw it up towards the middle, and let it hang there two dayes, then draw it within a foot of the top for two dayes more, then take it out, and stop it close, then roll it gently, and in two dayes broach it.

To make a good Hyppocras.

Some make it of Sack; some of White Wine, some of Rhenish Wine: Take to every gallon of White or Rhenish Wine two pound of Sugar, the worst is good enough, three ounces of Cinnamon, two ounces of Ginger, one ounce of Long Pepper, three ounces of Licoras, half a graine of Musk, half a pint of Damask Rose-water, two pennyworth of Orras, one pennyworth of Callamus Arromaticus, and three ounces of Anniseeds.

The use and preparation of Hyppocras.

You must beat all the said things like gross Pepper, save the Musk, and Rose-water, which use thus, Take the Musk, and with the back of a silver spoon, bruise it in a little of the Rose- water, then mingle it with the rest of the Rose-water and shake it well together, then if you will, you may boile the Spices with two gallons of the same Wine you purpose to make it of, and when it is cold, strain it into the rest of your Wine, and boile it almost an hour, ever stirring it, then after put in your Rose-water and Musk when it is bloud warm, then stop it close, and roll it well together, then take Raisons of the Sun and Figs, of each half a pound, out them into the bag, and hang it in the middle of the Butt till the Wine be out, and as the Wine shrinketh, let the bag downe. Or you may put the same into the Hippocras bag, and hang as aforesaid, then put the Rose-water and Musk by it self into that Wine, and roll it gently, and this is the easier and quicker way, but the other will be sooner and readier to broach.

Note that if it should want of pleasantnesse put to every gallon a pint of Spanish Cute, and that will help it, and make it perfect.

The Knowledge and Choice of Wines, with their Marks of their Countries.

Muskadine.

See that your Muskadine be sweet and strong, and of colour like Amber at first.

Malmsey and Bastard.

See that your Malmsey be perfect and pleasant, at the first well coloured, sweet, fine, quick and strong: But let your Bastard be only quick and strong.

White Wine.

Must be fair and short, and though that want colour, if it be quick and not full, it is not to be refused, for it is easily helped.

Clarret.

See that your Clarret be very well coloured, fair, fine and short, for if they belong at the fi[]st, meddle not with them, for they will not hold for the burnings.

Red Wine.

Your Red Wine you must use as you do with your White and Clarret.

Sherry Sacks.

Must be and are white at the first, and you shal know them by their work upon their Bung, where you shall see the picture of a Cock burned, and the longer they lye, the better they are.

Graves Wine.

Great Royston is the best take of them at Michaelmas. Perty Royston is the next, take of them at Bartholomew tyde, the Cask is hooped with half Hoops, and the mark of the Bung is like three O's, with a stroak through the middle, the first being greater then the other two, having a little stroak from the top to the middle, not much unlike three Diamonds.

Spain.

In Spain there is Bastard, Sacks, Hollocks and Spanish Cure, that is the best to keep for all the year.

Gascoyne Wine.

There goeth four Hogsheads to the Tun, and every Hogshead is sixty and three gallons, and observe how many pence the Gallon is worth, and so many pound the Tun is Worth.

Wines of Post Nellon,

Are good for all the year, and they are Red, White and Clarret, you shall know them by their round half hoops, and the Wines do grow in a dry high Country, and therefore the stronger and sounder.

Wines of Saint Martins.

Take no Clarret nor White, the Red is only good, and will not fail; for your Red is of a contrary nature to White and Claret, you shall surely know them by their Marks, they have Willow hoops, and the Tun is marked with three O's, and stroak through the middle.

Rave Wines.

They are sold for Sherries, of that sort of Wines Sack is the best to keep all the year, and they are full gage, and the Bung is marked with G having a little stroak thorow the head, being burnt in.

Wines Gatterel.

It is over against Bourdeux, of which take none except it be a very dry year, they have Willow hoops, and quarter bar[]ed, and they be faint and weak.

Boyning Wines the best for all the year.

They are extraordinary for all the year; you shall know it by the taste, for its sharp and tart, ready to edg the teeth, and they be three Punchons to a Tun, and are full gage; and Malmsey and Candy Cute very good is made there.

Wines of Steave.

Then have you Wines of Steave, very good Muskadine, and that Vessel is not like the other, for they are longer greater and broader, and more Gage by three or four Cisternes.

The Countries of Rhenish Wines.

There is a place called Beallefficer, that is the worst Wine, you shall know it by the Fat, for it is double barred over the head, and twenty six gallons make a Lyne.

Wines of Brabymast.

That is better than the former, and they be in certain stripes and Cressels, and they be three po[]tles & two gallons and that is called Vage, and nine gallons are a Lyne.

Rhenish Wines.

There is Rhenish Wine of Barba Muska, and that is the best, and is single barred in the fat, with a broad bar; they be full gage, and the Bars for the most part are marked at the edges, with five figures of 3, and a stroak through them neer the bottom.

If Rhenish Wine fail and grow faint, take a pound of Brimstone, melt it in a pint of Damask Rosewater, then dip linnen cloaths in it, and burn it in a empty vessel, then Rack your tainted Wine into the vessel so prepared, then take one ounce of Coriander seeds, Callamus Benjamin, Storax, Damask powder, of each three pennyworth, beat them all, and put them in a bag, and hang them four dayes in the Fat, and beat the Wine,and roll and stop it close, and at four days end, it will be perfect.

To shift Wines, and rid away your Lugs.

If you have any Lugs of White Wine, Clarret or Sac, that will not sell, take in two Butts of pleasant Malmsey, which you may make three with your Lugs, and the Malmsey will be pleasant and good.

Batew Wines.

They are in very long Pipes, and very hard, they are not very good to keep all the year, yet good for present sale, they want two Cisterns and a half of Gage.

Wines of Angway.

The most part of it is in Pipes, and that is very good Wine, and strong, and lacketh very little of Gage, and is quarter barred.

Wines of Orbions and Omegas.

Four Hogsheads make a Tun, they be good for half the year, they have half hoops, and one broad bar at the head, with four pins on either side towards the end of the bar, thus,

$$\begin{array}{cccc} \circ & \circ & \circ & \circ \\ \hline \circ & \circ & \circ & \circ \end{array}$$

The property of Gascoyn Wines.

It will be sick most part of the Summer, and ropeth long, when it so changeth, keep him close from vent, and fill him over, then stop him close, and turne him over in his Lees two or three times, and it will amend him.

Note that all such Wines that are so hooped with half hoops, grow in the dryest and highest Countries, and are the best and soundest, and those with the Willow hoops grow in the West Countries, and the smallest are unsound.

A Remedy for shifted Wines.

To every Butt take two gallons of Red Wine, for that will preserve the Malmsey, [] well as Cute doth the Bastard, and so you shall save the more. Or in stead of the R[]d, take three or four gallons of Cute, if it be Spanish Cute, one gallon is as good, and will go further then three of Candy Cute, so that you put into the Butt two gallons of Red Wine, and one gallon of Spanish Cute, you shall make it perfect; if it be not pleasant enough, you must put in the more Cute.

How to make or divide Malmseys.

If you have three Butts of Malmsey you may make four, of two you may make three, of one you may make one and a half with such Lugs as

you have of Clarret, White Wine or Sack that is old, with two gallons of
Spanish Cute to every Butt, and so you may rid away your Lugs and old
Sacks: and the Art followeth that must be used.

To every Butt six eggs, both yolks and whites, and one handful of Bay
salt, beat them well together mixing therewith a pint of old Sack, and put
them all to[]ether. If it want colour, then take two gallons of Red Wine,
and a quarter of a pound of Co[]iander seeds beaten very small, put them
well mingled together into the Butt, then give six or eight stroaks more
and stop it close, and in three or four days broach him.

To make Muskadine.

Take a pleasant Butt of Malmsey called Ratnew, and draw it half out,
and fill it up within four or five gallons with fat Bastard, then Parrel it with
six yolks of eggs, and one handful of Bay salt, and a pint of Conduit water,
beat them well together, and then put them into the Butt, and if the colour
be too deep or too high, th[]n take three gallons of sk[]mmed milk, and
eight whites of eggs, and mingle them well together with the milk, and put
them into the Butt and they will mend []t; and for the pleasant taste
thereof, take four pennyworth of Sugar, Long Pepper and Cloves, of each
two pennyworth, bruise them, and put them all into the Butt, then beat the
Butt an hour, and stop it close[] after lay it up three dayes, and then you
may broach it[] Or you may put the Spices into a little bag and sink it with
a piece of lead into the Butt.

For Allegant that growes hard and faint.

First draw it into fresh Lees, then take three gallons of stone Honey well
clarified, scum it well, and let stand till it be cold, and take four yolks of
Eggs, a pint of Rose water, and one ounce of Lemmons, beat them well
together with the honey, and then put them into the Pipe, and then roll or
beat the Pipe half an hour, and then stop it close, and three dayes after you
may broach it.

If Bastard Prick.

Draw him presently from his Lees, if he have any, and put the Wine into
a Muskadine Butt, to the Lees of Malmsey, and then put to the Bastard
three of four Gallons of the best wort of the first tap, but let it be cold
before you put it in, then take two handfuls of Fordy Almonds, blanch and
bruise them, and mingle them with a gallon of Cute and put them into the
Bastard, and roll it well for half an hour, and in two dayes, you may
broach it, and it will be perfect good.

A Parrel to the same Bastard.

First Parrel him with the whites of eight new laid Eggs, beat them wel with a handful of Bay salt, and a pint of the same Bastard, and put them into the Bastard then beat it an hour with a parting staff, then take one pennyworth of Allome, and burn it, and mingle it with a pin of running water, and put it into the Pipe, and then give it a stroak more, and roll it well, and a dozen upon the Bung, stop him close, and broach him, if you have occasion two hours after.

To make Tyre that is excellent.

Take a good Butt of Malmsey, and overdraw him one quarter, and then fill him with fat Bastard, and two gallons of Cute, then Parrel him as you did the Malmsey with the same things, and after the same manner, and so beat him and keep him clo[]e, and in two or three dayes you may broach him.

To make Muskadine of Jane.

Take a Butt of Jane or good Malmsey and fill him up with fat Bastard and Parrel him as you did with the Malmsey and beat him well one hour till he be fine.

A Parrel for the Muskadine.

When it comes to be fine, within four hours after, take six new laid eggs, beat them shels and all with one handful of Bay salt, put to them a quart of old Sack, one handful of white Sugar candy beaten small, then beat them all together very well, then overdraw the Butt eight or ten gallons, then beat the Butt an hour, then put in the Parrel, and then beat him again gently half an hour, and stop him close, and broach him within twenty four hours.

A Parrel for the Malmsey.

It must be Parrel'd as your Muskadine, saving only you must take yolks instead of Whites, [ ], use them all alike.

For a Malmsey that drinketh hard.

Overdraw him one quarter, and fill him up with pleasant fat Bastard, and four gallons of Red Wine, as much Sack, with two gallons of Cute, stop it close, and roll it wel, and it shal help it presently.

For Bastard that drinketh hard.

You must put in it three or four gallons of running water, and as much skimmed milk, then beat them wel, and give him a Parrel of the yolks of six eggs, with a pint of water, and put it into the Wine and beat the Butt well half an hour, and when he is fine, you shall rack him into a cleer Pipe, and put into him two gallons of Honey water, and stop him close and roll him, and within two dayes broach him.

To make a Pipe of Ossey.

Take a Pipe of Eager Bastard, then take a Butt of smal Sack, but first you must roll the Pipe of Bastard, and draw him half into [the other] Pipe, then take [ ] small Butt of Sack, fill up your Bastard therewith within ten of twelve inches; if your Bastard be but small, take the lesse Sack, for the Ossey must drink somewhat fat; then to take away the eagernesse which is a principal thing, take five gallons of new milk, and two gallons of water, and that shall make it white and well coloured, and wel in drinking, and then you must beat it, or else it wil faint in the Pipe; then take half an ounce of Orris, and two ounces of Cloves, and beat them smal, and hang them in a bag three dayes in the midst of the Pipe, and that shal give it a right sent and taste, and at three dayes end with-draw him from his Bastard Lees to good Sack Lees, and Parrel him thus; Take twelve whites of eggs, and a handful of White Salt well beaten together, with a gallon of White Wine, which is in the Trace, then put it into the Butt with your beating staff and fill him up, and let him lye til he shew fine, and then it wil seem for Ossey, which is excellent. Or with two Pipes you may make or draw, mingled together, four Butts of exceeding good Malmsey.

To shift Wines and Malmseyes, and put off your ill Wines.

If you have two principle good Butts of Malmseyes, you may make two and a half, with eight gallons of pleasant fat Bastard, and with the Lugs you have of Clarret, White and Sack, and if you put a gallon of Red Wine to every Butt it will do well,and you shall have the more Cute; or you may use Cute, (two gallons of Spanish Cute wil go further then five of Candy Cute; but Candy Cute is more natural for Malmesey then the other) then Parrel him with eight whites of eggs, and a handful of salt beaten together, then put them into the Wine, and beat the Butt half an hour, and stop him very close, and in two dayes you may broach him.

A pleasant Sent for Red Wine.

Take two ounces of Brimstone, half an ounce of Callamus, mix them together with half a pint of Burrage water, melt the Brimstone into a pan, and let the rest be with it therein, then put in so many Cloves as wil soak it up, and burne the Cloves in the Cask, throw away the ashes, then your Wine being rackt put into it a pint of Damask Rose water, then roll it wel half an hour; stop it close, and let it lye two dayes, then broach it. This shal give it or any other Gascoin Wine a most pleasant sent and taste.

For to make a Match.

Take one pound of Brimstone, half a pound of Coriander seeds, Anniseeds two ounces, of Cloves and Nutmegs one peniworth, Orris one penniworth, one penniworth of Cammomile, grate them, and beat all these together. Also for parrelling a Hogshead of White Wine, take two gallons of milk, and the whites of four eggs, and a handful of Bay salt, these being well parrelled, and put into the Hogshead, will do the work.

Also if you have a Butt of Sack that doth begin to be long, take two pennyworth of Roach Allom, burne it, then beat it smal with the whites of six eggs and one handful of Bay salt, if it begin to boile, give it the Parrel aforesaid.

Also if you have a Pipe of Malaga that pricketh, overdraw it ten gallons, [ ] put in Chalk, in this manner you may help it away: Roll it well, and put therein two gallons of Stone-Honey clarified and beaten , with a quart of Conduit water, and that shall fine the Wine again, and in two dayes close stopped it shal be perfect.

For Bastard that pricketh.

First draw it out into a fresh Pipe, and fresh Lees, then take three gallons of the best Stone Honey, clarifie it, and beat it with a quart of the same Bastard, then take a peck of Frumety well boiled, as for pottage, then mingle the Honey, and beat it together, then put it into the bag, and let the bag be long, that it may reach almost to the bottom, then put into another little bag, one pennyworth of Anniseeds, of Coriander seeds and Licoras, of each two penniworth, bruise them well, and put them into the little bag, then line him to the side of the other Bag, and sink them, and put into the Pipe a branch of Rosemary, then stop it close, and at two dayes end draw it up to the middle, and there let it hang two dayes, then leisurely take it out, and stop it close,and in one day after broach it.

PERFUMES.

The Kings Perfume boiled.

Take six spoonfuls of Rose water and as much Ambergreece as weigheth two Barly Cornes, as much Civet in weight, as much Sugar as weigheth two pence beaten in fine powder. All these boiled together in a perfuming pan, is an excellent Perfume.

The Queens Perfume.

Take four spoonfuls of Spike water, and four spoonfuls of Damask water, thirty Cloves, and eight Bay leaves, shred as much Sugar as weigh two pence, All these boiled together make a good perfume.

To keep your house apt to take Perfumes, and to take away grosse Aires.

Take Cypress wood, or Juniper in chips, and throw them on a fair pan of coales, deck your house with flowers, and brush and sprinkle it with vinegar and Rose water, and keep your windows and doors close till the house be perfumed, and then set up your Perfumes.

King Edwards Perfume to make your house smell like Rosemary.

Take three spoonfuls of prefect Rosemary, and as much Sugar as half a Walnut beaten in small powder. All these boiled together in the Perfuming pan upon hot embers with a few coales, is a very sweet Perfume.

Such Herbs as are good Perfumes.

Sweet Basil dryed in the Sun, Sweet Marjerom, young red Mints, the Pills of Lemmons dryed and powdered. All these are good for Perfumes, everyone will smell severally.

A sweet Perfume to burn.

Take Benjamin three ounces, Labdanum one ounce, Ambergreece three ounces, Civet one ounce, mingle all these together with Gumdragagant, and roll it, and make it three square with Fusses dissolved in Rosewater, mingle with the same.

Another Perfume to boil and burn.

Take Benjamin and Storax of each an ounce, Labdanum and Fusses, of each an ounce, and half a dram of Civet: to be burnt, beat them in a white Mortar; and to boil, put them in Rosewater. It is also a good Perfume for Gloves.

A fine and sweet Oyl.

Take Musk twelve graines, Civet six graines, Ambergreece eight grains, Benjamin six graines, A few Cloves, Storax, Callamint three grains. Grind all these together with the Oyl of Sweet Almonds. First wash your Gloves with Fusses dissolved a day in Damask water.

A Perfume for Gloves.

Take your Gloves, and wash them well in Damask water, then stretch them fair and softly, and lay them in a fair linnen cloth or sheet folded eight folds, that the Rosewater may dry in by leisure. Then take Oyl of Sweet Almonds upon a stone, and with your hands annoint your gloves, and rub them well over, and stretch them forth by little and little, and before they be throughly dryed take the powder of Sanders mixed with a little Ambergreece,and strow the powder finely searced upon them, and let them lye in a box in a sheet of white paper.

Another Perfume for Gloves.

Take your Gloves or any other leather, and wash them well in Rose or Damask water, then wring them out of the water,and dry them. Do so three or four times, then take Gumdragagant, & steep it in fine Damask water all night and so strain it, and mingle it with a quarter of an ounce of Ambergreece, and as much fine Musk. First, grind your Ambergreece with the Oyle of Trobyn, and mix them all together, within and without,and lay a paper betwixt the Gloves, Glove by Glove, and dry them under a feather bed.

A Perfume in Powder.

Take Ireos, Storax, Callamint, Lignum Aloes, Laudanum, graines or seeds of Juniper, as much of each sort as you will, beat together as much of one sort as of another. Cast the Perfumes into the fire, and then you shall see whether it wil smell well or not.

To make an Oyl Perfume for Gloves that shall never out.

Take Benjamin two ounces, of Storax and Calamint of each one ounce, the powder of Benjamin and Storax must be finely beaten by themselves; that done, take a pound of sweet Almonds, and mingle it with the Storax and Benjamin upon a Marble stone, and then put it into an earthen pot with more Oyle; then put in your gloves powdered, and so let it stand very close covered. And when you will perfume [] p[]ir of Gloves take a little fair water in a spoon, and wipe your Gloves very fine with it. Take another spoon, and dip it in your Oyl, and rub it on your Gloves, and let them dry: this is excellent.

Perfumes sweet and good.

Take Gumdragagant, and lay it in Rose-water, until it be dissolved and liquid, then powder the things hereafter written, Take Laudanum an ounce, Benjamin an ounce, Coles of Willowes two ounces and half, beat all these together, and make paste of it with the Gum, and make as many balls or cloves as you will, then dry it in the shadow.

A Receipt to make a Perfume to preserve mankind from the Infection of the Plague, and also to burn in Chambers, Chests, and Presses for preserving of clothes, bedding and hangings.

Take pure old Juniper, shave it thin as may be, one ounce, of the flower or herb of Saint Johns wort half an ounce, of the Gums of Olibanum, Mastick, and pure [ ] Mirrhe, of each one ounce, your Gums grind great, your Saint Johns wort hack it small, your shavings of Juniper in the like sort, then mix them all together, and put them in some convenient vessel; then add thereunto pure Venice Turpentine, as much as will make it like a piece of paste, then use it at your pleasure, taking quantity of halfe a Nutmeg at a time, and burn it on a tile stone in your Chamber when you go to bed, and in the morning when you rise.

A Receipt for a Perfume.

Take Musk, Ambergreece, and Civet, of each a quarter of an ounce, of Orange flowers one ounce, grind all these things very smal on a stone, then mingle them well together with half an ounce of Oyl of Beanes, and for the want thereof, one ounce of sweet Almonds, and then apply it to the leather or other use you will put it to.

FINIS.

GLOSSARY

Medical terminology of the mid-seventeenth century is a combination of popular lay health beliefs and scientific concepts based upon humoral and iatrochemical medicine. Hence, the meaning of these terms is often alien to the modern reader. Numerous disease terms have not been in common usage for at least one century, while many extant terms had significantly different meanings to the practioners and patients of that era. This glossary presents contemporaneous definitions of key medical terms found in *The Skilful Physician*. The original spelling and language have been preserved to convey both the denotation and connotation of the terms. When definitions vary between contemporary sources, the range of these definitions is presented. Since these terms are based upon etiologic mechanisms and nosologies that differ significantly from a modern view, no attempt is made to bias the reader by relating these definitions directly to modern terminology.

A brief note is in order regarding the spelling and typography from 16th and early 17th century texts. The reader will note the equivalence of letters the *i/y* and *u/v*, producing words such as *yf* [if], *receyue* [receive], *vnmouable* [unmovable], *vnquyete* [unquiet] and *vrine* [urine]. In addition, vowels followed by a nasal (m or n) are printed as ã, ẽ, õ and ũ, producing words such as secõde [second], chaũceth [chanceth], Elephãcia [Elephancia] and sodẽ [sudden]. Finally, spelling is phonetic, producing variants such as cole [coal], hote [hot], hyer [higher] and fyer [fire].

Glossary References

BILLINGS

Billings, John S. *The National Medical Dictionary: Including English, French, German, Italian, and Latin Technical Terms Used in Medicine and the Collateral Sciences, and a Series of Tables of Useful Data* (Philadelphia: Lea Brothers & Co., 1890).

BLANCARD

Blancard, Steven. *The Physical Dictionary. Wherein the Terms of Anatomy, the Names and Causes of Diseases, Chirurgical Instruments, and Their Use, Are Accurately Described* (London: John and Benjamin Sprint, 1726).

BORDE

Borde, Andrew *The Breviary of Helthe* (London, 1547) Facsimile edition of British Museum Shelfmark: C. 122.d.1., Da Capo Press, Amsterdam, 1971.

CULLEN

Cullen, William. *First Line of the Practice of Physic* (New York: Samuel Campbell, 1793).

DUNGLISON(1845)

Dunglison, Robley. *Medical Lexicon: A Dictionary of Medical Science* (Philadelphia: Lea and Blanchard, 1845).

DUNGLISON(1895)

Dunglison, Robley. *A Dictionary of Medical Science* (Philadelphia: Lea Brothers & Co., 1895).

ELYOT

Elyot, Sir Thomas. *The Castel of Helth Corrected and in some places augmented* (London, 1641) Facsimile edition, New York: Scholars' Facsimiles & Reprints, 1937.

GOEUROT

Goeurot, John *The Regiment of Life, Whereunto is added a treatyse of the Pestilence, with the Booke of Children Newly Corrected and Enlarged* (London, 1546) Facsimile edition of Bodleian Library (Oxford) Shelfmark 8°.P.24 Med., Walter J. Johnson, Inc./Theatrum Orbis Terrarum, Ltd., Amsterdam/Norwood, N.J., 1976

HARRIS

Harris, John. *Lexicon technicum: or, An universal English dictionary of arts and sciences.* (New York: Johnson Reprint Corp., 1966 [1704 edition]).

HOOPER

Hooper, Robert. *Lexicon-Medicum; or Medical Dictionary; Containing an Explanation of Terms in Anatomy, Physiology, Practice of Physic, Materia Medica, Chemistry, Pharmacy, Surgery, Midwifery, and the Various Branches of Natural Philosophy Connected with Medicine* (New York: Harper & Bros., 1847).

LOWE

Lowe, Peter. *A Discourse on the Whole Art of Chyrurgerie* (London: R. Hodgkinsonne, 1654).

MORTON

Morton, Richard. *Phthisiologia, or, A Treatise of Consumptions: Wherein the Difference, Nature, Causes, Signs, and Cure of all Sorts of Consumptions Are Explained* ... (London: printed for Sam. Smith and Benj. Walford, 1694).

OED2

OED2: Oxford English Dictionary II [database online] Available from: BRS Software Products, McLean, VA; BRS/Search Full-Text Retrieval System, Revision 6.1, 1992.

PARÉ

Paré, Ambroise. Translated by Thomas Johnson. *The Workers of that Famous Chirurgion Ambrose Parey: Translated out of Latine and Compared with the French* (London: Thomas Coates and R. Young, 1634).

QUINCY

Quincy, John. *Lexicon Physico-Medicum; or, a New Medicinal Dictionary. Explaining the Difficult Terms Used in the Several Branches of the Profession, and in such Parts of Natural Philosophy, As are Introductory thereto* (London: T. Longman, 1787).

AGUES

Blancard: "*Intermittens Febris*, is call'd a Fever or Ague that ceaseth and returns at certain times; 'Tis either Quotidian, Tertian, Quartan, and some add the Quintan.

Intermittens Morbus, a Disease which comes at certain times and then remits a little. Intermittent *Fevers* or *Agues* proceed not from any fictitious *Focus*, but only from a wrong assimilation of the Chyle."

Harris: "*Intermittent Feavers*, commonly called, *Agues*; have certain Times of Intermission, beginning for the most part with Cold or Shivering, ending in Sweat and running exactly at set Periods."

AGUE, BURNING or BURNING FEVER

Harris: "CAUSUS, or a *burning Fever*, is that which is attended with a greater heat than other continued Fevers, an intolerable Thirst, and other Symptoms, which argue an extraordinary accension of the Blood."

ANCOMB

OED2: An ulcerous swelling or whitlow.

BLASTING/BLASTING OF THE FACE

Blancard: "*Bletus, Ictus*, one who has a Blast or Stroke spreading upon the side of his Body, by reason of an internal and malignant Inflammation, as in the *Pleurisy, Peripneumonia*; especially just after Death, it is to be seen livid or spotted, as from a stroke or beating."
"*Anasthesia*, a Defect of Sensation as in Paralytick and Blasted Persons."

Dunglison (1895): -infection of anything pestilential; stroke of sudden plague

BLAST IN THE EYE

Borde: "Xrophthalmia is the greke word. In englysh it is named a blast or an impediment in the eye, the which may come certayne ways . . . This impediment doth come of an euyl wynde or els of some contagiouse heat or of an euyl humour or suche lyke, for the eye wyll neither swell, nor water nor droppe."

BLEAR EYES

Borde: "Liptitudo is the latyn word. In englyshe it is named blere eyes whiche is whan the underlyd of the eye is subuerted. Rasis doth say ye Liptudo is whan ye white of ye eye is turned to rednes."

BLOODSHOT

Borde: "Atarsati is the Araby word. In latyn it is named Macula. In englysh it is whan the eye is blodeshottē, & some say it is a blemyshe in ye eye . . . This impedyment doth come by a strype or a blowe or some other casuall hurt by some euyll chaunce, or els of some euyll humour . . ."

BOTCH

Borde: "The 58. Capytle dothe shewe of a Carbocle or a botche.

Carbunculus is the latyn worde. Altoin is the araby worde. In englyshe it is named a Carbocle or a botche. Carbunculus is deryued oute of a worde of latyn named Carbo the

which is a cole in englyshe, for this infyrmyte hath the propertie of a cole that is hote
burnynge, for a carbocle dothe burne & prycke . . ."

Blancard: "*Phlegmone*, or *Inflammatio*; a Tumour of the Blood in the Flesh or Muscles,
causing Heat, Redness, Beating and Pain."

BOYNING
OED2: swelling.

BRAINE, DISEASES OF
Elyot: "Brayne hot and moyste distempered hath:
   The head akynge and heuye [heavy].
   Fulle of superfluities in the nose.
   The southern wind greuous.
   The Northern wind holsome.
   Slepe deepe, but vnquyete, with often wakynges, and straunge dreames.
   The senses and wytte vnperfecte.

   Brayne hot and drye dystempered hath:
   None aboundaunce of superfluities, whyche may be expelled.
   Senses perfecte.
   Moche watchē.
   Sooner balde than other.
   Moche heare in chyldehoode and blacke or browne, and coutlyd.
   The head hot and ruddye.

   Brayne colde and moist distēpered hath:
   The senses and wytte dulle.

   Moche sleape.
   The head sone replenysshed with superfluouse moysture.
   Distillations and poses or murres.
   Not shortly balde.
   Soone hurte with colde.

   Brayne cold and dry distēped hath:
   The head colde in felynge and with out colour.
   The vaynes not appearynge.
   Soon hurte with colde.
   Often discrased.
   Wytte perfecte in childhode, but in age dulle.
   Aged shortly and bald." (p. 4)

STOPPING IN THE BREST
See LUNGS, OBSTRUCTION OF THE

CANKER
Borde: "Cancer is the latyn word. In englyshe it is named a canker the which is a sore the
   which both corode & eat the flesshe corruptynge ye Arters the vaynes & the sinewes coro-
   dyng or eatyng the bone and doth putryfy & corrupt it. And then it is seldome made
   whole."

"Carcinodes is the greke word. In latyn it is named Cancer in naso. In englyshe it is named a Canker in the nose."

Lowe: "Of Pustules and Ulcers in the mouth.

Those Pustules and Ulcers with oftentimes possesse the upper part of the mouth and gums, are namee by the Greeks *Apthe'* and by Avicen *Altolla*, in vulgar the Water Canker, and are of a white fiery quality, for the most part incident to young children, sometime to those of elder age.

The Signes are evident to the sight, and are known by the colour. Those which are doe proceed of blood, the colour is red, hot, the part tumified; if it proceed of Flegm, the colour is white, with little dolour; if of choller, it is jawnish [yellowish] colour, with som tumour, punction, and heat; if of Melancholy, the colour appeareth blackish, which is worst of all: thos which be black and scurfy like the crust of bread, it sheweth great corruption and adustion of humours, very dangerous, and for the most part deadly: those which be red or white, are not malignant: such as are superficial, are easily cured, those which penetrat more profunditie, are difficile . . ." p. 200

Pet. What are those six kindes of Ulcers?
Jos. The first is sanious, 2. virulent, 3 filthie, 4 cancrous, 5. putrid or stinking, 6 corrosive or rottenn away . . .

Pet. How take they their names of the accidents?
Jos. . . . of the cankers or hardnesse turned over it called cancrous . . ." p. 326

Quincy: "Eroding gingival ulcers, formed without a previous tumor."

CANKER IN THE NOSE

Borde: "Carcinodes is the greke word. In latyn it is named Cancer in naso. In englyshe it is named a Canker in the nose.

CARBUNKLE

Borde: "Altoin is the araby worde. In greke it is named Althaca. In latyn it is named Carbunculus. In englyshe it is named a Carbocle or a botch Carbunculus doth take his name of Carbo whiche is to say in englyshe a cole. For a cole beynge a fyre is hote, as so is a Carbocle . . . This vlceration & infyrmyte most comonly doth brede in the emunctory places, there where ye .iii. pryncypal members hath theyr purgynge places the whiche be under ye eare or throte, or els about the arme holes or brest, or els about the secret partes of a man or woman, or in the share, or thyghe or flanke. And of Carbocles there be .iiii. kyndes. The fyrst is blacke. The secōde is reed. The third is of a glase or grenyshe colour. And the fourth is of a swarte or dym colour . . ."

Lowe: "There is small difference betweene Anthrax and Carbuncle, saving that Anthrax is the greeke word, and Carbuncle the Latine, and is so called because it burneth the place where it is, like unto coales. Carbuncle is defined to be a pustule, inflamed, black, burning the place, it is sore with many blisters about it, as if it were burnt with fire or water. The cause is divers, according to the sundry kinds thereof; the cause of the simple Carbuncle is an ebulition of grosse blood, thick and hot, where it falleth in any place it burneth and maketh ulcers, with a scale accompanied with great inflammation and dolour.

The signes of the simple Carbuncle are these, there appeareth many little black pustules not eminent, sometime pale, which groweth sodainly red, with great inflammation about the place where it is, and is harder than it ought to be, the sick loseth appetite and coveteth sleep, accompanied with cold sweat and fevers.

The signes of the maligne, are vomiting continually, weak appetite, trembling, swe-unding, beating of the heart, the face wareth white and livid."

Harris: "CARBUNCULUS, the same with *Anthrax*."

"ANTHRAX, *Carbo*, *Pruna*, or *Carbunculus*, is defined to be a Tumour that arises in several places, surrounded with hot, fiery and most sharp pimples, accompanied with acute Pains, but without ever being separated, and when it spreads it self farther, it burns the flesh, throws off lobes of it when it is rotten, and leaves an ulcer behind it, as if it had been burnt in with an Iron."

CATARRHE

Blancard: ". . . But there are no such things as Catarrhs, for there is nothing falls from the Head to those parts [below]. But the glandules of the Nostrils, and those that are about the parts of the Mouth, are often obstructed, and hence, come those Disorders. It is thus distinguish'd if it fall on the Breast, the *Cattarh* is call'd *Rheum*; if on the Jaws, *Branchus*; if on the Nostrils, *Coryza*."

Cullen: "The cattarh is an increased excretion of mucus from the mucus membrane of the nose, fauces and bronchiae, attended by pyrexia." Frequently treated under title of tussis (cough) paragraph 1045, p.48.

Harris: "CATARRHUS, is a Defluxion of Humours from the Head towards the Parts under it, as the Nostrils, Mouth, Lungs, &c. Some distinguish it by the Name of *Loryza*, when it falls on the Nostrils, by that of *Bronchus* when on the Jaws; and by the word *Rhume*, when it falls on the Breast."

Quincy: "Catarrhus, . . . a defluxion of sharp serum from the glands about the head and throat, . . . commonly called a *Cold*." C. Bellinsulanus=mumps; C. Suffocatus (Barbadensis) =croup; C. Vessicae= "glus"="a kind of dysuria, called *dysuria mucosa*, purulent urine. It consists of a copious discharge of mucus with the urine."

CATHERICK (Cataract [*sic*])

Borde: "Catharacta is the barbarous worde. In greke it is named Ypechima. In englysh is is named a catharact the which doth let a man to see yfuely . . . This impediment doth come of a grosse and a wateryshe humour the whiche doth lye before the syght lettynge a man to se clerely, for he can nat deserne a far of, a crowe from a man, nor a beest from a bushe, and of one thynge he shall se .ii. thynges although it be but one thynge."

CHOLER

Lowe: "Pe. What is Choller? Jo. It is an Humour, hot and drie, of thinn and subtill substance, black coloured, bitter tasted, proper to nourish the parts hot, and drye, it is compared to the fire."

Harris: Bile. . . . BILE, or the *Gall*, is a Liquor partly Sulphureous and partly Saline, which is separated from the Blood of Animals in the Liver . . .

CLEANSE or PURGE (BACK, BRAINS, CHOLER, EVIL SAVOR OF THE NOSE, GUMS, GUTS, HEAD, MELANCHOLY, MELT, PHLEGME, STOMACH, TEETH, VEINS or WIND)

Borde: "Emunctoria is the latin word. In englishe it is named the emunctory or cleansing places of mans body. Here is to be marked that man hath .iii. principall mēbers the hert, the brayne, and the liuer, and euery one of these principall members hathe emunctory places to clense them selfe as the hertes emunctory places be under the arme holes there where ye heres dothe growe. The brayne hath many emunctory places to purge him selfe, as the eyes, the eares, the nose, the mouth, the heres, and the poores of the heed. The liuer hathe emunctory places, as the bladder, the foundment and the flanks or the share." (Extrauagantes section)

COLICK/COLLICK
(see STONE entry for differential diagnosis)

Goeurot: "Against disease of the raynes of the backe, and the loynes. Payne of the reynes is called nephretica passio, & cōmeth of some one or grauel, & it is most lyke vnto the colicke in cure, but in causes they be cleane contrarie: for the colicke beginneth at the lower partes on the righte side, and goeth vp to the hyer partes on the left side, of the belly, and it lyeth rather more forwarde then backewarde, but nephretica passio begynneth contrarywise aboue, descendyng downewarde, and euer lieth more towarde the backe.

Also nephretica is paynfuller afore meat, and the colicke is euer more greuous after. And often the colicke chaūceth sodenlie, but nephretica contrarie, for commonlie it commeth by litle and litle, for euermore before, one shal fele payne of ye backe wt difficultie of vrine.

Item there is more difference, for the colicke sheweth vrynes [urines] as it were coloured, but nephretica in the begynuinge is cleare, and white like water, & after waxeth thycke, and then appeareth at the bottom of the vessel leke red sande or grauel." (Fol. lxiii)

Harris: "COLICK, is a vehement pain in the Abdomen or lower Belly, and takes its Name from the part chiefly affected, *viz.* the Gut *Colon*, which is stretch'd, prick'd, and corroded by Winds or Excrementious Humours, either remaining within its Cavity or fixt to its very coat."

Quincy: Any disorder of stomach or bowels attended with pain
1. Bilious colic—abundance of acrimony or choler that irritates the bowels so as to occasion continual gripes
2. Flatulent colic—bowel pain from flatules and wind pent up therein
3. Hysterieal colic—arises from disorders of the womb
4. Nervous colic—convulsive spasms and contortions of the guts themselves, from some disorders of the spirits, or nervous fluid, in their component fibers.

COLLICK, STONE

Quincy: "There is also a species of this distemper which is commonly called the *stone colic,* which is also, like the hysterical, by consent of parts from the irritation of the stone or gravel in the bladder or kidneys: and this is most commonly to be treated by nephretics and oily diuretics, and is greatly assisted with the carminative turpentine clysters."

COLLICK, WIND
see Colic entry from Quincy: flatulent colic

CONSUMPTION
Borde: "Ptisis is the greke worde. In latyn it is named Consumpcio. In englyshe it is named a consūpcion or a wastynge, and there is .ii. kyndes, the one is natural and the other is vnnatural. The natural consumpcion resteth in aged persons in whom blode and nature dothe decrece and so consequetly wekenes foloweth, wherfore in old tyme old men were named wasted men consumed by age. An vnnatural consumpcion either it is with a feuer or without a feuer, yf it be with a feuer there is an other sicknes ronnynge in the body with it as the feuer hectycke or some other longe sicknes the whiche dothe consume the naturall moysture in man. Or els it doth come by some other feuer or sicknes the which dothe extenuate or make thyn the blode of man, so to conclude a consumpcion consumethe a man away out of this worlde. And some doth say that this empediment dothe come of an vlcerous matter in the longes."

Richard Morton: "A Consumption in general is a wasting of the *Muscular* parts of the Body, arising from the Subtraction, or Colliquation of the Humours, and that either with, or without a Fever, and it is either Original, or Symptomatical.
   An Original Consumption is that, which arises purely from a Morbid Disposition of the Blood, or Animal Spirits, which reside in the *System* of the Nerves and Fibres, and is not the effect of any other preceding Disease. Of which there are two sorts, to wit, an *Atrophy*, and a Consumption of the Lungs."

Quincy: "To waste, signifies wasting of muscular flesh, frequently attended by hectic (*definition: slow and almost continual*) fever; and is divided by physicians into several kinds, according to the variety of causes, which must carefully be regarded in order to a cure."

COUGH
Blancard: "*Tussis*, a Cough; 'tis a vehement Efflaition of the Breast, whereby that which is offensive to the Organs of Breathing is expel'd, purely by the Force of the Air."

CORNES
Lowe: "Of the little hard Tumour in the Feet, commonly called *Cornes*. Those hard callous tumours which commonly possesse the toes and soales of the feet, but chiefly the joynts and under the nayles, are called Cornes, and in Latine *Clavus*, of which there are three kindes, to wit, *Corpus, Callus,* and *Clavus*. The cause, is chiefly in wearing of strait shooes, superfluous excrements which cannot avoid, so remaineth in the nervous part, and requireth a certain hardnesse, according to the nature of the part where they are. The Signes are evident to the sight."

CRAMP
Borde: "Spasmos is the greke worde. Spasmus is the barbarous worde. In latyn it is named Conuulcio or Contractio neruorum. In englyshe it is named ye crampe whiche is attraction of sinewes, and there be .iiii. kyndes the fyrste is named Emprosthotonos the which is whan the heed is drawen downeward to the brest. The second is named Thetanos, and that is whan the foreheed and all ye whole body is drawen so vehemently that ye body is vnmouable The thyrde is named Opisthotonos, & that is whan the heed is drawen backewarde or the mouth is drawen towardes ye eare, for these thre kyndes loke in there

captyles. The fourth kynd is named Spasmos the which doth darwe [sic] the sinewes very strayt and sperusly in fete and legges."

"The .256. Capytle doth shewe of one of the kyndes of the crampe.

Opisthonos is the greke worde. In latyn it is named Conuulcio retrossa. In englishe it is named a crampe, the which doth draw the heed backwarde towarde the shoulders, some latynest dothe name it Rigor ceruicis, and some doth name it Spasmus retrossus."

"The .343. Capytle doth shewe of one of the kyndes of the crampe.

Thetanos is the greke worde. The barbarous worde is named Tetanus, out of whichd is vsurped a word named Tetanisi. Thetanos in englyshe is named a crampe the which doth pull ye head backewarde & dothe drawe the body so vehemently that for a space a man shalbe vnmouable, for this matter loke in the capytle named Spasmos, and vse the medecines that there be specified and beware of venerious actes after a ful stomake and beware of anger and feare."

"Tortura is the latyn worde. In englyshe it is named a drawynge vp of the mouth towarde the eare.

The cause of this impediment

This impedimente dothe come of a spasmouse cause, some dothe saye that it is a palsie, but it is a kinde of a crampe."

Paré: "*Of the flatulent convulsion, or convulsive contraction, which is common called by the French,* Goute Grampe, *and by the English, the Crampe.*

That which the French call *Goute grampe*, wee here intend to treat of induced thereto rather by the affinity of the name than of the thing, for if one speake truly, it is a certaine kinde of convulsion generated by a flatulent matter, by the violence of whose running downe or motion, oft-times the necke, armes, and legs are either extended or contracted into themselves with great paine, but that for a short time. The cause thereof is a grosse and tough vapour, insinuating it selfe into the ancles of the nerves, and the membranes of the muscles. It takes one on the night, rather than on the day, for that then the heat and spirits usually retires themselves into the entrailes and center of the body, whence it is that flatulencies may bee generated, which will fill up, distend and pull the part whereunto they runne, just as wee see lute-strings are extended. This affect often takes such as swimme in cold water, & causeth many to be drowned, though excellent swimmers, their members by this means being so straitly contracted, that they cannot by any meanes be extended."

Quincy: "Crampus so Helmont calls the cramp. It is a sort of convulsion, occasioning a sudden and painful rigidity of the muscle, which soon goes off; it principally affects the fingers, hands, feet, or legs."

CURNEL

Borde: "Amigdale is the latyn worde. In englyshe it is lytle cornels in the rote of the tonge as some saye, but I do saye it be .ii. fleshly peces of the whiche doth lye to ye .ii. vmiles lyke ye fashion of an almõ.

"Cherade is the greke worde. Some auctours do call it Strume. And some do call it in greke Antiades. The latyns call it Glandule. The barbarous people do name it Scrophule. In englyshe it is named Carnelles in a mannes flesshe . . ."

"Glandule is the latyn worde. In greke it is named Antiades or Cherade or Strume. In englysh it is named Carnelles in the flesshe. And there be .ii. kyndes the one is harde and the other is softe ... The cause of harde carnelles cometh of coloryke humours, and the softe carnelles doth come of corrupte blode mixt with fleume."

"The .317 Cpytle dothe shewe of carnelles in the necke.

Scrophule is the latyn worde. In englyshe it is named knotts or burres which be in chyldrens neckes."

DISTEMPER(S)
Blancard: General term/synonym for disease; used frequently in this context.

DROPSIE
Borde: "Hidrops, or Hidropis, or Hidropesis is deriued out of a worde of greke named Hidor, which is water, for the sicknes doth come of a wateryshe humour. The olde auncient grekes did name this sicknes Lencoplegmantia. In englyshe it is named the hiedropsy or the dropsy. There be .iii. kyndes of ye dropsies, the fyrst is named Ascites and some doth name it Alchites ... The seconde kynde of ye hidropsies is named Timpanites ... The thyrde kynde of ye hidropsies is named Sarcites, and some doth name it Iposarca and some doth name it Anasarca ..."

"Astites or Asclites be ye greke wordes. The barbarous men do name it Alchites or Alsclites. In englyshe it is one of the kyndes of the Hiedropsies, and ingēdred in the bely for the bely wyll boll & swel, and wyl make a noyse as a botel halfe full of water."

Blancard: "Hydrops, a stagnation of a water Humour in the Habit of Body, or some particular cavity; and 'tis either *general*, as an *Anasarca* and *Ascites*, to which some add a Tympany, but falsly; or *particular*, confin'd to one Part, as a *Dropsy*, in the Head, Breast, Hand, Foot, &c. of which in their proper Places severally. A Dropsy."

Quincy: "Hydrops ... a dropsy; thus named because water is the most visible cause of the distemper
Hydrops cysticus, the encysted dropsy. It is water enclosed in a cystis, that is in a hydratid.
Hydrops genu, a dropsy in the knee; when water is collected under the capsular ligament of the knee, this disorder is formed.

Hydrops ad matulam, from Matula, a chamber-pot or urinal, i.e. Diabetes, which see.
Hydrops medullae spinalis, i.e., spina bifida.
Hydrops ovariae, a dropsy of the ovaria.
Hydrops pectoris, i.e. Hydrothorax, or dropsy in the chest.
Hydrops pulmonum, dropsy of the lungs.
Hydrops sacculus lachrymalis, i.e., hernia lachrymalis
Hydrops scroti, i.e., hydrocele.
Hydrops testis vel testium, i.e., hydrocele.
Hydrops uteri, dropsy of the womb."

"Hydropic, one that is troubled with a dropsy; also a medicine contrived for that distemper"

EMRODS
Bord: "Haemorrhoides is ye greke word. In olde tyme the latyns dyd use this barbarous word named Emoroides. In englyshe it is named ye Emorodes or pyles the which be vaynes in

the extreme parte of the longacion to whom doth happen by diuers tymes .ii. sondry passions, the fyrsts is lyke pappes and teates, and they wyl blede, and be the very Emerodes, ye other be lyke wartes and they wyll yche, and water & smart, and they be named the pyles, and in the sayd place doth brede other infyrmytes, as Ficus in ano, Fistula in ano . . ."

Quincy: synonym of haemorrhoides.

EVIL OF THE NOSE
Quincy: "scrobula".

Dunglison 1839: evil was synonym for scrofula.

EYES THAT HAVE SKINS OVER THEM
Blancard: "*Pterygium* . . . a membranous Excrescence above the horny Tunic of the Eye, called *Unguis* and *Ungula*, growing for the most part from the inner corner towards the Apple of the Eye, and often obscuring it . . ."

FAINTNESSE ABOUT/AT THE HEART
Borde: "Cardiaca passio be the latin word. In englyshe it is named the Cardyacke passion, or a passion, about the hert, for the hert is depressed and ouercome with faintnesse."

FALLING SICKNES
Blancard: "*Analepsia*, or *Epilepsia*, Falling-sickness." "*Epilepsia*, or *Morbus Caducus*, or *Comitialis*, because that the persons affected fall down on a sudden. Or, *Hercules*, because it is hard to be cur'd; also *Lues Deifica*, *Sonicus*, *Sacer*, &c. And it is an interrupted Convulsion of the whole Body, which hurts all Animal Actions, proceeding from an Explosion of Animal Spirits in the Brain, whereby the Persons affected are suddenly cast upon the Ground. This explosion arises either from an irritation, or pricking in the Spirits, or when something *Heterogeneous* is intermix'd with the Animal Spirits. The *Epilepsy*, or *Falling-sickness*."

"*Cataptosis*, is not a Disease, but a Symptom of Epilepsies and Apoplexies, signifying a sudden or casual falling to the Ground, which is an involuntary Motion of some Organical Member, proceeding from a Palsie, and Relaxation of the Muscles and Tendons beyond Nature."

Quincy: "an epilepsia" "Epilepsia . . . it being sufficient to know that it is a convulsion, or convulsive motion of the whole body, or of some of its parts, with a loss of sense."

FEAVER CAKE
listed under AGUE in text

Dunglison 1839: Ague cake- A visceral obstruction (generally of the spleen) following agues.

FEAVERS, CONTINUAL
Borde: "Febris sinochos is the greke worde. In latyn it is named Fibris sinochus or Febris continua. In englyshe it is named a continuall fever. Synochus is derived of .ii. wordes, syn that is to saye without, & choos whiche is to say trauel, and that is as much to say as a feuer without rest."

Lowe: [Fever] "It is an extraordinary heat, beginning in the heart, sent through all the body with the spirit and blood, by the vaines and arteries, . . ." [p. 291]

Blancard: "*Febris*, a Fever, is an inordinate motion, and to great an Effervescence of the Blood, attended with Cold first, and afterwards with Heat, Thirst, and other Symptoms, wherewith the Animal *Oeconomy* is variously disturb'd. Fevers in general are divided in to Intermittent, Continued, Continent, and Symptomatical; as also into *Quotidien, Tertian, Quartan, Erratic, &c.* Agues or Fevers."

Harris: "FEAVER, is a fermentation or inordinate Motion of the Blood, and a too great heat of it, attended with Burning, Thirst, and other Symptoms, whereby the Natural Oeconomy or Government of the Body is variously disturb'd. . . . *Continual Feaver*, is that whole fit is continued for many Days, having its times of Remission, and of more Fierceness, but never of Intermission."

Quincy: "Fever, is an augmented velocity of blood. The almost infinite variety of causes of this distemper does so diversify its appearances, and indicate so many ways of cure, that our room here will not allow of any more than to refer to reverious, Willis, Morton, Sydenham, and Huxham for the practice, in all its shapes."

FEAVER, QUOTIDIAN
Borde: "Febris quotidiana be the latyn wordes. In englysh it is named a cotidiane, the which doth infest a man euery day."

FELLON (also see WHITLOW)
Borde: "Antrax is the latyn worde. In englyshe it is named a Felon, and is like a Carbocle, but nat so great in quantyte or substance."

Blancard: "*Paronychia, Panarium*, or *Reduvia*, a preternatural Swelling in the Finger, and very troublesome. It arises from a sharp malign Humor, which can gnaw the Tendons, Nerves, the Membrane about the Bone, and the very Bone it self. A *Whitlow*."

Quincy: "Felon, so the paronychia is called when its seat is in the periosteum at the beginning . . .
Paronychia, . . ., circum, about, and [greek], unguis, the nail is a tumor upon the end of a finger, commonly called a felon or whitlow."

FISTULA
Borde: "Fistula is the latyn word. In greke it is named Seruix. In englyshe it is named a fystle, the which is a corrupt appostumacion in a vayne, or a fystle is a depe ulceracion, long, and strayt, and most comonly it wyl be in a mannes foundement."

Blancard: "*Fistula*, a straight long Cavity, or a winding narrow and callous Ulcer, of difficult cure, proceeding for the most part from an Apostheme. *Fistula's* differ from winding Ulcers in this, that *Fistula's* are callous and hard, but Ulcers are not. Sometimes an Issue is call'd a *Fistula*."

Quincy: "so the Latins call a catheter." "Fistula, is any kind of pipe, and therefore, some anatomists call any parts that have any resemblance thereto in their figure, fistulae; . . . as the aspira arteria, fistulae pulmonis; the uretra, fistula urinaria . . . but its common use is for ulcers that lie deep, and ooze out their matter through long, narrow, winding passages; in which cases the bone are frequently foul, and the extreme parts callous."

FLUX

Goeurot: "In al fluxes of ye belly, cause the excremētes to be dulye serched, for if the disease be seuche, that the meate commeth out, euen as it was receyued, or not half dygested, ye sayde fluxe is called lienteria. Yf great aboundaūce of waterye humours haue their issue by lowe, the sayde fluxe is named diarrhea, whyche is a moch to saye as fluxe humorall. And yf bloode of matter appeare wyth the excrementes in the syckeness, then they call it dyssenteria, which is a gret disease and a daungerous for to cure."

Borde: Extrauagantes "The .19. Capytle doth shewe of the kindes of fluxes.

Fluxus ventris be the latin wordes. In englyshe it is named the flyxe, and there be .iii. kindes named in latyn Lienteria, Diarrhea and Dissiteria. In englyshe it is named the Lyentery, the Dyarrhy, and ye Dyssentery The Lientery egesteth or doth auoyde the meat in maner as it was eaten. The Dyarrhy is a common laxe. The Dyssintery is the blody flyxe, and some doth name these flyxes after this maner. Intestinal, Epatycall and Sãguine. Intestinall cometh of day and nyght with fretynge in the bely. Epatycke or Epaticall flyxe cometh without paine prycking or fretynge. The blody or Sanguine flux maketh excoriacion of the guttes with payne prickynge and freatynge."

Blancard: "*Fluxus Alvinus*, the same with *Diarrhoea, Fluxus Hepaticus*, a kind of Dysentery, wherein black shining Blood, and too long roasted as it were, is driven out of the Guts by the Fundament, but without Pain. It is sometimes taken for a Dysentery, wherein serous sharp blood is evacuated, and is often the Consequence of it."

Quincy: "Fluxion, . . . It also signifies the same as Defluxion or Cattarrh, from fluo, to flow. For which reason likewise *Fluxus Alvinus* is a *diarrhaea, Fluxus Hepaticus* a *dysentery*, from the contents of the stools, and the like."
"Dysenteria, . . . a dysentery. It is a painful discharge from the bowels by way of stool. It is often called the *bloody flux,* because blood sometimes appears in the stools; but this is not a common symptom nor essential to the disease. Dr. Cullen defines it to be a contagious fever, in which the patient hath frequent stools, accompanied with much griping, and followed by a tenesmus."

Cullen: under discussion of dysentery; ". . . the matter voided by the stool is very various. Sometimes it is merely a mucous matter, without any blood, exhibiting that disease which Dr. Rodererhas named the *morbus mucosus*, and others the *dysenteria alba*."

FRENCH DISEASE

Borde: "Morbus gallicus or Variole maiores be the latyn wordes. And some do name it Mentagra, but for Mentagra loke in Lichen. In englyshe Morbus gallicus is named the french pockes, whan that I was yonge they were named the spanyshe pockes the which be of many kyndes of the pockes, some be moyst, some be waterashe, some be drye, & some skoruie, some be lyke skabbes, some be lyke ring wormes, some be fistuled, some be festered, some be cankarus, some be lyke wennes, some be lyke bites some be lyke knobbes or knurres, and some be vlcerous hauing a lytle drye skabbe in the midle of the vlcerous skabbe, some hath ache in the ioyntes and no signe of the pockes & yet it may be ye pockes"

"Lichen is the greke worde. Lichenais the barbarous worde. In latyn it is named zarna or Impetigo, and some doth name it Mentagra, & some grecions doth name it Psora. For this matter loke in the capytles of the aforesayd names. But Psora in greke is taken for one of the kyndes of leprousnes which is a perylous sicknes & is infectiouse and so be at maner of kindes of skabbes wherfore I do aduertise al maner of persons ye which be vnfected nat to lye in bed w and person or psons the which be infected w these infyrmites or any other diseses lyke, as the pestylence, the sweatyng sicknes, or any of ye kyndes of the agewe or feuers, or any of the kyndes of the fallynge sicknes & suche lyke, and Meutagra is engendred of a grosse melacholy humour."

"Mala fratizoz is the araby word. In latyn it is named Morbus gallicus or Variole maiores. In englyshe it is named one of the fyrst kyndes of the french pockes the which be skabbes & pimples lyke to leprosyte, wherfore for this matter or sicknes loke ī the capytle named Morbus gallicus. The grecions can nat tell what this sickness doth meane wherefore they do set no name for this disease for it dyd come but lately into Spayne & Fraunce and so to us about the yere of our lorde .1470."

Paré: "The French call the *Lues Venerea*, the Neapolitane disease, the Italians and Germans [as also the English] terme it the French disease, the Latines call it *Pudendagra*, others name it otherwise. But it makes no great matter how it be called, if the thing it selfe bee understood. Therefore the *Lues Venerea* is a disease gotten or taken by touch, but chiefly that which is in uncleane copulation; and it partakes of an occult quality, commonly taking its originall from ulcers of the privie parts, and then further manifesting its selfe by pustles of the head and other externall parts; and lastly, infecting the entrailes and inner parts with cruell and nocturnall tormenting paine of the head, shoulders, joynts, and other parts. In processe of time, it causeth not an hard *Tophi*, and lastly corrupts and foules the bones, dissolving them, the flesh about them being oft-times not hurt; but it corrupteth and weakeneth the substance of other parts according to the condition of each of them. The distension and evill habit of the affected bodies, and the inveteration or continuance of the morbifick cause. For some lose one of their eyes, others both, some lose a great portion of the eye-lids, othersome looke very ghastly, and not like themselves, and some become squint-eyed. Some lose their hearing, others have their noses fall flat, the pallat of their mouthes perforated with the losse of the bone *ethmoides*, so that instead of free and perfect utterance, they falter and fumble in their speech. Some have their mouthes drawne awry, others their yards cut off, and women a great part of their privities tainted with corruption. Their bee some who have the *Urethra* or passage of the yard obstructed by budding caruncles, or inflamed pustles, so that they cannot make water without the help of a Catheter, ready to die within a short time, either by the suppression of the urine or by a Gangrene arising in these parts, unlesse you succor them by the amputation of their yards. Others become lame of their arms, and othersome of their legges, and a third sort grow stiffe by the contraction of all their members, so that they have nothing left them sound but their voice which serveth no other purpose but to bewail their miseries, for which it is scantly sufficient." pp. 723–4.

Blancard: "*Lues*, in the largest sense, is take for all manner of Diseases; sometimes 'tis restrain'd to contagious and pestilential Diseases, but more strictly signifies the *Venereal* or *French Pox*."

"*Lues Venerea, Morbus Gallicus, Italicus, Neapolitanus, Hispanicus* and *Syphylis* according to *Fracastorius*, the French Pox is a malignant and contagious distemper communicated from one to another by Coition or other impure Contact, proceeding from virulent Matter, and accompanied with fall of the *Hair, Spots, Swellings, Ulcers, Pains* and many other direful Symptoms."

GIDDINESS IN THE HEAD

Paré: "*Of the* Vertigo, *or Giddinesse*

The *Vertigo* is a sudden darkening of the eyes and sight by a vaporous & hot spirit which ascendeth to the head by the sleepy arteryes, and fils the braine, disturbing the humours and spirits which are conteyned there, & tossing them unequally, as if one ran round, or had drunk too much wine. This hot spirit oft-times riseth from the heart upwards by the internall sleepy arteries to the *Rete mirabile*, or wonderfull net; otherwhiles it is generated in the brain, its selfe being more hot than is fitting; also it oft-times ariseth from the stomack, spleen, liver and other entrals being too hot. The signe of this disease is the sudden darkening of the sight, and the closing up as it were of the eyes, the body being lightly turned about, or by looking upon wheels running round, or whirle pits in waters, or by looking down any deep or steep places. If the originall of the disease proceed from the braine, the patients are troubled with the head-ache, heavinesse of the head, the noyse in the ears and oft-times they lose their smell . . . But if such a *Vertigo* be a criticall symptome of some acute disease affecting the *Crisis* by vomit or bleeding, then the whole businesse of freeing the patient thereof must be committed to nature." pp. 639–640

GOUT

Lowe: "This disease (which commonly doth possesse the joynts, by the falling of some humor above nature betwixt the joynt bones) is called by the Latines *Morbus articularis*, and in vulgar the Gout, of the which there be divers kinds and names according to the joint which is diseased, as for example: that which occupieth the jawes, is called *Sciagonogra*: if in the Neck, it is called *Trahelagra*: in the Backe, it is called *Rachiagra*: that in the shoulders is called *Omogra*: that in the Clavicules, is called *Clersagra*: that in the elbow is called *Pethagra*, that in the hands is called *Cheiragra*, that in the foot is called *Podagra*, and that in the Haunch is called *Ischias*, and that in the knees is called *Gonagra*: here I shall content me to speak of he last two, because they be most common, the others I leave to the learned Physition, as matters more Physicall than Chyrurgicall. The disease which is called *Sciatica* proceedeth partly by the usage of such meats and ingendereth Phlegmatique humors, also a Defluxion of grosse congealed humor, which possesseth the joint of the hanch bone, which partly doth proceed for want of exercise, as also sometime by immoderate using of women, stopping of the hemorrhoides or monethly courses." pp. 264–5

Blancard: "*Arthritis*, or *Morbus articularis*, the Gout, which is a Distemper that exercises its Tyranny about two or three, or more Joints, and their Interstices, and it is defin'd to be a pain about the Joints, produced from an *Effervescence* of the Nervous acid Juice with the fix'd saline Particles of the Blood, whence the *Nerves, Tendons, Ligaments*, the thin membranes about the Bones are contracted, and miserably tormented; whence proceed Swellings, Redness, hard sandy *Concretions* in several Parts of the Body, and other Symptoms that accompany it. It is fourfold, *Chiragra*, the *Gout* in the Hands; *Ischias*, in or about the Bone that is connected to the *Os Illium*; *Gonagra*, in the Knees; and *Podagra*, in the Feet; almost and incurable Distemper . . ."

"*Arthritis Vaga*, or *Planetica*, the erratic or wandring *Gout*; a Disease in the Joints that creates pain, sometimes in one Limb, sometimes in another. It is call'd *Vaga*, wandring, because 'tis not constant to one and the same place, as the true *Gout* is. Its Cause is owing to a Fermentation of the *Acid* and *Alcali*; which as it happens in one Joint or other vellicates the Nervous Fibres, and produces that Pain; and this is also sometimes call'd the *Rheumatism*."

"*Coxarius Morbus*, the Hip-Gout."

GRAVEL IN THE BODY; GRAVEL (see also STONE)

Paré: Under heading "*Prognostickes in the stone.*"

". . . Women are not so subject to the stone as men, for they have the neck of their bladder more short and broad, as also more straight; wherefore the matter of the stone by reason of the shortnesse of the passage is evacuated in gravell, before it can be gathered and grow into a stone of a just magnitude." p.666

GREEN SICKNESS

Harris: "CHLOROSIS, or *Morbus Virginius*, commonly *Icterus Albus* or the *Green-sickness*, seems to be a kind of Phlegmatick Pituitus Dropsy, arising from an Obstruction of the Menses, want of Fermentation in the Blood and Detention or Deprivation of the Ferment in the Womb; whereupon the Muscular Fibres being obstructed, they become Lazy and unfit for *Action*."

GUMME IN THE EYE

Blancard: "*Achne* denotes Lint, or the gumminess of the Eye, or sometimes 'tis taken taken for the Spume of the Sea, or the subtle Froth of Water."

HEART, COOLING OF THE

Elyot: "The hart cold distempered hath:

The pulse very lyttell.

The brethe lyttell and slowe.

The breste narowe.

The body all colde, except the lyver doth inflame it.

Fearefulnesse.

Scrupulosite, & moche care.

Curiositie.

Slownesse in actes.

The breste cleane withoute heares." (p. 5)

HOT AND COLD [as qualities of disorders]

Lowe: "Pe. How many sorts of Aposthumes are there?

Jo. Two, hot and cold.

Pe. Which are the hot?

Jo. Those which proceed of blood and choller.

Pe. Which are the cold?

Jo. Those which come of phlegme or melancholy." p. 69.

IMPOSTHUME

Borde: "Flegmon is the greke word. In latyn it is named Appostema clidum or perticulare. In englyshe it is named an impostume or an inflacion ingendred in a perticuler place, and is very hote and burnynge, and doth swell."

Blancard: "*Aposthema* . . . is an Exulceration left after a *Crisis*; but *Apostasis* and *Metastasis* sometimes differ in this, That the former is meant of an acute *Crisis* the latter of the Translation of a Disease from one part to another, an Apostume, an Imposthume." (see also ULCER)

IMPOSTHUME OF THE EYES

Borde: "Algarab is the Araby word Auicen doth name it Algaras. In englyshe it is an impostume in the corner of the eye."

"Bcthor is ye araby worde. In latyn it is named Pustula or Appostema. In englyshe it is named a pushe a wheale or an impostume in a mans eye And there be some auctours sayth that it is a lytle whyte whelke or wheale in the face named as I do thynke an ale pocke. And some auctours say it is a wheale in the mouth or tonge."

"Ophtalmia or Hipophtalmia be the greke wordes The barbarus worde is named Obtalmia, and some say Hipopia. And the latyns doth name it Inflatio inconiunctiua of Apostema calidum in cõiuctina In englysh it is named a hote impostume in ye eye . . . This impediment doth come of a colde reumatike humour, or els of a corrupt blode mixte with choler as autentike doctours dothe declare, but I saye it maye come accidentally as by a strype or a blowe with a mannes fyst or such like matter, for & if there were no cause of an infyrmite there shuld be no sicknes, . . ."

ITCH

Borde: "Pruritis is the latyn worde. In englyshe it is a sprowtynge or burstyng out in ye secret places of a man and woman, an some dothe name it a ych for the pacient must crache and clawe."

"Prurigo is the latyn wode. In englyshe it a named itchynge of a mannes body skyn or flesshe."

Quincy: "Psora, a scab or tetter, a kind of itch."

JAUNDIES, BLACK AND YELLOW

Borde: "Hictericia is the latyn worde. The barbarous worde is Ictericia. In englyshe it is named the Jawnes or the gulsuffe, and there be .iii. kyndes of this infyrmyte which be to sayet he yelowe Jawnes the blacke Jawnes, and ye grene sicknes named Agriaca, and some do name it Penafeleon, & Melankyron or Melanchimon is ye black Jawnes
The cause of this infyrmyte
The cause of the yelow Jawnes doth come of reed coler myxte with blode, or els as I haue had experyence, the yelow Jawnes doth come after a great sicknes or a thought taken, the which hathe consumed the blode, and than the skyn & the exteryal parts must nedes turn to yelownes for lacke of blode, coler hauyng the dominion ouer it. The black Jawnes dothe come of coler adusted, or els of melacoly, the which putrifieng the blode doth make the skyn blacke or tawny, and comonly the body leane, for ye body or flesshe is arified & dryed up. The grene Jawnes dothe come of yelow coler myxt with putrified fleume, & corruption of blode."

Quincy: "Icterus, the jaundice. It is a vitiated state of the blood and humours, from the bile regurgitating, or being absorbed into it, by which the functions of the body are injured and the skin is rendered yellow."

Dunglison 1839: Melæna entry; "*Black jaundice* . . . name given to vomiting of black matter, ordinarily succeeded by evacuations of the same character. It seems to be often a variety of haematemesis. . . . Melæna also signifies hemorrhage from the intestines."

JAW FALLEN

Quincy: "*Jaw, (Falling of the.)* See *Trismus Nascentium* . . .

Trismus Nascentium, commonly, but improperly, called the *Falling of the Jaw*. It is a tetanic complaint which attacks infants in the course of the second week after their birth. Its chief symptoms is a locked-jaw, but the disorder does not appear to differ from the *Tetanus*, which see. It is generally fatal in two or three days, and is never expected after the child is a fortnight old."

KIBES

Borde: "Perniones is the latyn worde. Pernoni is the barbarous worde. In englyshe it it named ye kibes in a mannes heles."

Blancard: "*Pernio*, a preternatural Swelling caus'd by the Winter Cold, especially in the Hands and Feet, which at last break out. Kibes, or Chilblains."

LASK

Borde: Extrauagantes "The .19. Capytle doth shewe of the kindes of fluxes.

Fluxus ventris be the latin wordes. In englyshe it is named the flyxe, and there be .iii. kindes named in latyn Lienteria, Diarrhea and Dissiteria. In englyshe it is named the Lyentery, the Dyarrhy, and ye Dyssentery . . . The Dyarrhy is a common laxe. The Dyssintery is the blody flyxe, and some doth name these flyxes after this maner. Intestinal, Epatycall and Sãguine . . . Epatycke or Epaticall flyxe cometh without paine prycking or fretynge . . ."

OED2: looseness of bowels, diarrhea.

LEPROSIE (see also Sawcie Face)

Borde: "The .199. Capytle doth shew of leprousnes.

Lepra is the latyn word. In greke it is named Psora. In englysh it is named leprousnes, and there be .iiii. kyndes of leprousnes which be to say Elephãcia, Leonina, Tiria and Alopecia. These .iiii. kyndes beestes, for these .iiii. kindes of leprousnes hath the ppertes of ye bestes as it appereth playnly in ye captytles of ye sicknesses."

"Alopecia is the greke worde. Ophiasis, both ye grekes and the latyns dothe use that worde The barbarous worde, is Alopecia. The Araby worde is Albaras. In englyshe it is a sodẽ fallyng of a mans here of his heed & berde hauynge growynge upon the skynne under the here an humour lyke brane or otemel and betwyxt the fynger is a white drynes, it is named Alopocia for as muche as ye worde is deryued of a worde of greke named Alops which is in englyshe a Fox, for a Fox ones a yere hath that infyrmyte shedynge his here hauynge also a lytle skurfe under ye here upõ ye skyn . . . And then the skurfe is lyke otmel, but some loketh whytyshe & other blackyshe."

"Elephas or Elephantia be the greke wordes. In latyn it is named Cancer vniuersalis. In englyshe it is named the Elephancy, or the Olyphant sicknes, for an Olyphant is sturdy & hathe no ioyntes, and who so euer that hath this kynde of leprousnes cã not moue his ioyntes & is starke wherefore he is bedred and can nat helpe him self."

"Leonina is the greke worde. In englyshe it is named the lyons propertie, for this worde is deriued out of Leo Leonis whiche is in englyshe a lyon for as ye lyon is most fercest of al other bestes so is this kynd of leprousnes most worst of al other sicknesses, for it doth corode and eat the flesshe to the bones, and the desine doth rotte away."

"Tiria is the latyn worde. In englyshe it it named the tyre or the property of an adder whiche is full of skales, so is this kynde of leprousnes ful of skales and skabbes corodynge the fleshe."

Lowe: "This disease which is called *Elephantiasis*, if it be universally throughout all the body, it is called Leprosie, and by the Arabians *Malum sanctæ manus*: but if it be particular, it occupieth only one member, which spoyleth the form, figure and disposition thereof, and maketh it rough, scurfie, red and unequall, like the skinne of the Elephant, for the which it is called *Elephantiasis*: if it possesse the skinne and not the flesh, it is called *Morphæa* . . . The Signes, is great tumor possessing the whole member or some part thereof, and doth augment by little, and little unsensible, not dolorous, sometimes inflamed, the eyes troubled, the breath evill savoured, the skinne rough, knotty and unequall, hard and scurffy; at last the body becometh atrofied and leane, the bones tumified, the hands and fingers become swelled, and the feete deformed . . ." pp.270–271.

Blancard: "*Lepra*, the Leprosy, a dry Scab, whereby the Skin becomes scaley like Fish. It differs *Leuce* and *Alphus*, in that a Leprosy is Rough to the Touch, and causeth an itching, for the Skin is the only part affected, and therefore it being flea'd off the Flesh, underneath appears sound and well."

"*Elephantiasis*, five *Lepra* & *Leprosis*, is a cutaneous Distemper, appearing first of all with *Pustules* in the Face, Forehead, Breast, Arms, about the Hips. They are of a bluish colour, like a *Canker*, but without pain. *2dly*, Such like Pustules appear on the Tongue, and in the Throat. *3dly*, These exulcerations are broad, but not deep, never reaching below the skin, but their Extremities or Edges are hard; they are most frequently on the Fingers, Toes and Joints; and if they are remov'd from one place, they break out in another. *4thly*, By degrees they seize also on the Nose, which is often eat up, Bones and all, and at last fix on the Palate and Wind-pipe. *5thly*, there is a Swelling near the Extremity of the Nose and Ears. *6thly*, A thin Skin grows over the Apple of the Eye. *7thly*, The Skin is very rough, and chapt in many places, and covered with Scales. *8thly*, The Hairs fall off, the Nails grow crooked, like the Talons of Birds of Prey. The muscles appropriated to Inspiration lose part of their use, by reason of the many exulcerations, and in process of time the sanguiniferous Vessels are so straightened, that when you prick 'em with a Pin no Blood ensues, but you may see a purulent Matter. The *Leprosy*.

LIGHTS
OED2: Lungs

LIGHTS, CORRUPTION OF THE
Goeurot: "Pthisis is an ulceration of the longes, by the which al the body falleth into consūption, in suche wyse that is wasteth al saue the skyn. Ye maye knowe hym that hath a pthisicke, for from day to day he waxeth euer leaner and dryer, and hys hear falleth, and hath euer a cough, a spitteth somtyme mater and bloody stringes wythal. And yf yt [that] whyche be spytteth be put ito a basyn of water it falleth to ye bottome, for it is so heauye." Fol. xxix

Blancard: "*Phthisicus*, a Man in a Consumption, whose Lungs are spoil'd or corrupted."

"*Phthisis*, a Consumption of the whole Body, rising from an Ulcer in the Lungs, accompany'd with a slow, continu'd Fever, smelling Breath, an a Cough."

LIVER, COOLING OF

Goeurot: "Yf the lyuer be colde, for the phlegmatyke matter that is in it, the persō hath his water white, out of coloure, the face pale, and his mouth watry, lytle bloode, and feleth heuynesse aboute his lyuer." Fol. li.

LIVER, HEAT OF

Goeurot: "Yf the lyuer [liver] be to hote, bycause of to moch blood, the person hath red vrine hasty pulse, his veines great & full, and he feleth his spattle, mouth and tonge sweter then it was wont to be, wherfore it is good to be let blood of ye liuer veine on the ryghte arme . . .

Yf the lyuer be ouer hote by cholera the pacient hathe hys vryne cleare and yelowe, without measure, great thyrst without appetyte, & feleth great burnyng in his bodye, and cōmonly hath his bellye rounde, and hathe the face yelowe."

Borde: "Eper is the latyn worde . . . If the liuer be hote, payne and heat is felt in the ryght side . . ."

LIVER, OBSTRUCTION (STOPPING) OF

Goeurot: "Oppilation or stoppyng cōmeth sometyme in the holownesse of the lyuer [liver], and it is knowen by cōpasson [compassion] and payne of the stomacke, and is healed by medicines laxatiue, as it is declared before.
And sometyme the oppilation is in the veynes of the holowe parte of the lyuer, and is perceyued then by ye grefe which the pacient feleth in his backe, & in his reynes . . ." Fol. lii.

Borde: "Eper is the latyn worde . . . If the liuer be opylated the face wyl swel, and payne wyl be in the ryght side . . ."

LUNGS, STOPPING OF THE

Goeurot: "Shortness of the wind procedeth oftentymes of fleume, that is tough and clāmishe, hangynge vpon ye longes [lungs] or stoppinge ye conduits of ye same, being in the holowenes of the brest, or of catarrous humours yt [that] droppeth downe into the longes, and thereby cōmeth straitnesse in drawing of the breth, whych is called of phisitions dispnoea or asthma, & when ye pacient can not bend his necke down for drede of suffocation it is called orthopnoca . . ." Fol. xxviii

Borde: "Orthopnoisis is the greke worde. In latyn it is named Recta spiracio. In englysh it is named an euyl drawynge of a mannes brethe, for yf he do lye in his bedde he is redy to sound, or the brethe wylbe stopped . . . This impediment dothe come either of the malice of the lunges or of opilacions of the pypes or els it may come thorowe viscus fleume."

Blancard: "*Dyspnoea*, a difficulty of breathing, which proceeeds from vitiated, obstructed, or irritated Organs."

MEAZELS

Blancard: "*Morbilli*, the Measles, red Spots which proceed from and aerial Contagion in the Blood; they neither swell nor suppurate and differ only in Degree from the Small-pox."

MEGRIM

Borde: "Hemicrania is a compoūde of .ii wordes, of Hemi which is to say in englysh the mydle, and of craneum which is to say the skulle. In englyshe it is named ye megryme, which is a sicknes that is in the heed kepynge ye mydle part of the skull descendynge to the temples, and doth fetche a compas lyke a rayne bowe, and ye diuers tymes it wyl lye more at the one syde than ye other, the barbarus men doth name his sicknes Emigrania."

Paré: "*Of the* Hemicrania, *or Megrim.*

The Megrim is properly a disease affecting the one side of the head, right, or left. It sometimes passeth no higher than the temporale muscles, otherwise it reacheth to the tope of the crowne. The cause of such paine proceedeth eyther from the veynes and externall arteryes, or from the *meninges*, or from the very substance of the braine, or from the *pericranium*, or the hairy scalp covering the *pericranium*, or lastly, from putrid vapours arising to the head from the ventricle, wombe, or other inferiour member. Yet an externall cause may bring this affect, to wit, the too hot or cold constitution of the encompassing ayre, drunkennesse, gluttony, the use of hot and vaporous meates, some noisome vapour or smoake, as of Antimony, quick-silver or the like, drawne up by the nose, which is the reason that Goldsmythes, and such as gilde mettals are commonly troubled with this disease. But whence soever the cause of the evill proceedeth, it is either a simple distemper or with matter: with matter, I say, which againe is either simple or compound . . ." (p. 640)

Quincy: "a headache that affects only one part of the head at a time"

MELANCHOLY (MELANCHOLICK)

Lowe: "Pe. What is Melancholy?

Jo. It is an Humour cold and drye, thick in consistence, sour tasted, proper to nourish the parts that are cold and drye, and is compared to the earth or Winter."

Blancard: "*Melancholia*, a Sadness without any evident Cause, whereby Peoa[p]le fancy terrible, and sometimes ridiculous things to themselves. It proceeds from the degeneracy of the Animal Spirits from their own Spirituous saline Nature into an acid, like the Spirit of Vitriol, Box-tree, Oak, &c. Also 'tis called black Choler, or black Blood, Adust, and *Salinosulphureous*."

Quincy: ". . . thus called, because supposed to proceed from a redundance of black bile. But it is better known to arise from too heavy and too viscid a blood, which permits not a sufficiency to spirits to be separated in the brain to animate and invigorate the nerves and muscles. Its cure is in evacuation, nervous medicines and powerful stimuli."

MELT, THE

Corpus suprarenale (Suprarenal or adrenal gland) or spleen from the context: "The Kidneyes are fastned very strongly to the Back bone, and that on the left side is right under the Melt, and that on the right side a little higher . . ." The left corpus suprarenale rests on kidney; the right corpus suprarenale is displaced ventrally.

Paré: Heading *"Of the Spleene or Milt."* (p. 111)

OED2: lists quote for obscure usage: "To knock down, properly by a stroke in the side, where the [melt] or spleen lies."

MORPHEW

Borde: "Mophea is the latyn worde. In Englyshe it is named the morphewe. And there be .ii. kynds of the morphewe, the white morphewe, and ye blacke morphewe. The white morphewe is named Alboras for is loke in the capytle named Alboras."

Blancard: "*Alphus*, or *Vitiligo*, is thus described by *Celsus*; A Distemper wherein the white Colour of the Skin is somewhat rough, not continued, but rather like so many several Drops: sometimes it disperses it self wider, but with some Interstices. *Alphus* is likewise call'd *Morphæ*. It differs from *Leuce*, in that it penetrates not so deep."

MOTHER, THE

Goeurot: "Fyrst agaynst superfluous fluxe of the mother, in the which ye must cõsider whether it doo come of to greate quantitye of bloode, and thẽ it is good for to open the veyne saphena, and abstayne frõ all thynges that multiplye the bloode, as egges, wyne and flesshe. Or whether it cõmeth of cholere, . . ."

Borde: "Matrix is the latine worde. In greke it is named Mitra. In englyshe it is named the matryx or the moder, or the place of concepciõ the which hath divers tymes many impedimentes as suffocaciõs, lubrycyte, the mole of the matryx, the rysyng of the matryx, and the fallynge out or descendyng downe of the the matryx the which no mayd can haue for the orifice of that place in a mayd is very strayt considerynge there be .v. vaynes the which doth breake whan a maid doth lese her maydenheed."

Blancard: "*Mater*, the same with *Matrix*, or *Uterus*; it signifies also a Woman who hath brought forth a Child."

OBSTRUCTION OF THE MATRIX (see MOTHER)

Blancard: "*Obstructio*, a shutting up of the Passages of the Body, either by Contraction, or by some foreign body which has enter'd within them. An *Obstruction*."

"*Matrix*, the same with *Uterus* . . ."

Quincy: "*Obstruction*, signifies the blocking up of any canal in the human body, so as to prevent the flowing of any fluid through it, on account of the increased bulk of that fluid, in proportion to the diameter of the vessel."

"*Matrix*, the womb of a female. Some chemical philosophers thence figuratively apply to any thing that gives nourishment and increase to any bodies: so the earth is a *matrix* to the seed sowed in it. It is also the same as *Gangue*, which see."

Similar terms in text: stopping of the Liver, stopping of the spleen, stopping of the lungs, stopping in the Brest

PALSIE

Borde: "Paralisis is the greke worde. In latyn it is named Dyssolucio. In englyshe it is named ye Palsey, and there be .ii. kindes, the one is universal and the other is perticuler. The universal palsey doth take halfe the body either the ryghte syde or ye lefte syde. And what syde so ever is taken the sayd sicknes doth take away halfe the memory, the one eye is dymme, and halfe the spech or al is taken away the one legge and the one arme is benommed or astonned that can nat do thyr office, and the proper name of this palsey, amonges ye grekes is named Hemiplexia, and some grekes & latyns dothe name it Semiapoplexis. The barbarous worde is named Semiapoplexia. The perticuler palsey doth rest in a perticuler member or place whiche is to say, in the tonge, heed, arme, legge, and such lyke membres Ignorant persons doth say ye is whã a mannes heed, handes, or legges dothe shake trymble or quake, that it is the palsey for suche matter loke in the capytle named Tremor."

From text: "This shaking is a continual strife of natural powers, which are raised with out ceasing. It hapneth; first by looking from a great height, by sudden fear or sudden joy, or much cold or great heat, or much bleeding . . ."

Quincy: "is a privation of motion, or sense of feeling, or both, . . . joined with a coldness, softness, flaccidity, and, at last, wasting of the parts . . . the internal senses, and the motion of the heart and thorax, or the pulse and respiration, are not necessarily destroyed. It is wont to be called a particular paralysis."

"There is a three-fold division of a palsy worth taking notice of in practice: the first is a privation of motion, sensation remaining. Secondly, a privation of sensation, motion remaining. And, lastly, a privation of both together . . ." Definition includes paralysis, hemiplegia, paraplegia and apoplexy.

PEARLE IN THE EYES

Lowe: "The humor cristalline may suffer all sorts of diseases, but the most common is the intemperature dry, or when it goeth out of the own place; the dry temperature is cause by the withering & drying of the Cristallin called *Glaucoma*, and becometh all white."

OED2: "Thin white film or opacity growing over the eye."

PESTILENCE

Quincy: "the Plague"

PHLEGME

Lowe: "Pe. What is Flegme?
Jo. It is an Humour cold and humide. thinn in consistence, white coloured, when it is in the vaines it nourisheth the parts cold and humide, it lubrifieth the moving of the joynts, and is compared to water."

Blancard: "*Phlegma*, or *pituita*, a slimy Excrement of the Blood, caused often by too much nitrous air. 'Tis likewise a watery distill'd Liquor, opposite to Spirituous Liquor; also those Clouds which appear upon distill'd waters. *Hippocrates* uses it often for an *Inflammation*. 'Tis also the Disease of Hens, call'd the Pip, and is sometimes taken for a viscous Excretion."

PILES

Blancard: "The *Hæmorrhoides* or *Piles*"

PIN AND WEB (see also entry for Web)

Quincy: "*Pin and Web*, is a horny induration of the membranes of the eye, not greatly unlike the *Cataract*."

PISSING

Borde: "The .98. Capytle doth shewe of them that can nat kepe theyr water but doth pysse as much as they do drynke.

Diabete is the greke worde. And some grekes doth name it Dipsacos or Sipho. The latyns do name it Afflictio renum. The barbarus men do name it Diabetica passio. In englyshe it is named an immoderate pyssinge." (Marginal printed notation: "Inordinate pyssinge")

"Mictus or Mictura be ye latyn wordes. In greke it is named Vria. In englyshe it is named pissinge, and there be many impediments of pissing for some can nat holde theyr water & some can nat pysse or make water, some doth pysse blode, & some in theyr pyssinge doth auoyde gravel & some stones, and som whan they haue pyssed it doth burne in the issewe as well in woman as in man."

PLAGUE

Paré: "*Of the signes of such as are infected with the Plague*

Wee must not stay so long before wee pronounce one to have the Plague, untill there be paine and a tumour under his arme holes, or in his groine, or spots (vulgarly called Tokens) appeare over all the body, or carbuncles arise: for many dye through the venenerate malignity, before these signes appeare. Wherefore the chiefest and truest signes of this disease are to be taken from the heart, being the mansion of life, which chiefly and first of all is wont to be assailed by the force of the poison. Therefore, they that are infected with the Pestilence, are vexed with often swoounings and fainting; their pulse is feebler and slower than others, but sometimes more frequent, but that is specially in the night season; they feele prickings over all their body, as if it were the pricking of needles; but their nostrils doe itch especially by occasion of the malign vapours rising upwards from the lower and inner, into the upper parts, their breast burneth, their heart beateth with paine under the left dug, difficulty of taking breath, Ptissick, Cough, paine of the heart, and such an elation of puffing up of the *Hypochondria* or sides of the Belly, distended with the abundance of vapours raised by the force of the feverish heat, that the Patient will in a manner seeme to have the Timpany. They are molested with a desire to vomit, and oftentimes with much and painfull vomiting, wherein green and black matter is seen, & alwaies of divers colours answering in proportion to the excrements of the lower parts, the stomack being drawn into a consent with the heart, by reason of the vicinity and communion of the vessels; oftentimes bloud alone, & that pure, is excluded & cast up in vomiting; and it is not only cast up by vomiting out of the stomack, but also very often out of the nostrils, fundament and in women out of the wombe; the inward parts are often burned and the outward parts are stiffe with cold, the whole heat of the Patient being drawn violently inward after the manner of a Cupping glasse, by the strong burning of the inner parts; then the eye-lids waxe blew, as it were through some contusion, all the whole face hath a horrid aspect, and as it were the colour of lead, the eies are burning red & as it were, swoln or puffed up with Bloud or any other humour shed teares; and to conclude, the whole habit of the body is somewhat changed and turned yellow.

Many have a burning fever, which doth shew it selfe by the Patients ulcerated jawes, unquenchable thirst, dryness and blackness of the tongue, and it causeth such a phrensie by inflaming the braine, that the patients running naked out of their bed seek to throw themselves out of the windowes into the pits and rivers that are at hand. In some the joynts of the body are so weakned, that they cannot go nor stand from the beginning they are as it were buried in a long swoune and deepe sleep, by reason that the fever sendeth up to the braine the grosse vapours from the crude and cold humours, as it were from greene wood newly kindled to make a fire.

Such sleeping doth hold him especially while the matter of the force or carbuncle is drawne together, and beginneth to come to suppuration. Oftentimes when they are awaked out of sleep, their doe spots and markes appeare dispersed over the skin, with a stinking sweat. But if those vapours be sharpe, that are stirred up unto the head, instead of sleepe, they cause great waking, and alwayes there is much diversity of accidents in the urine of those that are infected with the Plague, by reason of the divers temperature and condition of the bodies: neither is the urine at all times and in all men of the same consistence and colour: For sometimes they are like unto the urine of those that are sound and in health, that is to say, laudable in colour and substance, because that when the heart is affected by the Venemous Aire, that entreth in unto it, the spirits are more greatly grieved and molested than the humours: but those, *i* the spirits, are infected and corrupted when these do begin to corrupt . . .

And to conclude, the variety of accidents is almost infinite, which appear & spring up in this kinde of disease, by reason of the diversity of the poyson, and condition of the bodies and grieved parts, but they doe not all appeare in each man, but some in one, and some in another." pp. 832–833

Blancard: "*Pestis*, the Plague, an epidemick contagious Disease, arising from a poisonous and too much exalted Nitre in the Air, which secretly and suddenly takes a Man, extinguishing the Spirits, clotts the blood, deadneth the sound Parts, and is accompanied with Blotches, Boils, and a train of other dreadful Symptoms."

PLURISIE

Goeurot: ". . . apostemes called pleuresie, & it may be knowen by iiii. manner of signes. Fyrst the paciēt [patient] hath a great burnyng feuer [fever]. Secondly, the ribbes are so sore within, as if thei were prycked continually wt nedylles. Thirdly, the pacient hath a shorte breathe. The .iiii. sygne is a strōg cough, wherewyth the sycke is vexed, and by these sygnes maye ye surelye knowe a ryght pleuresie, that is the skyn vnder the rybbes wythin the bodye.

But there is an other kynde of pleuresie wythout vpon the rybbes apostemed, but in that is nothyng so greatte daunger nor the fyeuer [fever] is not so strōg as is the other aforerehearsed." Fol. xxvii.

Lowe: "Plurisie is an inflammation and tumor, or a masse of blood, which turneth into a bilious matter, in divers parts, but chiefly of the membraines and muscles, which knit and cover the ribs, wherof there are two sorts, the false and true: the false is outward in the muscles of the short ribs, and the true, is that which happeneth in the membraines, which knitteth the ribs,

The Cause, is externe and interne: externe, is great heat or cold: the usage of strong wine or very cold water, violent exercise, and cold ayre after great heate: the internall cause, is great repletion of all the foure humors, but chiefly the blood and choller, which maketh the most subtill part of the blood ascend from the cave vein into the vaine *Asygos*, thereafter in the vaines and membrainee intercostalles.

The Signes are great dolour, from the shoulder unto the nethermost rib, punction in the side, continual fever, difficulty of respyring, coughing, hard pulse, great alteration, with want of appetitie, evil favored breath, heavines, and ponderosity of the sides, great fever chiefly in the night, little sleep, some sweats which happen through great pain." pp. 220–221.

Blancard: "*Pleuritis*, a Pleurisy, an Inflammation of the Membrane *Pleura*, and the intercostal Muscles, attended with a continual fever and Stitches in the Side, difficulty of

Breathing, and sometimes spitting of Blood; an it is either a true Pleurisy, this which we have describ'd, or a bastard Pleurisy."

PLURISIE, HOT (see also definition of HOT and COLD DISORDERS).

Definition in text: ". . . a pricking pain about the ribs with a cough and an Ague . . ."

POCKS (See entries for MEAZELS and SMALLPOX.)

PRICKING

Paré: ". . . they feele prickings over all their body, as if it were the pricking of needles . . ." p. 832.

PUSHES

Borde: "Bothor is ye araby word. In latyn it is named Pustula or Appostema. In englysh it is named a push a wheal or an impostume in a mans eye . . .

"Pustule is the latyn worde. In englyshe it is named wheals or pushes . . ."

QUINZIE

Blancard: "*Angina*, an Inflammation of the Jaws or Throat, attended with a continual Fever, and a difficulty of Respiration and Swallowing. It is twofold, either *Spuria* or *Exquisita*, a bastard or a true *Squincie*."

Harris: "ANGINA, a *Quinsy* or *Squinancy*, is an Inflammation of the Jaws or Throat, attended with a continual Feaver and difficulty of Respiration and Swallowing, and it is two-fold; either *Spuria* or *Exquista*, a Bastard or a True *Squinsie*: The latter is again four-fold, *Synanche*, or *Parsynanche, Chynanche* and *Parchynanche*: of all which in their proper places."

RAINS (or REINES) OF THE BACK

Goeurot: "Against disease of the raynes of the backe, and the loynes. Payne of the reynes is called nephretica passio, & cōmeth of some one or grauel, & it is most lyke vnto the col-icke in cure, but in causes they be cleane contrarie: for the colicke beginneth at the lower partes on the righte side, and goeth vp to the hyer partes on the left side, of the belly, and it lyeth rather more forwarde then backewarde, but nephretica passio begynneth contrary-wise aboue, descendyng downewarde, and euer lieth more towarde the backe.

Also nephretica is paynfuller afore meat, and the colicke is euer more greuous after. And often the colicke chaūceth sodenlie, but nephretica contrarie, for commonlie it commeth by litle and litle, for euermore before, one shal fele payne of ye backe wt difficultie of vrine.

Item there is more difference, for the colicke sheweth vrynes [urines] as it were coloured, but nephretica in the begynuinge is cleare, and white like water, & after waxeth thycke, and then appeareth at the bottom of the vessel leke red sande or grauel." (Fol. lxiii)

Borde: "Renes is the latin worde. In greke it is named Nephroi. In englyshe it is named the raynes of the backe ye whiche may haue many impedimētes as indacions, the stone, ache and such like. For this matter loke in the capitles of these infyrmites and in the Extrauagates in the ende of this boke."

(from Extrauagantes) "Renes is the latyn worde. In greke it is named Nephroi. In englyshe it is named the raines of a mannes backe the whiche may haue diuers impedumentes as ache, the crycke, and straininge &c."

Paré: "Of the Kidneyes, or Reines." p. 117

Blancard: Kidneys from entry for "Urine" ". . . We known Reins are affected by Caruncles, Blood, and *Pus*, coming away with the Urine; . . ."

RHEUME

Definition from text: "Rheume is nothing else but a defluxion that falls from the head into the throat or brest, which doth otherwhiles so stop the pipes of the Lights and throat that its ready to choak, also these Rheumes fall into the nose, and cause the pawse.

These Rheums are caused divers waies; as from gross meats which cause vapours, or of cold, or from a sharp North wind which bloweth suddenly after a South wind.

The cold Rheumes are knowne by these signes following, as wearinesse, heavinesse of the whole body, sleepiness, heavinesse of the head and forehead, palenesse with full vaines, stuffing of the head or nose, swelling of the eyes, pain in the throat, motion to vomit, swelling of the Almonds . . .

Hot Rheume, the signes thereof are these, viz. the face is red, mixt with a pale or black colour, great heat in the nose with itchings, when the mouth and the throat is full of bitternesse and sharpnesse, and if the head be hot in feeling . . ." p. 135

Blancard: "*Rheuma*, Rheum, a defluxion of Humours from the Head upon the Parts beneath, as upon the Eyes, Nose, &c."

Harris: "CATARRHUS, is a Defluxion of Humours from the Head towards the Parts under it, as the Nostrils, Mouth, Lungs, &c. Some distinguish it by the Name of *Loryza*, when it falls on the Nostrils, by that of *Bronchus* when on the Jaws; and by the word *Rhume*, when it falls on the Breast."

RICKETS

Blancard: "Rhachitis, . . . a Disease amongst the *English*, which is an unequal nourishing of Parts, accompanied with a Looseness of the same, softness, weakness, faintness, drowsiness, a great swelling Head, with Leanness below the same and Protuberences about the Joints, crookedness of Bones, straightness of the Breast, swellings of the abdomen, stretching of the Hypochondres, a Cough &c. The *English* call it the *Rickets* . . ."

RING-WORM

Borde: "Impetigo is the latyn word. And some latyns do name it zerna or zarma, this sicknes doth dyffer in the more and lesse, the grekes dothe name this sicknes Lichen, the barbarous word is Lichena. In englyshe it is named roughnesse of the skyn or scabbes in ye skyn, and there be .ii. kyndes the one is a dry scabbe and the other is wete or an vlcerous scabbe named in englysh a rynge worm or beynge of that sort."

Paré: "*Of the* Herpes; *that is Teatars, or Ringwormes, or such like.*"

Blancard: "*Herpes*, a spreading and winding Inflammation; 'tis two-fold, either *Miliaris* or *Pustularis*, like Millet-seed, which seizes the Skin only, and itches; or *Exedens*, consuming, which not only seizes the skin, but the *Muscles* underneath. The cause of it is, that the *Glandules* of the Skin are too much stuff'd with salt *Particles*, which, if the peccant Matter abount, grow into a Crust, and eat the *Parts* they lie upon. A *Ring-worm* or *Tettar*."

ROOF FALLEN
see entries for "Jaw fallen" and "Ufula".

RUPTURE
Borde: "Ruptura is the latyn worde. In greke it is named Epigozontaymenon. In englyshe it
is named a rupture, and that is whan the Siphac wich is a pellicle or skyn that doth compasse about the guttes is relaxed or broken then ye guttes doth fal into the codde. And
there be .iii. kyndes of ruptures, the first is zirbale, the second is intestinall, and the thirde
is nuterall, for he dothe take his originall of both the other . . . A rupture doth come of
cryĕg, or els of a great lyfte, or of a great fall or brose, or lepynge unesely upon an horse,
or clymynge ouer a highe hedge or style, or by a great strain or vociferation."

SAINT ANTHONIES FIRE
Goeurot: "In Greke herisipela, and of the Latines Sacer ignis, our Englysshe women call it
the fyre of Saynt Anthonye, or chingles, it is an inflammatiõ of membres wit excedyng
burnynge and rednesse, harde in the feelynge, and the most parte crepeth aboue the
skynne or but a lytle depe within the flesshe.

It is a greuous payne, and maye be lykened to the fyre in consumyng . . ." (The Booke of
chyldren)

Borde: "Ignis santi Anthonij, Ignis persicus and Pruna be the latyn wordes. In englyshe it is
named saynt anthonyes fyer, the be lytle wheales the whiche doth burne as fyre, how be
it Ignis periscus or saint anthonyes fyer is nat so vehement as is the infyrmyte named
Pruna, for Pruna is more grosser and greate, and dothe burne more than dothe saynte
anthonyes fyer."

Paré: "*Of a Gangreene and Mortification.*

Certainely the maligne symptomes which happen upon wounds, and the solutions of
Continuity are many, caused either by the ignorance or negligence of the Chirurgion; or
by the Patient, or such as are about him; or by the malignity and violence of the disease;
but there can happen no greater than a Gangreene as that which may cause the mortification and death of the part, and oft times of the whole body; wherefore I have thought good
in this place to treate of a Gangreene, first giving you the definition, then showing you the
causes, signes, prognostickes, & lastly the manner of cure. Now a Gangreene is a certaine
disposition, and way to the mortification of the part, which it seaseth upon, dying by little
and little. For when there is a perfect mortification, it is called by the Greekes *Sphacelos*,
by the Latines *Syderatio*, our countrymen terme it the fire of Saint *Anthony*, or Saint
Marcellus." p. 452.

Lowe: "We must here consider the difference betwixt Gangrene and Sphasell, and know that
Gangren is the latin word, [i]t is a mortification of the parts it happeneth in, except the
bones, and is curable: but Sphasell or sideration, is a mortification both of the soft and
solid parts, which is no way remedied but by amputation, som do call it S. Anthony or S.
Martials fire. . . . The signes are these, the member weareth black, like as it were burnt,
afterwards it becometh rotten, and in that time it overthroweth the whole body, in such
sort that the skin both come from the flesh . . ." p. 88.

Blancard: "*Erysipelas*, . . . St. *Anthony's* Fire, is a Swelling in the Skin or any fleshy or
membranous Part, red, broad, not spreading high, not beating with a Pulse, but attending
with a pricking sort of Pain, arising from a sharp and frequently sulphureous Blood. I take

the cause of it not to be the Blood so much a serous Sweating, which is sharp and sulphureous, and flows from the Fibres themselves."

SAWCIE FACE

Borde: "Salsum flegma be the latyn wordes. In englyshe it is named a saucefleume face which is a tokē or preuy signe of leprousnes."

"Gutta rosacea be the latyn wordes. In englysh it is named a sauce fleume face, which is a readnes about the nose and the chekes with small pymples, it is a preuy signe of leprousnes."

Blancard: "*Gutta rosacea*, a Redness with Pimples, wherewith the Cheeks, Nose and the whole Face is deformed as if it were sprinkled with red Drops; these Pimples or Wheals often increase, so that they render the Face rough and horrid, and the Nose monstrously big."

SCALD HEAD (see also entry for SCURF)

Paré: "*Of the* Tinea, *or Scalde Head.*

The *Tinea* . . . or scald head, is a disease possessing the musculous skin of the head or the hairy scalpe, and eating thereinto like a moth. There are three differences thereof, the first is called by *Galen* scaly or branlike for that whilst it is scratched it cast many branlike scales: some practitioners terme it a dry scall, because of the great adustion of the humour causing it. Another is called *ficosa*, a fig-like scall, because when it is despoyled of the crust or scab which is yellow, there appeare graines of quick and red flesh, like to the inner seeds or graines of figs, and casting out a bloudy matter. *Galen* names the third *Achor*, and it is also vulgarly termed the corrosive or ulcerous scall, for that the many ulcer wherewith it abounds are open with many small holes flowing with liquid *sanies*, like the washing of flesh, stinking, corrupt and carrion like, somewhiles livid, somewhiles yellowish. These holes, if they be somewhat larger, make another difference which is called *Cerion* or *Favosa* (that is, like a hony comb) because as *Galen* thinks, the matter which floweth from these resembleth hony in colour and consistence . . ." p. 638

Quincy: "Scalled head, see Crusta Lactea"; "Crusta Lactea, when the Tinea affects the face it is thus named. In the hairy scalp only it is called Tinea only, or scalled."

"Tinea, a sore or tetter that discharges a salt lymph. Tinea Capitis, scalled head, this and the Crusta Lactea are commonly described as distinct and unconnected diseases."

SCABBED HEAD (see entries for SCALLED HEAD and SCURF)

SCIATICA (see also entry for GOUT)

Borde: "Siatica passio is the barbarous worde. In latyn it is named Dolor scie. In greke it is named Ischias, the of whiche worde dothe come Ichiadici, and some doth name this infyrmyte Coxendrix or Coxendricis morbus.
The cause of this infyrmyte
This infyrmyte doth come of harde lyenge on the hokyll bones or lyenge on the grounde, or upō a forme, or such lyke harde thinges, it may come by a stripe or a great fall, and it wyll ronne from ye hokyll bone to the kne, and from the kne to the ancle and from

the ancle to the lytle too, & than it is past cure, and otherwhile this gout wyl haue a reflec-
tion to the raynes of the backe, and to ye flankes, and it may come of a grosse fleumaryke
humour, . . ."

Paré: "*Of the* Ischias, *Hip-gout*, or Sciatica

For that the hip-gout in the greatnesse of the causes, bitternesse of pain, and vehemency
of the symptomes, easily exceeds the other kindes of Gout, therefore, I have thought good
to treate thereof in particular. The pain of the *Sciatica* is therefore the most bitter, and the
symptomes most violent, for that the dearticulation of the hucklebone, with the head of
the thigh-bone, is more deepe than the rest, because also the phlegmaticke humour which
causeth it is commonly more plenteous, cold, grosse and viscid, that flowes down into this
joint, and lastly because the *Sciatica* commonly succeeds some other chronicall disease,
by reason of the translation and falling down thither of the matter, become maligne and
corrupt by the long continuance of the former disease. But the paine not only troubles the
hippe, but entering deepe, is extended to the muscles of the buttocks, the groines, knees,
and very ends of the toes, yea often times it vexeth the patient with a sense of paine in the
very vertebræ of the loines, so that it makes the patients, and also oft-times the very
Physitians and Surgeons to thinke it the wind or stone Collicke." pp. 719.

SCURF, WHITE (see also entry for SCALD HEAD)

Borde: "Acor or Acoris be the greke wordes, Furfur is the latyn word, Acora is the barbarus
word In englyshe it is named dandruffe or a skurfe in the heed lyke bran or otmell, the
which doth penetrate the skyn of the heed makynge lytle holes, dyfferinge from an other
infyrmyte in the skyn of the hed named Fauus . . ."

"The .290. Capytle doth shewe of a lytle skurfe in the heed.
     Porrigo or Porre or Furfures some latenyst dothe use these termes. The grecions dothe
use this worde named Pitariasis. In englyshe it be smal skales bygger than the skales of
dandruffe sprowting out in latitudes and longitudes lyke ye heed of a leke."

Blancard: "*Crusta lactea*, a Species of *Achor*, a Scurf, or crusty Scab, only with this difference, that an *Achor* infects only the Head, but this, not only the Face, but almost the whole
body of an Infant, at the time of its first sucking. *Crustea lactea* turns white, but *Achors*
have another colour."

"*Psora*, a wild Scab that makes the Skin scaly. A Scurf."

Hooper: "Small exfoliations of the cuticle, which take place after some eruptions on the
skin, a new cuticle being formed underneath during the exfoliation."

SHINGLES

Goeurot: "In Greke herisipela, and of the Latines Sacer ignis, our Englysshe women call it
the fyre of Saynt Anthonye, or chingles, it is an inflammatiõ of membres wit excedyng
burnynge and rednesse, harde in the feelynge, and the most parte crepeth aboue the
skynne or but a lytle depe within the flesshe.

It is a greuous payne, and maye be lykened to the fyre in consumyng . . ." (The Booke of
chyldren)

Borde: "Formica is the latyn worde. In greke it is named Mirmichia. In englysh it is named
a little wheale growynge out of the skyn, some doth call this sicknes in latyn Formica
milliara as who should say briefly bytinge of Amytes or Pysmars or Antes, for this

infyrmyte dothe take his name of an Ante or a Pysmare, or Emyt al is one thynge, & why this sickenes is so called is because the similitude is lyke the bytynge of an Ante &c. And there be .iii. kyndes of this infyrmyte, the fyrst is runnynge, the seconde is corodynge or eatynge and the thyrde is named Formica milliaris the whiche I do take it for the syngles . . ."

"Herisipulas is the greke worde. In latyn it is named Apostema calidum. Some latyns do name it Ignissacer. Auicen doth name it Spina bycause it doth prycke & burne. In englyshe it is named the shyngles or the shyngylls, and the barbarous worde is named Erisipule."

Quincy: "It consists of small pimples, which soon form little vesicles that dry and become scaly. This disorder usually spreads farther than its first limits."

SINGING IN THE BRAIN

Goeurot: "Sometyme there chaunceth deafnes by wynde, whyche is in the eare, the whyche causeth tynklynge in the head . . ."

Borde: "Tinnitus aureum be ye latin wordes. In englysh it is named syngynge or a sounynge in a mannes eares, and this doth prognosticate deefnes

                    The cause of this impediment

This impediment dothe come of a ventosyte or wynd the which is ing the heed and in the eares and can nat get out."

Marginal index note: "Piping in the eare."

SMALL POCKS

Blancard: "*Variolæ*, the Small-pox, consists in a contagious Disorder of the Blood, contracted from the Air or otherwise, accompany'd with a continued wandering fever, which sometimes encreases and sometimes decreases, with a Pain in the Head and Loins, Anxiety, and Inquietude, also a breaking forth of Pimples or Wheals, which swell and suppurate."

SPLEEN and STOPPING [OPPILATION] OF THE SPLEEN

Goeurot: "The splene is a mēbre lōge softe, and spongy, beinge in ye lefte syde ioyned unto the holownesse of ye stomacke, and to the thycke endes of ye rybbes, & to ye backe, the whiche is ordeyned fo to receyue the melācholy humours, & to cleanse the blood of the same, for by that meane ye blood remayneth pure & nette. Wherfore it is good nourishyng for al the membres, and is the cause that maketh a bodye merye, but oftentymes there happeneth oppilatiō or debilitie wherof commeth the blacke iaundys.

And somtymes it is greater, fuller, or grosser then it ought to be, by ouermuche melancholie that is not natural, caused of the dregges of the blood engendred in the lyuer, & doth hyndre generacion of good blood, wherthrough the membres become drye, for defaute of good nourishynge. And therfore the pacient is called splenetycke, which ye maye knowe by that, that after meate they haue payne in theyr left syde, and are alwayes heuye, and hath theyr faces somwhat enclynyng unto blaknesse." fol. lvi.

Blancard: "*Splenetica*, such Medicines as are good against the Disease called the Spleen."

"*Hypochondriacus Affectus*, or *Affectio Hypochondriaca*, a pure flatulent and convulsive Passion, arising from flatulent and pungent Humours in the Spleen, or Pancreas, which afflicts the Nervous and Membranous parts. The Hypochondriack Disease."

Dunglison 1839: "Hypochondriasis . . . *Spleen* . . . This disease is probably so called, from the circumstance of some hypochondriacs having felt an uneasy sensation in the hypochondriac regions."

SPOT IN THE EYE (see also PUSHES)

Borde: "Tarphati is the barbarous word. In latyn it is named Macula in oculo. In englyshe it is named a spot or a pusshe in the eye."

STINKING BREATH and STINKING NOSTRILS

Borde: "The .154. Capytle dothe shewe of the stenche or euyl savour that may come out of a mannes mouth or nose or the arme holes.

Fetor oris or Fetor narium or Fetor assellarum be the latyn wordes. In englyshe it is named stench of the mouth, stench of the nosethrilles, and stench of the arme holes . . . This infyrmyte dothe come diuers wayes, yf it do come out of the mouthe or nosethrylles, either it do come out frõ the heed or stomake, or by some roten tothe . . ." Printed margin note: "Stynkynge breth."

STITCH

Quincy "Pleurodyne, pains in the pleura, usually a rheumatism" "Pleurodyne rheumatica, rheumatism in the muscles of the thorax, or bastard pleurisy."

Dunglison 1839: "Pleurodynia"
"A spasmodic or rheumatic affection, generally seated in the muscles of the chest."

STOMACH, COLD IN THE

Elyot: "The stomach cold distempered
He hath good appetite.
He digesteth yll and slowely, specyally grosse meates and harde.
Cold meates dothe waxe soure beinge in him undigested.
He delytethe in Meates and drynkes, which be Cold, and yet of them he is indammaged." p.7

STOMACH, HEAT IN THE

Elyot: "The stomacke hot distempered
He digesteth welle, specially harde meates, and that wyll not be shortly altered
Lyght meates, and soone altered, be therin corrupted.
The appetite lyttell and slow.
He delytethe in Meates and drynkes, whyche be hotte, for euery natural complexion delyteth in his semblable." p.7

STONE; STONE IN THE KIDNEYES

Borde: "Nehpresis or Nephritis be the greke wordes. Nefresia is the barbarous worde. In latyn it is named Dolor renum, and some doth say it is Calculus in renibus. In englyshe it is named the stone in the raynes of the backe.

The Cause of this impediment

This impediment doth come of many wayes, as by great lyftynge, or great straynynge or to much medlynge with a woman, and it may come by kynd of eatynge of euyl meates ingendrying ye stone."

Paré: "*Of the causes of the stone.*

The stones which are in the bladder have for the most part had their first originall in the reines or kidneys, to whit, falling down from thence by the ureters into the bladder. The cause of the these is two-fold, that is, materiall and efficient. Grosse, tough, and viscide humours, which crudities produced by the distempers of the bowels and immoderate exercises, chiefly immediately after meat, yeeld matter for the stone; whence it is that children are more subject to this disease than those of other ages. But the efficient cause is either the immoderate heate of the kidneyes, by meanes whereof the subtler part of the humours is resolved, but the grosser and more earthy subsides, and is hardened as we see bricks hardened by the sun and fire; or the remisse heat of the bladder, sufficient to bake into a stone the *fæces* or dregges of the urine gathered in great plenty in the capacity of the bladder. The straightnesse of the ureters and urinary passage may be accounted as an assistant cause. For by this meanes, the thinner portion of the urine floweth forth, but that which is more feculent and muddy being stayed behind, groweth as by scaile upon scaile, by addition and collection of new matter into a stony masse. An as a weeke often-times dipped by the Chandler into melted tallow by the copious adhesion of the tallowy substance presently becomes a large candle, thus the more grosse and viscide fæces of the urine stay as it were at the barres of the gathered gravell and by their continuall appulse are at length wrought and fashioned into a true stone." p. 664

Quincy: "Is an aggregate of many of the harder parts of the urine, pent up by reason of the straightness of the ducts."

The Skilful Physician: Differential diagnosis of stone and colic

"For the Stone in the Kidneyes.

There is great pain in the raines of the back, which draweth downwards; stirring encreaseth the pain, they are much inclined to vomiting, the body is bound, Urine raw and watrish, often provoking to pisse, but not without pain, the Urine avoids with gravel, sand and slime, yea sometimes mixt with blood.

To know it from the Chollick, first its not so sharp as the paine of the Chollick.

Secondly, The Chollick doth appear beneath on the right side, and stretcheth from thence upwards toward the left side, but the pain of the Kidneyes begins above, and stretcheth downwards, and a little more towards the back.

Thirdly, the pain is most of the Kidneyes fasting, the Chollick otherwise.

All Saxifrage and other things good for the Stone, are good for the Kidneyes, but not for the Chollick.

Lastly, there is found in the Urine gravel or sand, and not in the Cholick or pain of the guts."

STRAINE

Quincy: "a sprain, or strain, of the parts about a joint".

STROKE OR STROAK

Lowe: in a description of the causes of luxation, wrote:

"*Pet.* Which are the Extern [causes of luxation]?

Joh. Falls or stroaks, and too violent extending of the member violently against the figure naturall." p. 362.

STRONGURION

Borde: "Stranguria is the greke word. In latyn it is named Stillicidum vrine. In englyshe it is named the strangury, the which is a dystyllynge or droppynge of a mannes water diuers tymes in one houre with great payne & burnynge in the issewe of man of woman, or els it is an opylacion in the necke of the bladder, and thorowe the stone ore elles by some imposthumous humour . . . This infyrmyte doth come of some ulceracion in the bladder or raynes of the backe, or els it may come thorowe acredyte or sharpnes fo the water, as it may come also of to much heat or to much coldnes in the backe and bladder."

Blancard: "*Stranguria*, the Strangury; a difficulty of Urine, when the Urine comes away by Drops only, accompany'd with a constant inclination of making water."

SURFET

Borde: "Crapula is the latyn worde. In greke it is named Crepalæ. In englyshe it is named a surfyt, and some saye it is an heed ache . . . This impediment doth come of a euyll dyet eatynge and drynkynge late, or takynge of rawe or contagious meates, or taken of euyll drynkes drynkynge."

Blancard: "*Cræpale*, vel *Crapula*, an Headach, proceeding from the drinking of too much Wine."

SWEAT

Borde: "Sudor is the latyn word. In greke it is named Hydros. In englyshe it is named sweat, & there be diuers sweates the one doth come by labour, the other may come by sicknes and payne, and those be hote or colde, and there is an other sweat the which is vehement, and that sweat is named ye sweatynge sicknes, and some sweates dothe stynke and some dothe nat . . . The cause of sweates either it doth come of heat or corrupcion of the ayer, or it may come by one person infectynge another or as I sayde by labour or some sicknes."

SWELLING, WHITE

Dunglison 1839: "The French surgeons apply the term hydrarthrus to dropsy of the articulations. White swelling is an extremely formidable disease. It may attack any one of the joints, but is most commonly met within the knee, the haunch, the foot, and the elbow, and generally occurs in scrofulous children. It consists, at times, in tumefaction and softening of the soft parts and ligaments which surround the joints, at others, at swelling and caries of the articular extremities of bones; or both these states may exist at the same time."

TERMES IN A WOMAN

Borde: "Menstrua is the latyn worde. In greke it is named Roufgynechios. In englyshe it is named a womans termes, the which most comonly euery woman and mayden hath, yf they be in good helth and nat with chylde, nor geuynge no chylde sucke, from , xv. yeres of there age to .l. nat .ii. yeres vnder or aboue, and where I dyd saye that the womans termes in latyn is named Menstrua that worde of latyn is deriued out of a worde named Mensis whiche is a month, for euery month they ye hath theyr helth hath theyr termes or flowers. And there be iiii. kyndes of womans flowers, reed, tawny, white and blackyshe, the reed is natural, and the other be unnatural and nat perfyte and they betoken infyrmyte or sicknes to come whan they be nat reed."

TETTER

Borde: "Herpes or Herpethe be the greke worde. In latyn it is named Herpera and some do name it Flaua bilis. In englyshe it is named a tetter, and some doth name it Lupus or Lupie bycause a wolfe hath oftymes such impedimentes, it dothe crepe and corode and eateth the skyn and waxeth broder and broder."

"Serpigo is the latyn worde. And some auctours doth name it Ignis volatilis. And some saythe that this sicknes doth by lytle dyffer from a sicknes of skabbes named Impetigo, but that the one is bygger than the other, and some doth name Impetigo zarna as it doth appere more playnlyer in this boke before this matter and after as it is spec[i]fied in the capytles of these infyrmytes, but I do saye that this sicknes or disease named Serpigo is a burnynge skabbe, and doth ronne in ye skyn infectynge it more or lesse, and is named in englyshe a tetter."

Blancard: "*Herpes*, a spreading and winding Inflammation; 'tis two-fold, either *Miliaris* or *Pustularis*, like Millet-seed, which seizes the Skin only, and itches; or *Exedens*, consuming, which not only seizes the skin, but the *Muscles* underneath. The cause of it is, that the *Glandules* of the Skin are too much stuff'd with salt *Particles*, which, if the peccant Matter abount, grow into a Crust, and eat the *Parts* they lie upon. A *Ring-worm* or *Tettar*."

TRAVEL, WOMAN THAT IS IN

Travel== var. sp. of travail, syn. for labor

TYMPANY

Paré: "*Of the Dropsie*.

. . . First that Dropsie which fils that space of the belly, is either moist or dry . . . The dry is called the *Tympanites*, or Timpany, by reason the belly swolne with winde, sounds like a (*Tympanum*), that is, a Drum . . ."

Blancard: "*Tympanites*, *Tympanias*, or *Aqua intercus Sicca*, a Tympany, is a fix'd, constant, equal, hard, resisting Tumour of the *Abdomen*; which being beat, sound. It proceeds from a stretching Inflammation of the Parts, and of the Membraneous Bowels, whose Fibres are too much swoln with animal Spirits, and hinder'd from receding by the Nervous Juice which obstructs the Passage; to which Distemper there is consequently added, as the complement of all, an abundance of flatulent Matter in the places that are empty."

Quincy: "Tympanites . . . is the particular sort of dropsy that swells the belly up like a drum and is often cured by tapping."

UFULA (FALLING OF THE UFULA)

Lowe: "Of the Inflammation and relaxation of the *Uvula*, or *Columella*.

Nature hath placed and hung in the roof of the mouth, a piece of spongious flesh named by the Greeks, Gargarion, and by the Latines, Gurguleo, in vulgar the pape or chap of the mouth, the which being augmented, and lengthened above Nature, through distillation of humors, is caled Schion in Greek, and in Latine Columella, and Uva, for it being tumified in length, it is like a pillar, or collume, somtime the nether part of it is round, and then it is called Uva, through the similitud it hath with the blacke vine berrie: it is placed in the roofe of the mouth for divers reasons: First, it helpeth to pronounce the sound, and to speak cloer by dividing the ayre which cometh from the lights, for the which it is called *Plectrum vocis*: Also that the ayre which cometh by the Mouth and Nose, entreth not in the lights by the Trahe-Arterie, till the coldnesse of it be correded, so that the lights be not offended by cold. Such as want the pape or pellet, hath ordinarily deformitie in speech, with refrigeration of the loines: it doth impath that neither dust nor rhume enter the trahe arterie with the ayre . . .

The Signes are evident to the sight, by pressing down of the tongue, accompanied with dolour, feaver, difficulty to swallow the meat. The sick thinketh ever to have something in his mouth redie to go over with great hast by the continuall distilling of the humor, impassing to sleep but with open mouth; Sometime it hangeth so long that it falleth on the tongue, and so grieveth the sick, that sometime he is constrained to put his finger in his mouth to help the over-going of the meat, as saith Avicen." pp. 206–207

Blancard: "*Cion, collumella, gargareon, gargulio, uva, uvula, uvigena, uvigera, epiglottis, sublinguium, pensilis de palato Isthmus, gutturis operculum*, the Palate which hangs betwixt the two glanules call'd *Amygdale*, above the chink of the *Larynx* . . . Sometimes this *Uvula* sticks out too far occasioned by the Humours that fall upon it, which can't return by the Lymphatick Vessels, whence proceeds the Fall of the *Uvula*, which we call Roof of the Mouth."

ULCERS

Borde: "Aphtæ is the greke worde. Alcola is the barbarous worde. And Ulceratio in palato be the latyn wordes. In englyshe it is named a hote ulceration in the rough or palat of the mouth."

Lowe: "*Pet*. What are those six kindes of Ulcers? *Jos*. The first is sanious, 2. virulent, 3 filthie, 4 cancrous, 5. putrid or stinking, 6 corrosive or rotten away. . . . " p. 326.

Blancard: "*Exulceratio*, a Solution of continuity proceeding from some gnawing Matter, and in soft Parts of the Body, attended with a loss of their substance. It differs from an *Abscess* in this, that an *Abscess* is occasion'd by a *Crisis*. An Exulceration is either great, little, broad, short, narrow, straight, transverse, winding, equal, unequal, deep, &c. An Exulceration."

URINE, STOPPING OF THE (see also PISSING)

Borde: "The .192. Capytle doth shewe the suppression of a mannes vryne.
Ischuria is ye greke worde. In latyn it is named a Suppressio vrine. In englyshe it is named supression of the urine, that is to saye that whan a man wolde pysse and can nat."

WEB (IN EYE) (see also PIN AND WEB)

Borde: "Lencomata or Lencoma is the greke worde as some do say. In englyshe it is a webbe the whiche is rooted in and upon the eye or eyes."

"Pterygion is the greke worde. In araby it is named Sebel. In latyn it is named Vnguis. The barbarous word is Vngula. In englyshe it is named the webbe in ye eye, whiche is a neruus matter bred upon the eye, and dothe cover the pupyle of the eye."

Paré: "The *Ungula, Pterygion* or Web is the growth of a certaine fibrous and membranous flesh upon the upper coate of the eye called *Adnata*, arising more frequently in the bigger, but sometimes in the lesser corner towards the temples. When it is neglected, it covers not onely the *Adnata*, but also some portion of the *Cornea*, and coming to the pupill it selfe hurts the sight thereof. Such a Web sometimes adheres not at all to the *Adnata*, but is onely stretched over it from the corners of the eye, so that you may thrust a probe betweene it and the *Adnata*: it is of severall colours, somewhiles red, somewhiles yellow, somewhiles duskish, & otherwhiles white. It hath its originall either from externall causes, as a blow, fall, and the like; or from internall, as the defluxion of humours into the eyes . . ." p. 647.

Lowe: "Of the web in the Eye, called *Suffusio Cataracta* and *Hypochyma*.

Suffusio is a maladie called by the greeks *Hypoxima*; and by the Arabs *aqua* and *gutta*; in english, the Cataract or Tey, which is an abstruction of the Prunall, by a gathering together of a thick hardned of congealed humour betwixt the membrain *Cornea* and humour Christalline, directly upon the prunall empassing the sight . . . The Signes when it beginneth, the sick both imagine to see before his Eyes little things like flies or moats, like the dust of the sunne, threads of wool, haires, spiders webs, or as it were a circle about a candle when it is lighted, thinking one candle to be two . . ." p. 166.

Blancard: "*Hypochyma*, a depraved Sight, whereby *Gnats, Cobwebs*, little *Clouds*, &c. seem to swim before the Eyes. The cause of it seems to consist in turbid Humours, or sometimes in the Optick Nerves, whos little pores are obstructed by the Matter that is thrust into them."

"*Cataracta* is two-fold; either *beginning*, or a *Suffusion* only, or *confirm'd*, or a Cataract properly so call'd; the *incipient* is but a *Suffusion* of the Eye, when little clouds, motes, and Flies seem to fly the Eyes, but the confirm'd Cataract is when the Pupil of the Eye is either wholly or in part cover'd and shut up with a little thin Skin, so the the Sunbeams have not due admittance to the Eye . . ."

WEN

Paré: "A Wen or *Ganglion* is a tumour sometimes hard, sometimes soft, yet always round, using to breed in dry, hard, and nervous parts. And seeing that some of the tumours mentioned before in the former Chapter, sticke immoveable to the part to which they grow, because they are contained in no cyste, or bag; othersome are moved up and down by the touch of your fingers, because they are contained in a bag or bladder, it commonly comes to passe that Wens have their bladder wherein to containe them, and therefore we think fit the rather more freely and particularly to treat of their cure, because they are more difficultly cured, especially where they are inveterate and of long standing . . .

The description formerly set downe, will furnish you with the signes by which you may know when they are present; certainly from very small beginnings they grow by little and little to a great bignesse, in the space of six or seaven yeares, some of them yeeld much to the touch, and almost all of them are without paine." p. 272.

Quincy: "Wen, a soft, insensible and movable tumour under the skin."

WHITES or WHITE MENSTRUES

Blancard: "*Fluor Albus*, or *Fluor Uterinus*, is a a continual evacuation of corrupt Humours from the Womb, or Pores in the *Vagina*. The *Whites* in Women." Another synomym: Fluor Mulibris.

Quincy: "Fluor Albus, is a distemper common to the female sex, called by them the *Whites*. It arises from a laxness of the glands of the uterus, and a cold pituitous blood, that, instead of the menstrual discharges, issues out a slimy yellowish matter, not much unlike the running off of a gonorrhoea, and which it is so near akin to, as hardly to be distinguishe; and sometimes is attended too with such a sharpness, as to make it dangerous to men to have

any venereal intercourse with them at those times. . . . This is also called by some writers
Fluor Muliebris, and Uterinus."

WHITLOW (also see FELON)

Borde: "Perioniche is deriued out of .ii. wordes of greke of Peri which is to say about, and
Onix which is to say a naile which is an impediment about nayle. I do take it for a white
flawe or suche lyke do name it Paronichius."

from Extrauagantes:

"The .56. Capytle dothe shewe of a white flawe or blowe. Reduuie is the latyn worde.
And some dothe name it Rediuia. The barbarous worde is named Redimie. In englyshe it
is named a white blowe, or a white flawe, the which doth grow about the rote of the nayle,
the grekes dothe name in Paranochia, medecines may be had in this cause but my counsel
is nat to medle with no chirurgy matters, for as muche as phisicions wyl nat medle with it."

WIND

Borde: "Iectigacio is the latyn word. In englyshe it is named a wynde the which may be in
many mēbers of a man specially and most comonly under the skynne . . . This impedi-
mēbet doth come of a vaporous ventosyte or winde intrused vnder the skynne and can nat
gette out, it may also be in many other members."

WORMS

Borde: "Astarides is the greke worde. In englyshe it is lytle small wormes the whiche most
comonly doth lye in ye longacion other wyse named the ars gutte. And there they wyll
tycle in the fundement."

"Cvrcurbiti is the latyn worde. In englyshe it is square wormes in a mannes mawe and
guttes.

"Lumbrici is the latyn worde. In greke it is named Elmthia. In englyshe it is named longe
white wormes in the maw of the stomake and guttes."

"Sirones is the latyn worde. In englyshe it be wormes that doth brede under the skyn. And
there be .ii. kyndes the one kynde doth brede in the handes and wrestes, and the other
dothe brede in the fete and they be named degges."

WORM THAT EATETH THE TEETH

Paré: "Wormes breeding by putrefaction in the roots of the teeth, shall be killed by the use
of causticks, by gargles or lotions made of vinegar, wherein either pellitory of Spain hath
been steeped, or treacle dissolved also; Aloes and Garlik are good to be used for this purpose." p. 658.

The ingredients listed in *The Skilful Physician* are representative of the wide variety of simple and compound pharmaceuticals available in the mid-seventeenth century. This Table contains an alphabetical list of ingredients in the classification format used by the College of Physicians in the 1653 edition of the *Pharmacopœia Londinensis: or the London Dispensatory*.[1] This system divided medicinal preparations broadly into simple and compound medicines (see Introduction). These categories were then subdivided further in to categories such as roots, woods, barks, herbs and seeds for the Simples and types of medications for Compounds. Synonymous terms are listed after the main entry. To facilitate a comparison of these ingredients with other seventeenth century texts, footnotes have been added to indicate ingredients used in the 1633 edition of Gerard's *The Herbal* ([G]Gerard, John *The Herbal or General History of Plants. The Complete 1633 Edition as Revised and Enlarged by Thomas Johnson.* (Facsimile of Edition published by Adam Aslip, Joice Norton and Richard Whitakers, London, 1633) Dover Publications, New York, 1975), Culpeper's *Herbal* ([C]Culpeper, Nicholas. . . .) or the 1656 edition of the *Pharmacopœia Londinensis* (Culpeper, Nicholas *Pharmacopœia Londinensis: or the London Dispensatory: further adorned by the studies and collections of the Fellows, now living of the said Colledg.* Printed for Peter Cole, London, 1653). Two different symbols are used for the latter reference. The Old List, an English translation of the 1618 Latin edition of the *Pharmacopœia*, is indicated by *, while the modified New List is indicated by [+]. Selected ingredients are also described from the following sources:

AN: Nicolaus, Salernitanus *Eene-mittelnederlandische vertaling van het Antidotarium Nicolai met den latijnschen tekst der eerste gedrukte uitgave van het Antidotarium Nicolai* Leiden: W.S. van den Berg, 1917.

Bate's Dispensatory: Salmon, William *Pharmacopœia Bateana or Bates Dispensatory. Translated from the last Edition of the Latin copy . . .* Fifth Edition, William and John Innys, London, 1720.

Blancard: Blancard, Stephen *The Physical Dictionary. Wherein the Terms of Anatomy, the Names and Causes of Diseases, Chirurgical Instruments, and their Use are Accurately Described* London: John and Benj. Sprint, 1726.

Ges: Gesner, Conrad *The Treasure of Evonymus, cotyninge the vvonderfull hid secretes of nature, tochinge the most apte formes to prepare and destyl Medicines, for the conseruation of helth: as Quintessēce, Aurum*

---

[1]Culpeper, Nicholas *Pharmacopœia Londinensis: or the London Dispensatory: further adorned by the studies and collections of the Fellows, now living of the said Colledg.* Printed for Peter Cole, London, 1653.

*Potabile, Hippocras, Aromatical wynes, Balmes, Oyles, Perfumes, gar-
nishyng waters, and other manifold excellent confections. Wherunto are
ioyned the formes of sondry apt Fornaces, and vessels, required in this
art. Translated (with great diligence, & laboure) out of Latin, by Peter
Morvving felow of Magdaline Coleadge in Oxford.* (Iohn Daie, London,
1559) Fascimile edition of copy from Beinecke Rare Book and
Manuscript Library, Yale University. Da Capo Press/ Theatrum Orbis
Terrarum Ltd., Number 97, The English Experience, New York, 1969.

OED2: OED2: Oxford English Dictionary II [database online] Available
from: BRS Software Products, McLean, VA; BRS/Search Full-Text
Retrieval System, Revision 6.1, 1992.

Salmon: Salmon, William *The Compleat English Physician or, The
Druggist's Shop Opened.* Mathew Gilliflower, London, 1693.

SIMPLES

ROOTS

Angelica, roots of$^{G^*+C}$
Aron roots [Aron=Wakerobbin or Cuckoo-
    Pint^G]$^{G+C}$

Beats, roots of white$^{G^*+G}$
Betony roots^{GC}
Bur-roots [Butter-bur?*]^G
Burrage roots [Borrage]$^{G+C}$
Butchers broom roots$^{G^*C}$

Callamus arromaticus [*calamus aromaticus,
    calamus aronatics, callamus, Callamus
    benjamin*]$^{G^*+}$
Camock roots [or Red Harrow]^G
Caper roots$^{G^*}$
Cellendine roots$^{G^*+C}$
Comfry roots $^{G^*+C}$
Cowcumber roots, wild [wild
    cucumber^G] $^{*+}$

Daisies, roots [*Daisies, wild with roots*]$^{G^*C}$
Dock roots [*red Dock roots, yellow Dock
    roots*]$^{G+C}$
Dragon root$^{G^*+C}$

Elicampane root [*Enulacampana root,
    Enula campana roots*]$^{G^*+C}$
Eringo roots [*Erinringo roots*]$^{G^*+C}$

Fennel root, red$^{G^*+C}$
Fern roots$^{G^*+C}$

Gallingal and Great Gallingal [Galanga
    lesser and greater]$^{*+}$
Gallingale roots, garden [=Cyperus^G]$^{G^*+C}$
Garlick$^{G^*+C}$
Gentian roots$^{G^*+C}$
Ginger [*green Ginger, white Ginger*]$^{G^*+}$

Hermodactilus [*Hermodactulus*, bulb of
    Meadow Saffron$^{G, p. 164}$]^G
Horse rhadish root^{GC}

Ireos ["that is the roote of the white
    flowerdeluce" [iris]^G]^G
Ivy roots^G

Leeks, roots of unset$^{G^*+}$
Liquorice [*Licoras, English Licoras*]$^{G^*+C}$
Lilly, root of white [*Lilly roots, white*]$^{G^*+C}$
Lilly, root of a blew^G
Lyons claw [=Black Hellebore^{OED2}]$^{G+}$

Madder roots^{G+C}
Mallows, roots$^{G^*+C}$
Marigold roots$^{G^*+C}$
Marsh mallow roots$^{G^*+}$
Michocanum [probably Mechoacan]$^{G^*+}$
Morsus diabili roots [Devil's-bit]$^{G+}$

Onions^{G*C}
Orpine roots^{GC}
Orris roots, white [Fleur de Luce]$^{G*+C}$

Parsley roots [*Meadow Parsley root*]^{GC}
Peperitis roots [Horse rhadish]^{GC}
Philip pimperlow roots [?var. of Filipendula]
Pimpernel roots^{GC}
Plantane roots^{G*+C}
Predalian [Pedelion is synomym for Black
    Hellebore^{G}]$^{G+}$

Reeds, roots of small [=Calamus]$^{G*+}$
Red roots [probably Rose root or Rose-wart^{G}]
Rhadish roots^{G*+C}
Rhubarb, roots of monks^{G*+}

Sassaparilla roots^{G*+C}
Saxifrage root^{G*+C}
Setwal-roots^{G*}
Smallage roots^{G+C}
Sparage roots, Sparragus [Asparagus]^{G*C}
Spica of the Indies [Blancard: "*Spica Indica*,
    see *Nardus Indica*" p. 319 and ". . . Indian
    Spikenard," p. 242]$^{G*+}$
Squills [*squils*]$^{G+C}$
Spiknard^{G*+}
Succory roots [*sallets of Succory roots*]$^{G*+C}$

Tormentile root^{G*+C}
Tussilage, roots of

Wakerobbin root [Arum=Aron=Cuckoo-
    pint^{C}]$^{G*+c}$
Water lillies^{G*+}

BARKS

Ash trees [*ashen tree, Green Ash*]^{G*C}

Cassia^{G*}
Cinnamon^{G*+}

Elder [*green bark of Elder, inner bark of
    Elder, middlemost rind of Elder*]$^{G*+C}$

Guacum, Bark [Guaiacum^{G}]

Sassafrasse^{G+}
Sloe-bush, bark of^{G+C}

WOODS

Balsome wood^{G}

Cypress wood [*Cipresse, Ciprus*]$^{G*+C}$

Juniper, chips or shavings [for perfume]$^{G+C}$

Lignum aloes^{G*+C}
Lignum vitea [=wood of Guajacum]$^{G*+}$

Red-wood [(?)Red Rosewood= Rhodium^{G+}]

Sanders [*White Saunders, Powder of
    Sanders*]$^{G*+}$

Tamariscus^{GC} [Tamaris (?)$^{*+}$]

HERBS

Acatia^{G}
Adderstongue^{G*+C}
Aleberry
Alehoofe [= ground ivy]$^{G*+C}$
Alge epatum
Alkanite [Alkanet or Spanish Bugloss^{GC}]^{G*C}
Ambrosia [Ambrosie, that is Demigod's
    food^{G}]
Angelica, wild^{G*+C}
Archangel [*Archangel leaves, white
    Archangel*]$^{G+C}$
Aristologia [Aristolochia=hartwort or
    birthwort^{OED2}]^{G}
Aron [obs. for Arum=Wakerobbin or
    Cuckoo-Pint^{OED2}]$^{G+C}$
Arsemart^{G+C}
Astrology rotunda [= Gallingall meke^{G}]^{G}
Athanatia^{G} [context unclear, may also be a
    preparation of opium^{AN}]
Avens [=Colewort=Herb Bennet^{C}]$^{G+C}$

Balm [*balme*]$^{G*+C}$
Basil, sweet^{G*+C}
Bay-leaves [*Bayes*]$^{G*+C}$
Beanes^{GC}
Beets^{G*+C}
Betony^{G*+C}
Borrage leaves^{G*C}
Bove wort
Box leaves $^{G*+}$

Bramble [*Bramble leaves, red Bramble leaves, red Brambles*]$^{G+C}$

Briars [=Nep tree^G]^G

Brooklime^{G+C}

Buglos^{G*C}

Burnet [*Burnet leaves*]$^{G+}$

Burrage [Borrage]$^{G*+C}$

Bursa pastoris^{G*}

Butchers broom^{G*+}

Cabbage [=Coleworts^G]$^{G*+C}$

Calamint [*callamint aromaticus*]$^{G*+C}$

Camomile [Cammomile]$^{G*+C}$

Carduus balsam [*carduus balsom*; ?Gum thistle is English term for Euphorbium^G]

Carduus benedictus^{G*+C}

Catapusia [Cataputia or Common Garden Spurge]^G

Caunapitum [possibly Chamepitys or ground pine^G]

Cellendine^{G*+C}

Cene [*Cene Alexandria, cene Alexandrina*; probably Senna, which grew in Syria and had a trade route through Alexandria^{Blancard}]$^{G*+}$

Centory [Centaury]$^{G*+C}$

Cetrach [Ceterach]$^{G*+C}$

Chickweed^{G*+C}

Chives^{G+}

Cinqfoil^{G*+C}

Cipresse leaves^{G*+C}

Clary [*Clary leaves*]$^{G*+C}$

Clivers [*Cliver, Clivers artico*;cleavers]$^{G*+C}$

Clover^G

Cole, red [*red Cole leaf*; red cabbage]$^{G*+C}$

Colewort leaves [*red Coleworts*; (red) cabbage]$^{G*+C}$

Collombine leaves^{G*+C}

Colts foot [*coltsfoot*]^{G*C}

Comfrey [*Great Comfrey*, Great Confound^G]$^{G*+C}$

Costmary [=Alecost^G]$^{G*+C}$

Cuckoe sorrel [Cuckow's meate, or cuckow sorrel, that is, wood sorrel^G]^G

Curraline [Corrallina*, = Coral moss; "Sea moss, that is Corralline"^{G}]^{G*}

Daisie leaves [*Daisies*]$^{G*+C}$

Dandillion^{G*+C}

Dill^{G*+C}

Diptamnus cretius [Diptam^G, Diptany is obs form of Dittany^{OED2}; probably ==Dittany of Crete^C]^{GC}

Dithander [Dittander]$^{G+C}$

Dittony [*Dittony leaves*]^{G*C}

Dock leaves, garden [*red dock*]$^{G*+C}$

Dodder [or Thyme]$^{G*+C}$

Dothet, white ["The white Dothet doth grow in moorish grounds where Rosasolis growes, and groweth very neer the ground like a Plantane, but a more yellowish greene leaf, it beareth a blue flower on a tall stem and smal; no Herbal maketh mention of this Dothet." p. 110]

Dragon^{GC}

Elder [*Elder leaves*]$^{G+C}$

Elland leaves

Elme tree^{GC}

Egrimony [Agrimony]$^{G*+}$

Endive [*Endive leaves*]$^{G+C}$

Enula campane [Elicampagne]^{G*C}

Ewfrace [Euphrasia==Eyebright^G]^G

Eyebright^{G*C}

Fennel [*brown Fennel, red Fennel, Fennel spout, sweet red Fennel*]$^{G*+C}$

Fern^{GC}

Fetherfew [Fedderfew, Featherfew or Feverfew]$^{G*+C}$

Flax^{GC}

Folefoot ["... that is Coltes foote"^{G}]$^{G*+}$

Fumetory^{G*+C}

Gallingale [*French Gallingal*="Cyperus"^{G}]^{G,C}

Germander^{G*+C}

Goose-grasse [=Cleavers^G]$^{G*+C}$

Grasse, three leaved^G

Groundsel^{G*+C}

Harts-horn [Buckthorn^C]$^{G*+C}$

Hartstongue^{G*+C}

Hemlock [*white Hemlock*]$^{G*+C}$

Henbane^{G*C}

Herb Bennet [=Hemlock^G;Avens^C]

Herb canapitis [?Chamepitys=ground pine^G]

Herb Christopher^C [St. Christopher Herb^G]

Herb eve [=Buckthorn^C; Herb Ivie that is Buckes horne Plantaine^G, Buckthorn$^+$]

Herb-grace [Herb-grace that is Rue[G]][G+C]
Herb Robert[G+]
Heyhowd ["Heihow or *Hedera terrestris*[G]"=Alehoofe][G+C]
Hillwort [Hilwort is Puliall mountaine (pellamountaine)[G]][G+]
Hiperico
Hollioaks[G]
Holly without prickles[G]
Honey suckle leaves[G+C]
Horehound[G+]
House-leek [*houseleek*, houseleek or sengreen[+]][G+C]
Hysop[G+C]

Ivy, ground [Alehoofe][G+C]

Knot grasse [*knotgrass*][G+C]

Ladies mantle[G+C]
Lavender[G+C]
Lavender cotton[G+]
Leeks [*Unset Leeks*][G+]
Lettice[G+C]
Lilly leaf, white[G+C]
Liverwort [*liver-wort*][G+C]
Long wort [Longwort is Pellitory of Spain[G]][GC]
Lovage[G+C]

Madder, English[GC]
Madder, Great[GC]
Maidenhair [Bed-straw (Ladies')[C]][G+C]
Maiden wort
Mallowes [*Mallow leaves, Mallow stalk*][G+C]
Mallowes, garden[G]
Marigold leaves[G+C]
Marjerom[G+C]
Marjerom, sweet[C]
Marsh mallows[G+]
March [Marche is smallage[G]]
Mastratia [probably Mastricaria, or common featherfew]
Mastick[G+C]
Maudlin[G+]
Mellilot [*melilot, mellilot herbs, mellilote*][G+C]
Mercury[G+C]
Mint[G+C]
Mint, Lake [possibly water mint]

Mint, red[G]
Mint water[GC]
Mint, white
Mirtle leaves[G+]
Morsus diabili herb [Devil's-bit[G]][G+C]
Mosse of a Crab tree[G+]
Mother time [*Mother-time, wild time,* Mother of Thyme[C]][G+C]
Mousear[G+C]
Mugwort[G+C]
Mullet leaves [possibly var. sp. of Mellilot(?)]
Mustard[G]

Nep [*Nepe*, Cat-mint][G+C]
Nettles[G+C]
Nightshade [*night shade*][G+C]

Oak fernes[G+]
Oaken leaves[G+C]
Oculus Christie [wild clary[C]][G+C]
Orpine[G+C]

Parsley [*Parsly, Parslye, garden Parsley, mead Parsley*][G+C]
Peach leaves[G+C]
Pearlwort
Pellamountain[G+]
Pellitory of Spain [*Pelitory of Spain*][GC]
Pellitory of the wall [*pellitory of the wal, pellitory on the wall*][G+C]
Peniroyal[G+C]
Periwinkle[G+C]
Petty morral [Morrell or petie Morrel, that is Nightshade[G]][G+C]
Philippendula [*phillipendola*,filipendula=dropwort][G+C]
Pimpernel[G+C]
Plantane[G+C]
Plantane morrel
Polipodium of the oak [*pollipodium of the oak*][G]
Primrose leaves[G+C]

Ragweed [Iacobea sp.=seggrum=Coniza montana = Stagger-wort =Staner =wort =Cineraria =Egrigeron marinum or Sea groundsell=Prosper Alpinus= Artemesia alba; all are listed as varieties of St. James wort[G]]

Rew [*green Rew*, Rue]$^{G*+C}$
Ribwort^G
Rosasolis ["This Herb groweth in the
    Meadows in low Marish grounds, and in
    no other places; it is of Horseflesh colour,
    and groweth very long and flat to the
    ground with a main long stalk growing in
    the midst of six branches springing out of
    the roots round about the stalk with a hoar
    colour, and a main breadth and length; and
    I do warn you in any wise not to touch this
    Herb when you gather it, with your hands,
    for then the vertue is gone. . .", p. 137;
    Ros solis, that is Sundeaw^G]$^{G+C}$
Rose cake
Rose-leaves [*red Rose leaves*]^{G*C}
Rosemary^{G*C}
Rubarb^{GC}
Rye^{GC}

Sage [*brown Sage, red Sage, vertue Sage,
    wild sage*]$^{G*+C}$
Sage of Jerusalem^G
Saint Johns Wort^{G*+}
Saint Peters Wort^G
Sanacle^{G*+}
Savory [*winter Savory*]$^{G*+C}$
Saxifrage^{G*+C}
Scabious^{G*+C}
Scala coeli [Narrow leaved Solomon's seal]^G
Scolopendria^G
Scurvigrass [*Scurvey grasse, scurvigrasse,
    garden scurvigrass*]^{G*C}
Seagreen [*seagreene*, misspelling of
    Sengreen^G(?)]
Setwal^G
Shepherds purse [*Bursa pastoris*]$^{G*+C}$
Shee Holm [holm=hollioak^G]
Sickwort [possibly Sickle wort^{GC}]
Skivers
Smallage^{G*+C}
Sold mella [Soldanella or Scottish scurvy
    grass^{GC}]
Solomons seale^{G+C}
Sorrel^{G*+C}
Sowthernwood^{G*+C}
Sowthistle^{G*+C}
Speedwel [=vervain in text]$^{G*+C}$
Spiere Mint [=Mentha romana^G]^G
Spike [Lavender spike^G, Common spike$^+$]

Spinage^{G*+C}
Spurge [*garden Spurge*]$^{G*+C}$
Steches [Stœchas citrina^G]^{G*}
Stitchwort^G
Stone crop [Sedum acre; Stone crop, that is
    houseleek^G]$^{G*+C}$
Strawberry leaves [*wild Strawberry
    leaves*]$^{G*+C}$
Succory^{G*C}

Tansie [*garden Tansie*]^{G*C}
Wild Tansie [Silverweed]$^{G+C}$
Tarragon^{GC}
Thime [*garden Time, running Time^G,
    standing Time, unset Time*]$^{G*+C}$
Tobacco leaves^{G*+C}
Tormentil [*tormentile, tormentill,
    turmentile*]$^{G+C}$
Toutswaine leaves [Tutsane is *Clymenum
    Italorum^G*]^{GC}
Turbit [*turbith*]^G

Vervain [*vervaine*]$^{G*+C}$
Violet leaves^{G*+C}

Water mints^{G+C}
Water trifoil^G
Water-cresses [*watercresses*]^{G*}
Waybred [Waybread is
    Plantago^G=plantain]^{G*C}
Wheat chessel, course^{GC}
White wort [Whitwort, that is feaverfew^G]
Willowes, coles of^{GC}
Withy leaves^G
Wood-betany [*Wood-betony leaves*]$^{G+C}$
Woodbind [=Honeysuckle^{G+}]$^{G*+C}$
Wormwood [*wormewood, French
    Wormwood^G*, Roman Wormwood^{GC+}
    Romane Wormwood]$^{G+C}$
Wortwort [Sea Wartwort^G]

Yarrow^{G*+C}

FLOWERS

Bugloss flowers^{G*+}
Broom flowers^{G*+C}

Camomile flowers^{G*+C}
Centory, flowers of^{G*+C}

Cowslip flowers[G*+C]

Damask roses (red and white)[G+C]
Daisies, blossoms[G]
Dandillion, yellow flower like to[G]

Gilliflowers [*gilly flowers*][G*+]

Lavender spike [*Spike of lavender*][G*+C]
Lavender tops[G*+C]
Lillies[G+C]

Mallow flowers[G*+C]
Marigold [*marygold*] flowers[G*+]
Mellilot flowers[G*+C]

Orange flowers[G+]

Rose flowers, red[G*+C]

Saffron[G*+C]
Saffron, English[G]
Shepherds-flowers
Sticardue, flowers of [Stickadoue, French Lavender or stœchas[G]][G]

Woodbind flowers[G+]

FRUITS. BUDS.

Almonds, bitter [for oil][G*+]
Almonds, fordy
Almonds, Jordan [or sweet; "long sweet almond, vulgarly termed Iordan almond"[G]]
Apple[G+]
Apple of Colliquintida [Coloquintida, or coloquint and his kinds[G]; colocynthis][G*+]

Bay berries[G*+C]
Bramble buds[G]

Cassia fistula[G*+]
Cap dates
Cloves[G*+]
Costard [apple][G+]
Cubebes [*cubebs*][G*+]
Currans [*currants*][G*+C]

Damask pruins[G+]

Dates[G*+]
Dog berry["... they have no vse in Medicine."[G.]][G]

Elder berries[G+C]
Elder buds[G]
Figge[G*+C]

Fusses [stalks of cloves: "Some have called these *Fusti*, whereof we may English them Fusses"[G, p. 1535]][G]

Gooseberries[G+C]
Grapes, green[G+]

Hasel Nut [Hazel nut][G+C]
Hawes (berry of Hawthorne[C])
Hawes, berry of[C]
Hawthorn buds[G+]
Hips [probably Brier rose or Hep tree[G], Hip Rose[C]]

Ivy berries[G+C]
Ivy berries, black[G+C]

Juniper berries[G+C]
Lemmons, pills of[G+]

Mace[G]
Mirabilans, pills of the five kinds of [Myrobalans, Bellericks, Chebs, Emblicks, Citron and Indian[+]][G*+]
Mirabilans, yellow [var. of yellow or citron Myrobalan][G*+]
Nutmegs, powder of[G*+]

Nux vomica [Vomiting nuts[G], Vomiting nuts[+]][G+]

Oaken buds[GC]
Oranges [*Orange pils*][G+]

Pease cod [Pea pods[G]][G]
Pepper, brown [prob. black pepper, Piper nigrum[G*C]]
Pepper, Long [Piper longus[G*+C]]
Pepper, white [Piper album[G*+C]]
Pippin[G+]
Pomgranat pill[G+C]
Pompuleon [OED2: Name for *Citrus*

decumana or *Citrus pompoleum*, the
shaddock or pompelmouse (a tropical fruit)]
Poplar buds^{G+C}

Quince^{G*+C}

Raisons^{G*+}
Raisons of the sun^{G*+}
Reb [Probably Ribes or red curran[t]s^G]
Rose buds, red^{GC}

SEEDS

Ameos, seed of [Bishop's Weed^C]^{G*+C}
Angelica seeds^{G+}
Anniseeds [*Annis*]^{G*+}
Anodinum, seed of
Ashen keyes^{G*+}

Balsome seeds^G
Barley, apothecary
Barley, French^{*+}
Bean flower [flour ground from beans^C]

Cabbage seeds [coleworts]^{G+}
Callamint stones^G
Caraway seeds [*carraway seeds,
caraway*]^{G+C}
Cardomons^{G*+}
Coriander seeds [*Coriander*]^{G*+}
Cumin seeds [*Commin*]^{G*+}

Dill seeds^{G*+C}

Fenicreek [Fenugreek]^{G*+C}
Fennel seed [*Fennelseeds*]^{G*+C}

Graines of paradise [cardamons that grow in
"Ginny"^{G.}]^{G*+}
Gromel seeds [*grommel seeds*]^{G*+}

Hollioaks, seeds of^G

Lapis dactilus [date stone (seed)^G]^G
Linseed [flax seed]^{G*+C}

Mustard seed^{G*+C}

Nettles, crops of red^{G*+C}
Nettles, tops of^{G*+C}

Oats [*Oaten bran, Oatmeal, Oatmeal
grets*]^{G+C}
Orange seeds, reddish^{G+}

Parsley seeds^{G+C}
Pease, monks⁺
Pine apple kernel [pine cone kernels^{GC}]
Piony seed^{G*+C}
Poppy seeds^{G*+C}
Poppy seeds, white^{G*+C}

Quince kernels^{G+C}

Rice^{G+C}

Sassafras seed^G
Savory seed, winter^{GC}
Savory seed, summer^{GC}
Silver mountain seeds^G
Spurge seeds^{G+C}

Tansie seeds^{GC}
Time, seeds of unset^{GC}

Wheat [*Wheat bran, wheaten bran, wheat
flower/flour, Wheat flowers, wheat
meal*]^{G+}

GUMS, ROSINS

Aloes, Alloes sicatrina [a type of aloes
yielding juice]^G and Aloes hepatica^{G*+}
Amoniacum [*Armoniacum*, Gum from
Herbe Ferula or Fennell Gyant^G]^G

Bdelium^{*+}
Benjamin [benzoin^{OED2}]^{*+}
Birdlime [classified as a rosin ^{+, p. 48}]

Camphire^{*+}

Diagridy [=scammony^C]^{G*+C}

Euforbium castorium [gum from Euphorbia
plant^G]^{G+}

Frankinsence [*Frankisence, white*]^{G*}

Galbanum ["Gum from Herbe Ferula, or
Fennell Giant"^G]^{G*+}

Gum arebeck [gum of the Acacia tree[G]][G*]
Gum dragon [*Gum traganthum,*
  Gumdragagant; gum from Goats Thorne
  or Tragacantha[G]][G*]

Labdanum [*Gums of labdanum*; Ladanum*;
  "There be divers sorts of Cistus [Ledon],
  whereof that gummy matter is gathered
  called in shops *Ladanum*, and *Labdanum*,
  but vnproperly."[G, p. 1283]]*+
Lees [of wine]+

Manna [". . . Frankincence, in whom is
  found sometime certaine small grains like
  vnto grauell, which they call the Manna of
  Frankincence."[G, p. 1435]][G*+]
Mirrh [*Gum of mirrh, mirrhe*]*+

Olibanum [*Gums of olibanum*;"The Rosin
  carries the same name [Frankincence]; but
  in shops it is called *Olibanum*, of the
  Greek name and article put before it."[G, p. 1436]][G*+]

Opium ["condensed iuice of Poppie heads"[G, p. 370 [misnumbered 400]G+C]]

Opoponax [resin of; yellow gummy juice
  from the Hercules All-heale or Wound-
  wort[G, p. 1003]][G*+]

Perosen [*perrosen*, "resin of some kind,
  appl. the dry resin obtained from pine
  trees[OED2]]+
Pitch ["Pitch of the Cedars of Greece"+, p. 48;
  Blancard: "*Colophonia*, Rosin-Pitch", p.
  98; colophonia is the residue from
  distilling oil of turpentine+]]G+
Pitch, stone ["And when it [pine tar] is boiled
  is made a harder Pitch . . . because it is
  boiled the second time. A certaine kinde
  hereof being made clammie or glewing is
  . . . in English, Ston Pitch."[G, p. 1362]]G

Rosen ["Liquid and dry, rozin of firr tree,
  Larch tree, Pine tree"+, p. 48; Gesner: "Put
  .iiii pounde of Turpentin Rosin or larix in
  a larg crooked still . . ." p. 29.]]G+

Sanguis draconis [a gum/rosin from the
  Dragon tree[G]][G*+]
Starch, white [*Stirch, white*[OED2]; Salmon

(listed with Gums, Rosins and Balsams):
  "*Amylum, White Starch* . . . is made
  either out of *Wheat Bran* or *Wheat Meal*,
  by soaking it in water . . ." p. 949]
Storax [*Storax cremitie*; Gum of the Storax
  tree[G, p. 1526]; Blancard: "see *Styrax*", p.
  323; Styrax calamita (resin)][G*+]
Sugar [The iuyce of this Reed [sugar cane]
  is made the most pleasant and profitable
  sweet, called Sugar . . ."[G, p. 38]]G+
Sugar, brown
Sugar candy, white
Sugar, white

Turpentine [*Best Turpentine, good
  Turpentine, Gore Turpentine, Ordinary
  Turpentine, Venice Turpentine*; Blancard:
  "*Terebinthina*, Turpentine; 'tis twofold,
  Vulgar and *Venetian*; the *Venetian* is also
  call'd *Chious* or *Cyprian*; the best is clear,
  pellucid, white and of a Glass-colour; it
  comes from *Chious, Cyprus, Libya* and
  many other places . . ." p. 335][G*+]

JUICES

Avens, juice of

Betony, juice of
Brooklimes, juice of
Broom flowers, juice of[C]

Cellendine, juice of
Coleworts, juice of[C]

Daisies, juice of
Daisie roots, juice of

Fennel, juice of
Fennel, juice of red

Ground ivy, juice of

Hemlocks, juice of
Houseleek, juice of

Juniper berries, juice of

Lake mints, juice of
Lemmon, juice of*+

Liverwort, juice of

Mallowes, juice of[C]
Mints, juice of

Nettles, juice of red[C]

Onions, juice of[C]
Oranges, juice of[*+]

Parsley, juice of[C]
Pimpernel, juice of[C]
Plantane, juice of[C]
Plantane, juice of Broad[C]
Pumpkin, juice of the inner parts of

Ribwort, juice of
Rue, juice of[C]

Sage, juice of[C]
Scala coeli, juice of
Scurvigrass, garden, juice of
Scurvigrass, juice of[C]
Sider [cider]
Slowes, juice of[C]
Smallage
Sorrel[C]

Verjuice [a condiment made with sour,
    acidic juice of unripe grapes, crab apples
    and other fruit[OED2]]
Vervain juice
Vinegar[+]
Vinegar, White Wine
Vinegar, Wine

Watercresses
Wood-betony and Egrimony, juice of[C]
Woodbind leaves, juice of
Wormwood, juice of[C]

LIVING CREATURES

Cantharides [Blancard: Spanish flies][+]
Cat, fat
Cat, sucking
Capon
Chicken
Cock
Cock, red

Dog[+]

Earth-wormes[+]

Spider
Swallowes, young [fledged][+]

Tessers [possibly a variant of Tessar, a 17th
    century term for a silkworm from
    Italy[OED2]; silkworms are in the New
    Dispensary[+, p. 52]][+]

Whelp[+]
Wood-lice [millipedes][*+]
Worms, church yard[*]
Wormes, garden[*]

PARTS OF LIVING CREATURES

Ashes from unwashed sheeps wool
Auxungium poecati [sic, Auxungia
    porcati=lard][+]

Barrowes grease
Bears suet[*]
Beaver codd
Bee wax
Bezar stone [Bezoar stone= concretion from
    animal GI tract[OED2]][+]
Blood, dog
Blood, dove
Blood, fox
Blood, hares[+]
Blood, lamb
Blood, pigeon[+]
Boares grease [*Boars grease, bores grease*]
Boares pisle
Bones
Bores tooth[+]
Butter[+]
Butter, Ewes

Calves curd[+]
Calvs feet
Capons grease[*]
Civet
Cobwebs[+]
Cow-dung[+]
Cream
Cream, raw

Dung, goose [see also turd, goose]
Dung, green goose
Dung, of a white goose
Dung, sheeps

Egg [egge]+
Egg, treddle of an+

Fat of a Beare*+
Fat of a Fox*+
Fat of a Goose+
Fat of a graye+
Fat of a Heron+
Fat of dryed bacon+

Gall of a hare+
Gall of a hart
Gall of a lamb
Gall, ox [Oxe Gall]
Gall of an ox bladder
Gall of a raven
Goose
Grease, goats*+
Grease of a fat cat+
Grease of a fat pullet
Grease, hens+
Grease, hogs+
Grease, swines

Hair of a hare [wool of hares+]
Hair, thine own
Honey [hony, English Honey, Stone Honey]+
Harts horn [harts horne]+
Horses haunch bone, marrow of a dead

Ising-glasse ["Fish-glew",gelatin from fish:
    Salmon pp. 684–685]+
Ivory*

Lambs head
Leather, sheeps
Leather, white sheeps
Leg bones of a male deer
Lobsters shell

Marrow bones+
Marrow of an ox leg+
Milk*+
Milk, cowes [milk of a browne cow]+
Milk, Ewes+

Milk, goats+
Milk, womans+
Musk
Mutton, roasted rib of

Oystershels

Pike, neather jaw of a great+
Pith of a young Bief
Poison of a toad
Pork

Scull of a man that died through violence*+
Sheeps head, newly killed
Sheeps heads, black
Spanish Balls newly gathered from a horse
    [probably dung]
Sperma caeti [sperma ceti]+
Suet, bears*+
Suet, deers
Suet, harts+
Suet, mutton+
Suet of a loyne of mutton
Suet, sheeps+
Suet of kidney, sheeps

Tallow, harts+
Tallow, sheeps+
Trecklings, sheeps [probably sheep
    treddlings, pellets of dungOED2]
Turd, goose+
Turd, dogs white+

Unicorns horn*+
Urine, childs+
Urine of a man-child+
Urine of the party grieved+

Veal, Leg of

Wax (Beeswax)+
Wax, virgin (Beeswax)+
Wax, white (Beeswax)+
Whey+
Wool [Shank Wool carded in flakes; Wool
    newly taken from the sheep; Black wool
    newly plucked from sheeps neck; Wool
    from flanks and codds; flank wool; black
    Wooll]

BELONGING TO THE SEA

Amber[*+]
Ambergreece[*+]

Coral [*Curral*][G,*+]
Coral, red[G*+]
Curral, white[G*+]

METALS AND STONES

Allome[*+]
Allome, Roach [*allome,roch*; Blancard:
    "*Rochum Alumen*, or *Rupeum*, Rock-
    Alum", p. 298][+]
Alumen (alum)[+]
Alumen Plumosi [plumose alum]
Alabaster dust[+]

Bole armoniack[+]
Borus [=white lead[OED2], white lead[*+]]
Bloodstone,prepared ["Blood-stone is a kind
    of Jasper of diverse colors, with red spots
    in it like blood, stops the Terms and
    bleeding in any part of the Body." [+, p. 54]][+]
Brimstone[*+]

Calaminaris [*callaminaris stones, Lapis
    calaminaris*][+]
Cerus [=white lead[OED2]. white lead[*+]]
Chalk[+]
Christal [synonym of Sandifer[G pp. 536-7];
    "Christal being beaten into very fine
    powder a a drachm of it taken at a time helps
    the bloody-flux, stops the whites in women,
    and increaseth milk in Nurses."[+, p. 54]][+]
Copperas, white
Coppereas [*coperas*]
Cremer tartary

Gold[*+]

Iron[+]

Lapis tutiae [rock tutty][+]
Lead, red[+]
Lead, white [*lead, white-*][*+]
Limestones (for wine purification)
Littarge of gold[*+]
Littarge of silver[*+]

Littargy[*+]

Powder of steel[+]

Quicksilver[+]

Red stone from a swallow ["Young
    swallows of the first brood, if you cut
    them up, between the time they were
    hatched, and the next full Moon, you shall
    find two stones in their ventricle
    [ventriculus=stomach[Blancard]], one reddish,
    the other blackish . . ." [+, p. 34]; "the Stone
    found in the Maw of a Swallow" [+, p. 54]][*+]

Sal gemmi [[+], p. 53; *salgemmi*; Salmon:
    synonym for Rock salt; Blancard:
    "*Gemmæ sal* or *Sal Fossile*, a sort of
    common Salt taken out of Pits, which
    shines like Crystal, whence it hath its
    denomination, *Sal Gem*." p. 169][+]
Salt, Bay [Salmon: Rock Salt]
Salt of India [Salmon: Rock Salt]
Salt peter
Sandifer [*Sandyfer,powder of*; Gerard 1633,
    p. 535 describes preparation from ashes of
    the Glass saltwoort: "Stones are beaten to
    pouder, & mixed with the ashes, which
    being melted together become the matter
    wherof glasss are made. VVhich while it is
    made red hot in the furnace, and is melted,
    becomming liquide and fit to work vpon,
    doth yeeld as it were a fat floting aloft;
    which, when it is cold, waxeth as hard as a
    stone, yet it is brittle, and quickely broken.
    This is commonly called *Auxungia vitri*. In
    English, Sandeuer . . ."[G]][G]

Terra sigillata [*terra sigillatum*]
Tuttie [*tucia, tutia*, tutty, Blancard: ". . . is
    nothing but the Soot of Brass sticking to
    the Furnace in the fusion of that Metal."
    p. 348][+]

Verdigrease[+]
Vermillion [Blancard:"*Vermilion* is Cinabar,
    or red Lead"][+]
Vitriol, white[+]
Vitriol, Roman[+]

Whetstone[+]

SIMPLE DISTILLED WATERS

Angelica water

Betony, Water of[+,Ges p. 47]
Broom flowers, Water of[+]
Burrage water[+]

Damask rose water [*Damask water*][+]
Dragon water[+]

Morral water [Gesner, p. 44: "The water of
    Solanum or Morella is good against all
    agewes . . ."; OED2, Morel entry:
    ATTRIB. 1544 T. PHAER, Regim. Lyfe
    (1553) Cijb, "Seeth it in nightshade or
    morell water."][+,Ges p. 44]

Parfoliata, Water of
Plantane water [+,Ges pp. 34, 48]

Rose water, red [*rosewater, red*][+,Ges p. 48]
Rose water, white[+,Ges p. 48]

Sage water[+,Ges p. 42]
Scabious water [Water of scabious][+,Ges p. 43]
Succony [prob. misspelled Succory],
    Water of[+]
Spike water
Spinage water

Wormwood water+,[Ges pp. 24,47]

COMPOSITA OR COMPOUND MEDICINES

SPIRITS AND COMPOUND DISTILLED WATERS

Aqua coelestis[+]
Aqua composita [formulations in text]

Balme water[+]

Hipporcras [Hippocras, formulations in text]
Hungaria [Hungary water: Bate's
    Dispensary, p. 15]

PHYSICAL VINEGARS

Rose vineger[+]

DECOCTIONS

Lac virginis[+] [formula in text attributed to
    Dr. Walmesley]

ALTERING SYRUPS

Blackberries, Sirrup of

Candied Sugar, Sirrup of [formulation in text]
Corticibus citri, Syrrup de[+]

Damask roses, Sirrup of

Endive, Syrrup of

Ingibus sirrup [misspelling (?) of Intibus ==
    Intubus or Intybus -Garden succory,
    garden endive, wild endive or chicory[G],
    sirrup de Chichorio cum Rhabarbaro[+] or
    =*Endivia intubum* "'tis a cooling herb and
    the water of it is used in Fevers and in
    Inflamations. Endive"[Blancard]]

Jaunbes, Sirrup of [probable misspelling of
    Syrupus Iuiubinus (Jujubinus)[+], a
    decongestant]

Mulberries, Sirrup of

Roses, Sirrup of [formulation in text][+]

Scorbuttical Sirrup, Dr. Deodates
    [formulation in text]
Steches, Sirrup of[+]

Violets, Julip of ["Julep of Violets is made
    of the water of Violet flowers and sugar
    lide Julep of Roses"[+, p. 109]][+]
Violets, Sirrup of[+]

SYRUPS MADE WITH VINEGAR AND HONEY

Mell rosarum [*Honey of Roses*][+]

Oximil [*Oxymel*]+

Sirrup of mulberries+
Sirrup of poppy seeds+

CONSERVES AND SUGARS

Betony, conserve of

Raspices, preserved [raspberries[G]]
Roses, conserve of+
Roses, conserve of red+

POWDERS

Diatria papira or Piperion [Diatrion
    piperion+]
Diatragacanth [species Diatragacanthi
    frigidum[+, p. 123]]

Manus Christi [Diamargaritum simplex;
    Diamargariton frigidum[+, p. 122]]

ELECTUARIES

Mithridate [*mithridatum*][+, p. 131]

Succo rosarum [Electuarium è Succo
    Rosarum [+, p. 136]]

Treakle [Theriaca][+, p. 132]
Treakle, London [Theriaca Londenensis[+,
    p. 132]]

PURGING ELECTUARIES

Confectionum de Hameck [Confectio
    Hamech[+ p. 135]]
Diacatholicon [Catholicon[+, p. 135]]
Hiers, confection of [Hiera[+, pp. 135–6]]

PILLS

Cochia aurea [Pilula aurea[+, p. 140]]
Cochia pills[+, p. 140]

OILS

Simple Oils by Expression

Oyl of almonds+
Oyl of bayes [*Oyle of bayes*]+

Oyl of bitter almonds+
Oyle of cream [formula in text]
Oyl of eggs+
Oyle of lawrel [Laurel or baie tree[G]]
Oyl of linseed+
Oyl olive [*Oyle olive*]+
Oyle, rape+
Oyl of sweet almonds+

Simple Oils by Infusion and Decoction

Oyle of Adderstongue [formula in text]
Oyle of camomile+
Oyl of crastorum [*sic* castorum]+
Oyl of dill+
Oyl of lillies+
Oyle of white lily
Oyle of mallows [formula in text]
Oyle of marsh mallows [formula in text]
Oyl of mirtle
Oyle of poplar buds [formula in text]+
Oyle of roses [*Oyl of roses*][+, Ges pp. 347–50]
Oyle of scorpions ["is made of thirty live
    scorpions, caught when the sun is in the
    Lyon, Oyl of bitter almonds two pound,
    let them be set in the sun, and after fourty
    daies strained." [+, p. 160]][*+,Ges pp. 357–9]
St. John's Oyle [formula in text]
Oyl of wild cowcumbers+

Compound Oils by Infusion and Decoction

Nerve Oyle [possibly oil form of
    Unguentum Nervinum[+, p. 170]; e.g., *The
    New Dispensatory* contains formulations
    for both Oleum Pupuleum and
    Unguentum Populeum+]

Oyl of Exeter [*Oyle of Exceter*, Oleum
    Excestrense[+, p. 162], "Take the leaves of
    Wormwood, Centaury the less,
    Eupatorium, Fennel, Hysop, Bays
    Marjoram, Bawm, Nep, Penyroyall,
    Savin, Sage, Time, of each four ounces;
    Southernwood, Bettony, Chamepitys,
    Lavender, of each six ounces; Rosemary
    one pound; the flowers of Chamomel,
    Broom, white Lillies, Elders, . . ."]+

Oyle of hypericon [formula in text, *Oyl of hypericon*, Oil of St. John's wort][+,Ges pp. 342-4]

OINTMENTS

Unguentum populeum [Unguentum populneum[+]]

CERECLOTHS

Red Cerecloth

PLAISTERS

Oxicrotium [Emplatrum oxycroceum[+, p. 178]; Blancard: Oxycroceum-"a plaiser . . ." or (more likely from context) Oxycratum-a mixture of vinegar and water][+]
Stipticum Paracelsi equivalent formulation appears as Emplastrum Sticticum[+, p. 178]; Blancard: *"Sticticum Emplastrum,* . . . is commonly called *Paracelsus* plaister." p. 322][+]

CHEMICAL OILS

Oyle of broom flowers
Oyle of camomile flowers
Oyl of camphire
Oyl of juniper berris[+ Ges pp. 242-6]
Oyl of licoras
Oyle of linnen [formula in text]
Oyle of mastick[+ Ges p. 248]
Oyl of mints[+]
Oyl of Peter
Oyle of roses [*Oyl of roses*][+ Ges pp. 347-50]
Oyle of rue[+ Ges pp. 236-240]
Oyl of spike [Oil of Lavender: "I shall instance here only Oyl of Lavender, commonly called Oyle of Spike . . . [+, p. 181]][+ Ges pp. 232-4]
Oyl of sulphur[+]
Oyle of tarter[+]
Oyl of Vitriol[+]

CERTAIN SIMPLE MEDICINES

May butter [preparation of unsalted butter taken in the latter weeks of May, placed in an earthen crock, and clarified twice by melting in the sun and straining through rags][+]

COMPOUNDED OR PREPARED MEDICATIONS

Diareticum

OTHER PROCESSED HERBALS

Ashes
Damask powder
Laudanum
Spirits of frombois

PLANT OR ANIMAL FIBERS (FOR CERECLOTHS, PLAISTERS, ETC)

Cotton, black
Cotton wool
Plaister of Pitch
Scarlet cloth

WATERS OF MINERALS

Allome water

OILS OF ANIMAL PRODUCTS

Oyle of cream
Oyle of a goose wing
Oyle, neatsfoot [oleum bubulum]

FOODS/DRINKS

Ale

Bacon
Barley meal
Barme [leaven,froth from beer]
Bay salt
Beere
Bisket made without salt

Bread, brown [*browne*]
Bread, white
Bread, soure wheat
Brine
Broth
Broth, mutton
Browne wine

Caraway comfits

Leaven
Loaf, white

Malt
Marmalade
Manchet crumbs [manchet=finest wheaten
    bread or cake^{OED2}]
Mutton broth
Mutton, juice of roasted
Mutton pottage

Pastionel [". . . which is made of Sugar and
    yolks of Eggs, fine flower and butter,
    these work together into paste", in text]
Posset ale [*Posset curd made of strong ale*;
    "A drink composed of hot milk curdled
    with ale, wine other liquor, often with
    sugar, spices or other ingredients^{OED2}]
Pottage
Pottage, mutton

Sallet oil [sallet=salad^{OED2}]
Salt
Salt, Bay
Salt bief
Salt grease
Salt, white
Sowr leaven
Sowre bread
Sweet Barly Wort [liquid for making beer/ale]

Veal Broth

Yeest

WINES

Allegant [wine from Alicante, Spain]

Bastard

Bastard, eager
Bastard sirrup
Batew wines

Canary wine
Candy cute
Claret
Claret wine

Deal wine

Graves wine

Hollocks

Malaga
Malmsey
Muskadine
Muskadine of Jane

Sack [*Old Sack*; *Sherry Sacks*]
Spanish Cure
Spanish cute

Wine, French
Wine, French White
Wine, gascoin
Wine, gascoyne
Wine, red
Wine, Spanish
Wine, white

MISCELLANEOUS
NON-MEDICINAL ITEMS

Barrel soap

Incense

Shoomakers oil
Shoomakers wax
Snow water [*snow-water*]
Soap, black
Soap, gray
Soap, white
Soot
Spring-water

Tow
Turnsil [context: as treatment for red wine.

== Salmon, p. 757: Turnsole. *Claret-Rags*
"I. This is a Drug which was wholly
unknown to the Ancient Greeks, nor has it
any other Name in Latin but *Turnsole*, or
Tornsole which is a made word, which we
have Englisht *Claret-Rags*, more from
Color than the matter.

II. That which is sold in the Shops, is
nothing but old *Rags*, or old Linnen, dipt
in either the Juice of the *blood-red
Grape*, or the Juice of *Mulberries*, and
so dried in the Sun; or rather (which is
the most common), the *Feces* or *Lees of
Red or Claret Wine*, and dried for
Vulgar sale, and are brought to us out of
France.

III. But this is a Cheat, or an Abuse of
the first design, for the true *Turnsole* or
Claret-Rags, ought to be dipt in the
Juice of the Berry of the Herb called
Turnsole . . ."]

Whiting [from context, probably "a
preparation of finely powdered chalk[OED2]]

UNCERTAIN

Angel gold

Calcithers [possible misspelling of
   Colcothar or Colocynth]
Charnel [unclear from context: Either (1)
   Cornel = Cornelian cherry[G+], (2) the
   stone Sardius = The Cornelian =
   Carneolus = Corneolus (Salmon, p. 219)
   or (3) the fleshy-leafed plant carneol or
   Acesi[OED2]]
Clerk Robert [probably herb from context;
   possibly Herb Robert]

Epaline or Alge Epatum [probably variant
   spelling of "aloe hepatica"]

Juice of clestocks ["a worm so-called" p. 73]

Niprial

Possen ale [probably misspelling of Posset
   ale]
Powder imperial [possibly *Katarticum
   imperiale* from *Antidotinarium Nikolai*, p.
   86, fol. r.a.]
Powder of Holland [*Pulvis Hollandi*]

Veinfrage
Normandy glass

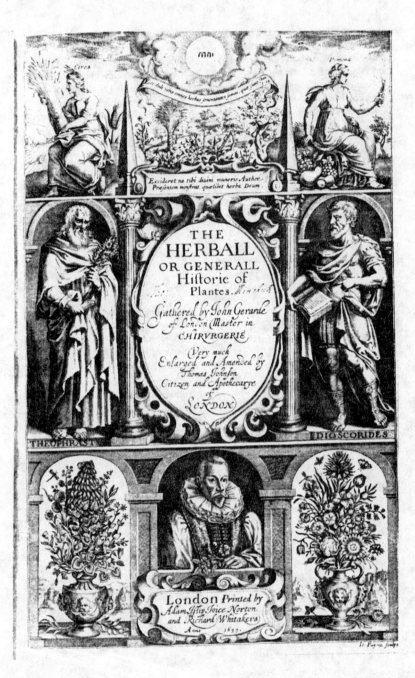

Hedera terrestris.
Ale-hoofe

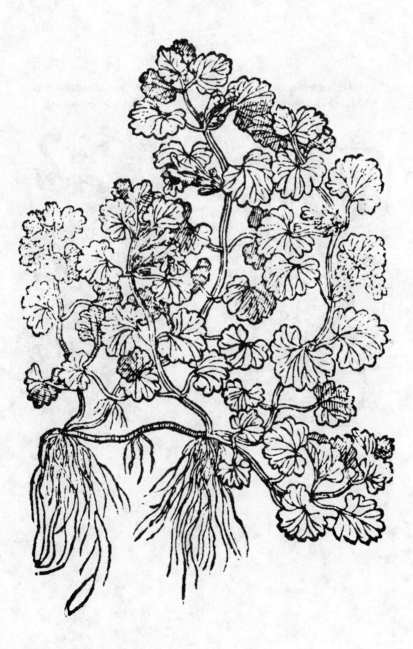

1 *Aristolochia longa.*
Long Birthwoort.

2 *Aristolochia rotunda*
Round Birthwoort.

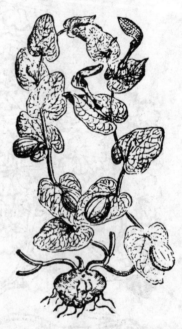

Arum vulgare.
Cockow pint.

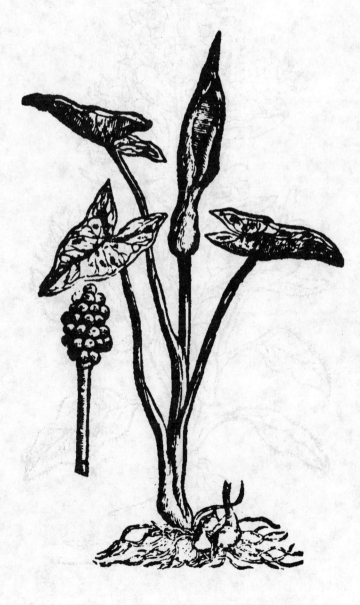

Borago hortensis
Garden Borage.

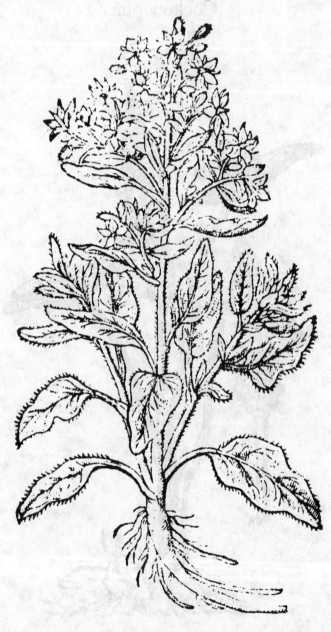

Carduus Benedectus.
The blessed Thistle.

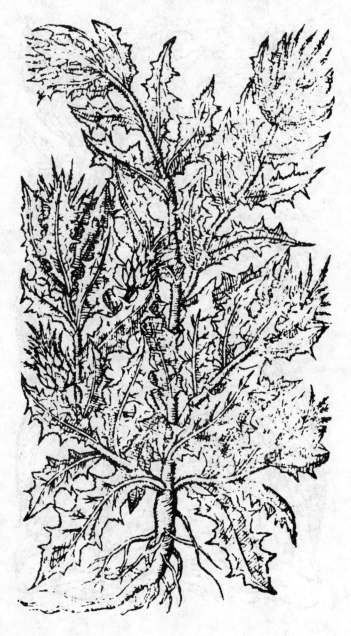

Consolida maior flore purpureo.
Comfrey with purple floures.

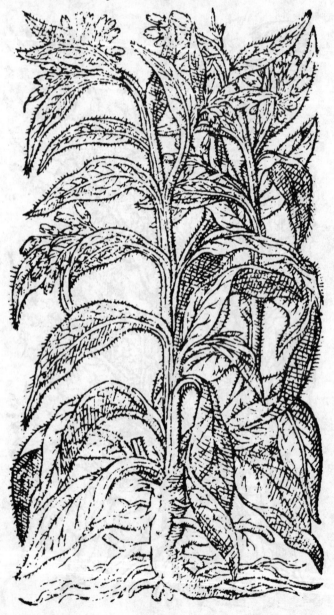

Cyperus longus.
English Galingale.

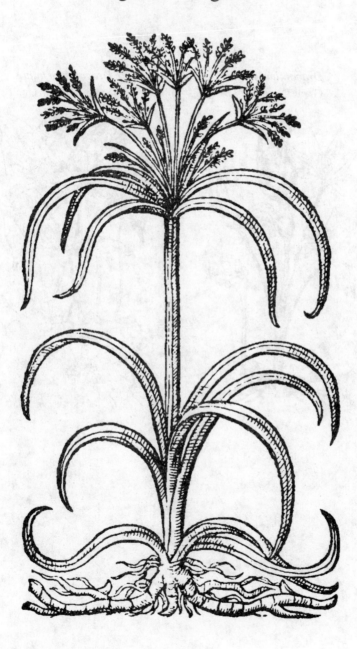

1 *Dracontium maius.*
Great Dragons.

2 *Dracontium minus*
Small Dragons.

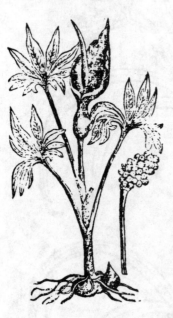

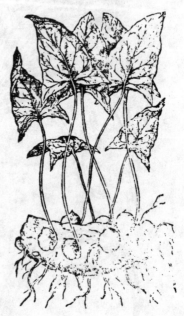

Euphorbium.
The poysonous gum Thistle.

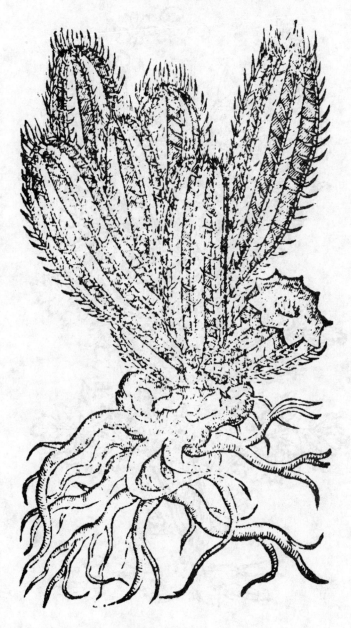

Matricaria.
Feuerfew.

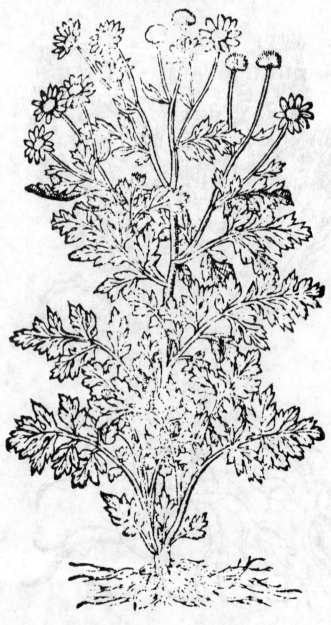

Iris alba.
White Floure de-luce.

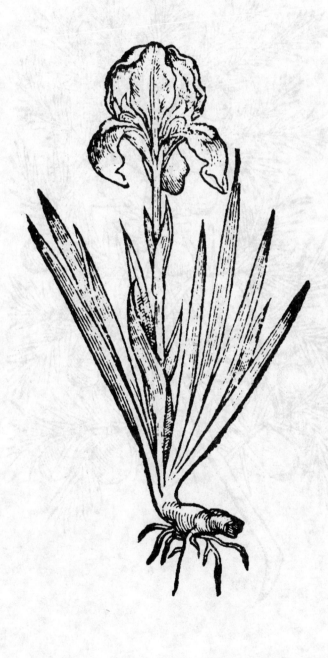

Juniperus maxima.
The great Juniper tree.

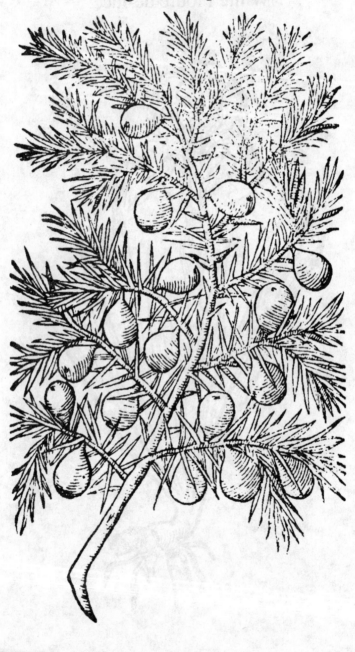

Polygonum mas vulgare.
Common Knot-grasse.

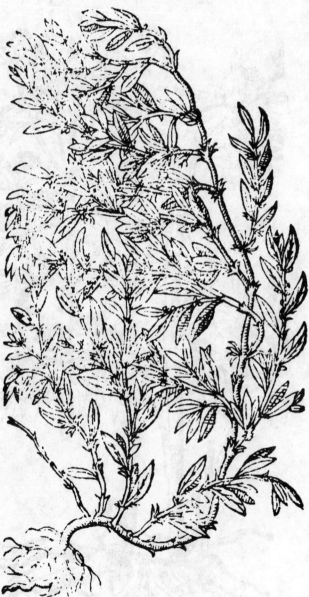

Leuisticum vulgare.
Common Louage.

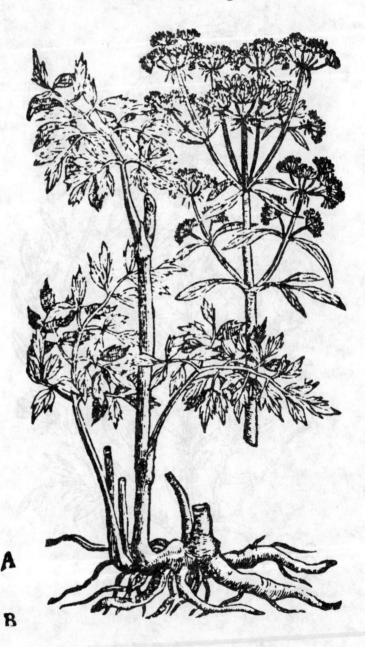

A

B

1 *Mercurialis mas.*
Male Mercurie.

2 *Mercurialis femina*
Female Mercurie.

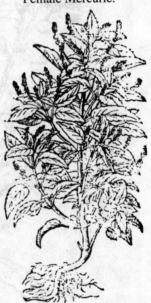
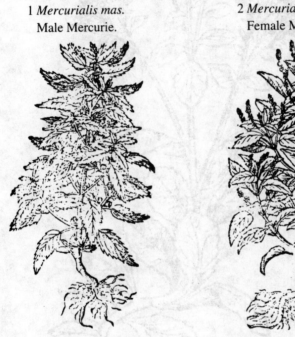

Telephium floribus purpureis.
Purple Orpyn.

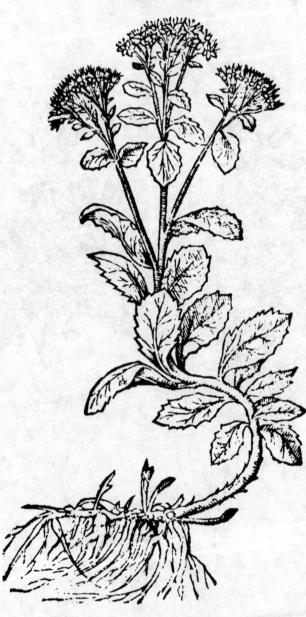

Polium montanum lateum.
Yellow Poley mountaine.

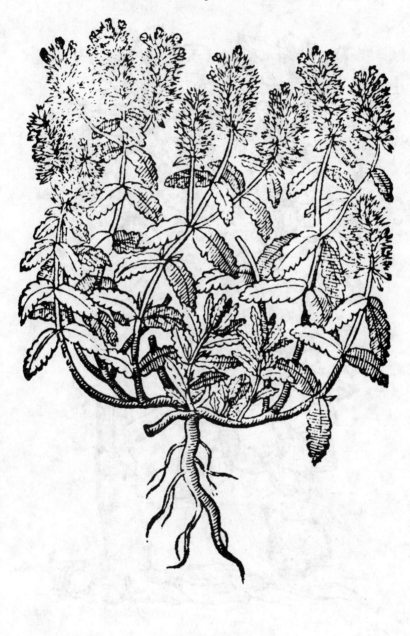

Malus Cotonea.
The Quince tree.

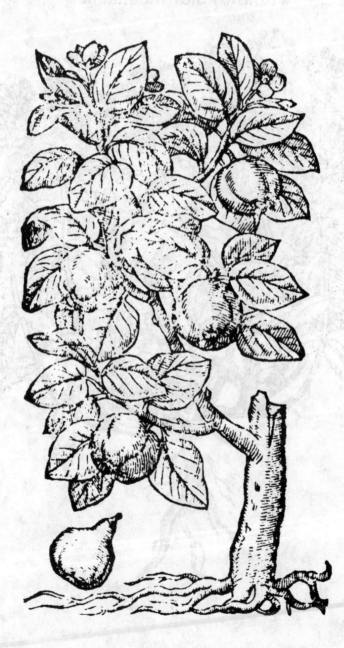

Ros Solis folio rotundo.
Sun-Dew with round leaues.

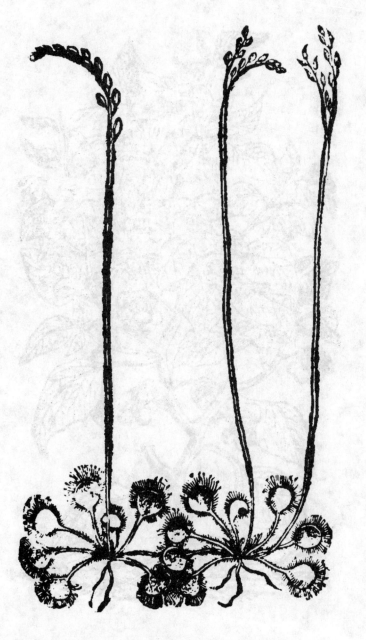

Solanum Hortense.
Garden Nightshade.

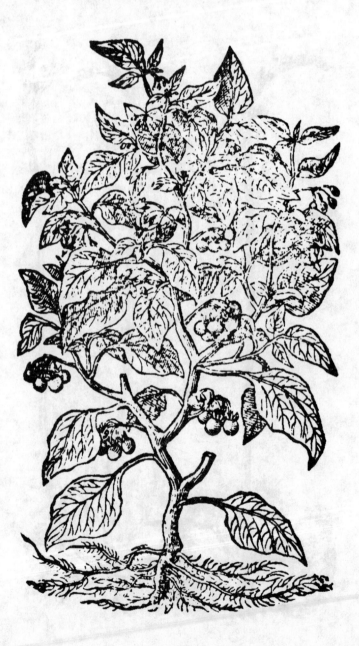

Polygonatum angustifolium ramosum.
Narrow leaued Solomons seale.

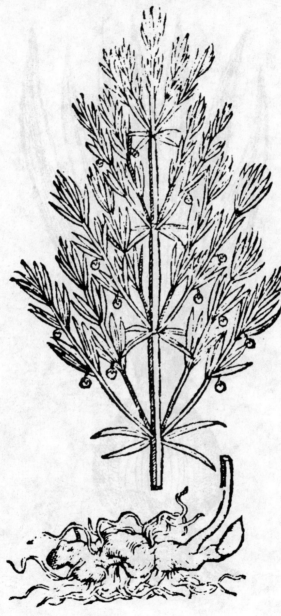

Pancratium Clusij.
Great Squill, or Sea Onion.

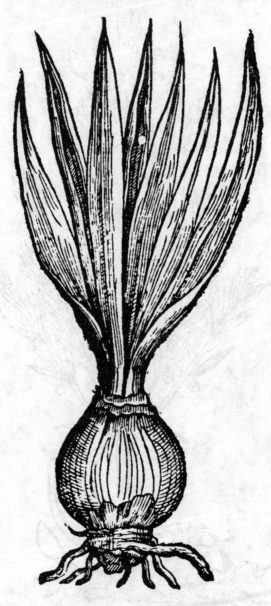

Heliotropium maius.
Great Torne-sole.

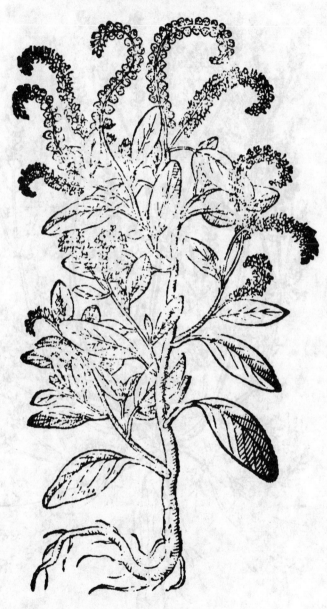

Verbena sacra.
Common Veruaine.

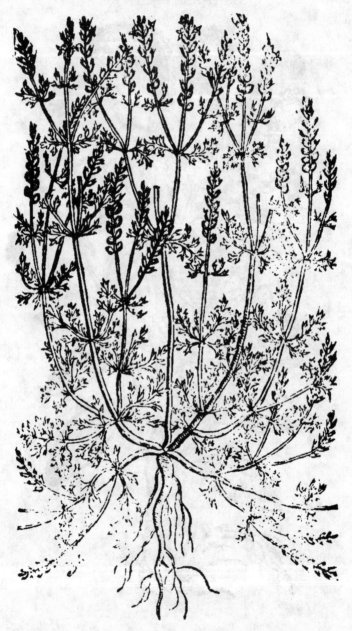

Millefolium terrestre vulgare.
Common Yarrow.

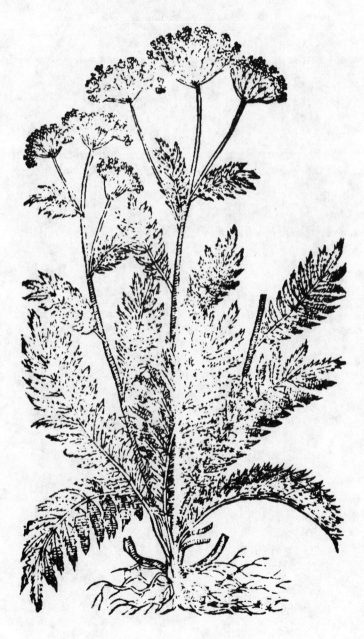

INDEX

Maudlin, 28
Meadow parsley, 119
Meals, frequency of, 4–5
Measles, 117, 134–135, 214
Meats
  and constitution, 6
  eating of, 3
  with salt, 6
Melancholy, 91–92, 153, 215
  purging of, 131–132
Mell rosarum, 36
Mellilot, 25, 67, 111, 154, 209
Melt, 215
Menstruation, 172–173, 228
  white, 231–232
Mercury, 24, 82, 93, 146, 147, 265
Metals, 244
Michocanum, 129
Migraine, 62, 75, 104–105, 215
Milk, 53, 54, 68, 75–77, 83, 100, 125,
     128, 130, 135, 155, 176,
     178–180, 188
  breast, 40, 134
  cow, 26, 36, 42, 48, 49, 98, 104, 146,
     154, 171
  ewe, 26
  goat, 33
  woman, 61, 67, 68, 74, 76, 77, 158,
     159
Mint, 19, 21, 24, 25, 33
  water, 165, 175
  white, 101
Mints, 60, 73, 87, 89, 95, 106, 137,
     164, 167, 168, 171, 190
Mirabilans, 79
Mirrhe, 29, 80, 84, 114, 123, 141, 148,
     173, 192
Mirtle leaves, 80
Mistletow, 156
Mithridatum, 37, 58, 59, 86, 117, 153
Morphew, 216
Morral water, 68
Morsus Diabili root, 20
Mosse of a Crab tree, 31
Mother, 216
Mother as a ailment, 105

Mother-time, 23, 50, 52, 145
Motherwort, 52, 168, 171
Mousear, 138, 157
Mouth
  canker, 46
  palate of, 166
  soreness of, 105–106
Mugwort, 23, 52, 60, 94, 110, 118
Mulberries, 137
Mullet leaves, 121
Musk, 25, 141, 179, 181–182, 191, 193
Muskadine wine, 27, 37, 117, 169, 182,
     187
  making of, 186
Mustard, 39, 88, 118, 120, 143
Mutton, 60, 153, 164
  broth, 129, 130

N

Navel, 106
Neats foot oil, 17, 44, 51, 99, 109
Nep, 16, 24, 28, 152, 166
Nettles, 20, 31, 57, 95, 102, 131, 164
Nightshade, 30, 68
  garden, 270
Nipple, chapped, 106
Niprial, 99
Normandy glass, 146
Nose, 106, 205
Nose bleed, 31–33
Nose canker, 46
Nostrils, smelly, 106
Nutmeg, 19, 22, 25, 27, 37–39, 70, 90,
     92, 101, 105, 117, 125, 135,
     153, 160, 164–167, 172–173,
     176, 181, 189, 192

O

Oak buds, 61
Oak ferns, 131
Oak leaves, 26, 43, 175
Oatmeal, 42, 53, 85, 97, 127, 128, 145,
     154
Oats, 18